Synopsis of
GYNECOLOGY

Synopsis of
GYNECOLOGY

DANIEL WINSTON BEACHAM, M.D., F.A.C.O.G.

Professor of Clinical Obstetrics and Gynecology,
Tulane University School of Medicine,
New Orleans, Louisiana

WOODARD DAVIS BEACHAM, M.D., F.A.C.O.G., F.A.C.S.

Emeritus Professor of Clinical Obstetrics and Gynecology,
Tulane University School of Medicine,
New Orleans, Louisiana

TENTH EDITION

with 228 illustrations, including 1 color plate

The C. V. Mosby Company

ST. LOUIS · TORONTO · LONDON   1982   144

A TRADITION OF PUBLISHING EXCELLENCE

Editor: Carol Trumbold
Manuscript editor: Ann Calandro
Design: Susan Trail
Production: Jeanne A. Gulledge

TENTH EDITION

Previous editions copyrighted 1932, 1937, 1946, 1956, 1959, 1963,
1967, 1972, 1977 (Volume one copyrighted 1932)

Printed in the United States of America

The C.V. Mosby Company
11830 Westline Industrial Drive, St. Louis, Missouri 63141

Library of Congress Cataloging in Publication Data

Beacham, Daniel Winston.
  Synopsis of gynecology.

  First ed.: Synopsis of gynecology / Harry
Sturgeon Crossen. 1932.
  Includes bibliographies and index.
  1. Gynecology—Outlines, syllabi, etc.
I. Beacham, Woodard Davis. H. Crossen, Harry
Sturgeon, 1869-   . Synopsis of gynecology.
III. Title.   [DNLM: 1. Genital diseases, Female.
WP 100 B365s]
RG112.B4   1981   618.1   81-18845
ISBN 0-8016-0526-1   AACR2

C/CB/B   9   8   7   6   5   4   3   2   1   01/B/064

PREFACE to tenth edition

The first edition of *Synopsis of Gynecology* was published in 1932 under the authorship of Harry Sturgeon Crossen. The second, third, and fourth editions were written with his son Robert James Crossen. The latter served as senior author of the fifth edition. The sixth edition title included their name as a grateful memorial to them. In accordance with the usual practice we have agreed to the resumption of the original title.

The edition is presented as a concise, orderly record of up-to-date information and concepts of disorders of the female reproductive system. Its organization will allow the rational assimilation of new knowledge by the medical student and will allow rapid review for those with a knowledge of gynecology. The description and discussion of examination are rather detailed in order to promote proficiency in this phase of gynecology.

Revised information is presented about infectious agents and therapy, problems in therapies of cervical intraepithelial neoplasia and diagnosis of occult invasive squamous carcinoma, use of more sensitive pregnancy tests, prolactin, banding of chromosomes, limits of ultrasonography, and decisions in infertility management. Selected references have been changed to provide recent sources.

Grateful appreciation is again expressed to Professor Don Alvarado of the Department of Medical Illustration of the Louisiana State School of Medicine for his valuable suggestions and excellent illustrations in this synopsis.

Daniel Winston Beacham
Woodard Davis Beacham

PREFACE to first edition

In the various medical and surgical specialties such a mass of facts and working information has developed that a large and expensive textbook is required for each. Obviously the medical student cannot purchase all of these. His funds are too limited to buy them and his time is too limited to read them. This growing difficulty in medical education must be recognized and overcome.

Regarding gynecologic instruction and study, medical students may be divided into two groups—first, those who expect to practice gynecology or closely allied branches and, second, those who expect to follow distant branches of the profession. Each member of the first group needs detailed working knowledge of the subject and hence requires a standard textbook, and the more thorough it is the better. It is a wise investment to purchase this as soon as he begins work in gynecology, for the convenience of frequent reference and study will double and treble the returns from his clinical work.

To the members of the second group gynecology is just one of a number of subjects which they need to know in a general way. Knowledge of the general principles and salient features is necessary to a rounded medical education which enables intelligent cooperation in the handling of patients. But there is no necessity for the detailed knowledge required by those who expect to treat gynecologic or allied conditions.

This synopsis is intended primarily for the students of the second group. It will be found useful also by the members of the first group who desire to supplement the large textbook with a pocket outline, for study at odd moments and memorization of the leading points in gynecologic examination, diagnosis, and treatment. No doubt the practicing physician will find it helpful as a guide to the understanding of the pelvic disturbances he may encounter or as a compact presentation of the outstanding features of this interesting department of medical knowledge.

H. S. Crossen

CONTENTS

Synopsis of
GYNECOLOGY

Chapter 1

ANATOMY AND PHYSIOLOGY

The genital tract in the female changes continuously from the time that its development begins until its function ceases. An associated structure, the anatomic region at the lower end of the trunk between the thighs, is the *perineum*. Superficially it is limited by the mons veneris anteriorly, by the gluteal and coccygeal regions posteriorly, and by the femoral regions laterally. Deeply its upper limit is the pelvic diaphragm, and its boundaries are the pubic arch and the arcuate ligament, the coccygeal tip, the ischiopubic rami, the sacrotuberous ligaments, and the ischial tuberosities. A line connecting the tips of these tuberosities would divide the perineum into an anterior, urogenital region and a posterior, anal region.

VULVA
Anatomy

Also called the pudendum or the external genitals, the vulva consists of the mons veneris, the labia majora, the labia minora, the clitoris, the urogenital vestibule and its glands, the urethral meatus, and the vaginal introitus (p. 56).

The *mons veneris* is a pad of subcutaneous fat lying over the symphysis pubis. The triangular area that it forms is covered with hair after puberty.

The *labia majora* compose the lateral boundaries of the vulva. The external surfaces present the ordinary characteristics of integument. Each labium is limited externally by the genitocrural fold and corresponds to the side of the scrotum in the male. The vestibular cleft between these labia corresponds to the scrotal raphe. The round ligament, passing through the inguinal canal of each side, terminates in the upper part of the labium majus of that side. When a distinct canal remains along the round ligament, it is called the canal of Nuck. If a cystic tumefaction develops at this location, it is termed a hydrocele of the canal and must be differentiated from a hernia, which might include not only bowel and omentum but also fallopian tube and/or ovary. Although coarse hair grows on the lateral sides of the labia majora, their inner surfaces are nonhairy. Sebaceous and sweat glands are numerous.

1

In children the labia majora are very small, and the labia minora project between them. As puberty is approached, the external labia become larger and meet in the median line. At puberty they, in common with the mons veneris, become covered with hair. A little later in life, particularly in married women, the labia minora become enlarged so much that they project forward, separating the labia majora. In old age the labia undergo marked diminution in size and prominence, the shrinking being due largely to absorption of the fat. The veins are numerous and large and become much distended when there is intrapelvic pressure, as in pregnancy or as a result of a tumor. Under such circumstances a wound of the labium may lead to serious and even fatal hemorrhage.

The *labia minora*, or nymphae, are two delicate mucocutaneous folds lying on the sides of the vaginal opening. Each labium minus apparently grows from, or is a secondary fold of, the upper and inner portion of the labium majus of that side. The labia minora begin just below the anterior junction of the labia majora as double folds, which pass above and below the clitoris. The folds that join above the clitoris form the prepuce. The labium minus of each side then descends along the inner side of the labium majus and blends with the labium majus, near the junction of the middle and lower thirds. The posterior extremities of the labia minora are united by a delicate fold that extends between them, just within the posterior margin of the vulvar orifice, and forms the fourchette. When the labia are separated, the fourchette is made tense, and between it and the hymen is a small depression called the fossa navicularis. This delicate fourchette is torn at childbirth, except in rare cases; in some females it is even obliterated by sexual intercourse.

The labia minor are very rich in blood vessels, especially veins; consequently behavior of the structures may be much like that of erectile tissue. They are rich also in lymphatics and nerves.

The *clitoris* is the analogue of the penis. During sexual stimulation the clitoris fills with blood, becoming larger and firmer. Although it is richly supplied with nerves, it is not essential for orgasm if the patient has developed a normal sexual reaction pattern. At the symphysis its two lateral halves separate to form the crura.

The *urogenital vestibule* is the remnant of the lower portion of the embryonic urogenital sinus. It is fissurelike when the labia are approximated and a shallow, triangular-shaped cavity when they are spread apart. The vaginal introitus inferiorly and posteriorly and the urethral meatus superiorly and anteriorly open into the vestibule. Openings of the major and minor vestibular glands and some of the paraurethral ducts in some women empty into the vestibule.

The two *major vestibular glands* are homologous with the bulbourethral glands and are called the vulvovaginal or Bartholin glands. They correspond to the Cowper glands in the male and lie, as a rule, behind the urogenital diaphragm. Each gland is very close to the lower end of the vestibular bulb of that side (Fig. 2-6, *B*). The gland is a small reddish body about the size of a small pea and is of the racemose variety. It produces a crystal-clear mucoid secretion that serves as a minor lubricant for coitus, during which the major lubricant is a transudate from the vaginal mucosa. The opening of the duct from each gland is external to the hymen, at about the junction of the lower and middle thirds of the vaginal orifice. The glands are not palpable unless they are or have been the site of infection, which may be either nonspecific, which is much more common, or gonorrheal. Acute infection may result in a very painful abscess. Cysts of the glands or ducts are the results of infection or trauma and are frequently seen by physicians. Although rare, malignant neoplasms may develop as squamous cell ductal or adenomatous carcinomas.

The *minor vestibular glands* are numerous, minute, tube-like depressions frequently seen about the urethral meatus, particularly between it and the clitoris. They are homologous to the glands of Littré and, rarely, may be the site of an infection.

The *urethral meatus* and the distal urethra for a variable distance are lined with stratified squamous epithelium continuous with that of the vestibule. In 1880 Skene described the two small tubular glands that are located on the posterior surface of the urethra at the meatus and that now bear his name. It was believed for many years that these were the only urethral glands. Huffman, however, after studying the development of such glands in the embryo and their number and location in the adult, found that they are numerous, forming extensive ramifications throughout the tissue around the distal portion of the urethra, and that they may extend back to within a short distance of the bladder.

The *hymen* is usually a circular fold of mucosa that partially occludes the vaginal introitus. It is subject to marked variations in thickness, elasticity, and vascularity, as well as in the number and size of the openings in it. Infrequently there is an imperforate hymen that prevents the escape of the menstrual fluid. Obviously this condition must be treated surgically; otherwise, repeated menstruations will result in hemocolpos, hemometra, hemosalpinx, and eventually hemoperitoneum. In some cases there are multiple small openings, resulting in a cribriform pattern. The hymen may have been ruptured in some cases as the result of trauma sustained in a fall or other accident. It is usually ruptured at the first sexual intercourse; however, the alteration may amount to nothing more than a stretching. In some cases the hymen is so rigid that it prevents coitus. In other instances there is distinct tearing, with considerable pain and some bleeding. In rare cases bleeding persists and may assume serious proportions. Carunculae myrtiformes are irregular tags of tissue surrounding the vaginal orifice that result from parturition.

Blood supply. Blood for the perineum comes principally from the internal pudendal arteries, which are terminal branches of the anterior trunk of the internal iliac artery.

Lymphatics. The perineum—including the integument, the vulva, and the low-ermost portion of the vagina—and the anal canal external to the mucocutaneous junction are drained by lymphatics that empty into the superficial and deep in-guinal nodes and, later, the iliac nodes. Drainage of the clitoris is into the inguinal and the external iliac nodes.

VAGINA
Anatomy

The vagina is a musculomembranous passageway that has its lower opening, called the introitus, at the midportion of the vulval vestibule. It lies between the urinary bladder and the rectum. The uterine cervix, around which the vagina is attached, protrudes into its upper end. Its size and shape are variable and it is capable of great distention, as is evidenced when the baby passes through it. The length of the vagina is ordinarily 7.5 to 10 cm along its anterior wall and 12.5 to 15 cm along its posterior wall. Normally the anterior and posterior vaginal walls lie in contact, and on cross section the cavity is represented as a slit shaped somewhat like an **H**. The wide diameter of the vagina, some distance up the canal, is the transverse one, but that of the vulval cleft is the anteroposterior one.

Relationships. Fig. 1-1 shows the angle that the axis of the uterus and the axis of the vagina normally form. That portion of the cervix within the vagina is known as the portio vaginalis. The vagina is lined with squamous epithelium. Its mucosa is arranged in transverse folds, or rugae, that branch outward from longitudinal ridges or rugous columns, extending along the midline of the anterior and posterior walls. The term "urethral carina" is applied to the rugous column beneath the distal urethra. The lower part of the vagina, which passes through the pelvic diaphragm and the perineum, is supported by the tissues around it. Above the pelvic floor its walls are easily dilatable. The upper end of the vagina is termed the vaginal vault, or fornix, which is divided into anterior, posterior, right, and left fornices. The urethral vaginal septum is a dense connective tissue partition separating the ante-rior vaginal wall from the distal urethra. Beneath the latter this septum becomes the thinner vesicovaginal septum. The proximal urethra and the bladder lie upon the vagina, being separated from it by the thin layers of firm connective tissue representing the lower borders of the endopelvic fascia. These layers usually result in an avascular cleavage plane between the bladder and the vaginal wall.

Laterally the lower vagina is surrounded by its connective tissue, which attaches it to the muscular fascial structures of the pelvic diaphragm and the perineum. The ureters pass medially and obliquely near the upper lateral sides of the vagina. The upper third of the vagina is supported by paravaginal and parametrial subperitoneal connective tissue that is continuous with the bases of the broad ligaments. The upper fourth of the posterior wall is separated from the rectum by the rectouterine

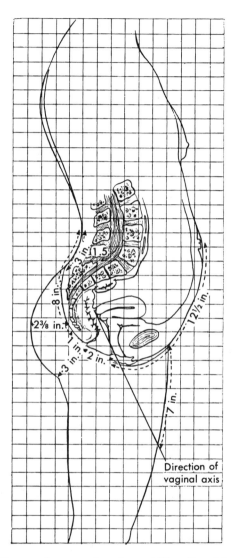

Fig. 1-1. Artist's model, 28 years of age, mother of two children (6 and 8 years old), has practically never worn a corset, is in good health, and is fairly muscular. Height 5 feet 7 inches, weight 140 pounds, bust measure 36 inches, waist 27 inches (2 inches above umbilicus), circumference at umbilicus 30 inches, hips 39 inches, thigh 22½ inches (2 inches below gluteal crease), anteroposterior diameter of body at waist 6¾ inches, anteroposterior diameter of thigh (2 inches below gluteal crease) 6⅝ inches. The other data are given on the outline. To conform to the so-called perfect form the hips should be a trifle large and the weight somewhat more.

Redrawn from Crossen, R.J.: Diseases of women, St. Louis, The C.V. Mosby Co.

pouch known as the cul-de-sac of Douglas. The pelvic viscera—particularly the large intestine, sometimes the ovaries, and (if it is retroplaced) the uterus—are immediately above the posterior vaginal wall; consequently they are easily palpable. At a lower level the vagina lies on and is separated from the anterior rectal wall by the thin, fibrous endopelvic fascia. Posteriorly these fibrous layers usually form an avascular plane between the vagina and rectum. Continuing inferiorly, the pelvic diaphragm and dense connective tissue support the wall posteriorly. The perineal body separates the vaginal and anal canals and in its maximum dimensions separates the vulval vestibule and the anus.

Blood vessels and nerves. The blood supply to the vagina comes from the anterior trunk of the internal iliac artery through the vaginal, uterine, middle hemorrhoidal, and internal pudendal branches. The lymphatics of the lower vagina drain into the same nodes as those of the vulva, and those of the upper vagina drain into the same nodes as those of the cervix. They have innumerable anastomoses. The nerve supply comes from the pelvic plexus on each side. The uterovaginal or cervicouterine ganglia, also known as the Frankenhäuser ganglia, innervate the vagina, uterus, and clitoris.

Histology and cytology

Cyclic changes of the vaginal epithelium are under control of the ovarian hormones. Layers in this membrane have been termed the (1) basal, (2) intermediate, and (3) superficial layers.

Estrogens cause an increase in the rate of cellular division in the basal layer, as evidenced by increased mitotic activity and a greater number of cells. As the basal layer grows, the intermediate zone emerges with development of granular cells containing more darkly staining nuclei. The intermediate zone cells, with continuing estrogen influence, become the large, thin, superficial zone cells with small, densely staining nuclei. Since the cells of the intermediate and superficial zones appear similar to corresponding layers of the skin, the terms "precornified" and "cornified" are commonly used. Progestogens tend to oppose the estrogenic effects. The superficial and intermediate layers are shed with menstruation to leave the basal layer for cyclic regeneration of the vaginal epithelium.

Papanicolaou followed the cyclic changes in the vaginal epithelium by the vaginal smear technique and found that he could recognize changes associated with ovulation and early pregnancy. Fig. 1-2 depicts the changes in vaginal smears during the various phases of the cycle.

The thickness of the vaginal epithelium and the amount of glycogen present in the cells depend on the presence of estrogen in the circulating blood. In the neonate some of the maternal estrogen is carried over into the fetal circulation. As would be expected, this stimulates the growth of the vaginal epithelium and causes glycogen deposits to appear in the epithelial cells, so that the adult type of epithelium is present when the child is born. This state persists for about 5 days, after which there is a gradual decrease in the thickness of the epithelium as well as a decrease in glycogen. At the end of the first month the epithelium is only a few layers thick, and the glycogen is absent.

In prepubescent girls the vaginal epithelium consists of an inactive basal layer three or four cells deep. There is no glycogen in these cells during this period. With the onset of puberty the three layers are promptly established, and glycogen appears. After the menopause the vaginal epithelium returns to the prepuberty state with no glycogen and with a basal layer only two or three cells deep. Alkaline phosphatase is found chiefly in the basal layers, and its highest concentration occurs during the last half of the cycle.

There are two other factors of importance in the physiology and pathology of

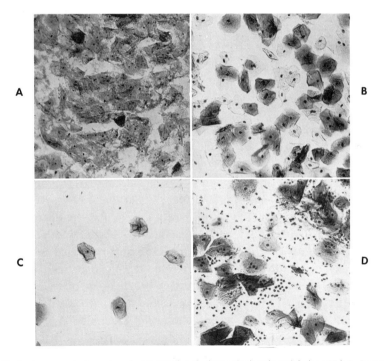

Fig. 1-2. Vaginal smears during normal menstrual cycle (Papanicolaou's stain). (× 165.) **A,** Postmenstrual phase: early estrogen effect (cornified cells appear darker). **B,** Late proliferative phase: good estrogen effect. **C,** Preovulatory phase: marked clearing of cells. **D,** Preovulatory phase: marked mucus and leukocytic flush.   *Continued.*

Modified from Goldhar, A., Grady, M.H., and Masters, W.H.: Fertil. Steril. **3:**376, 1952.

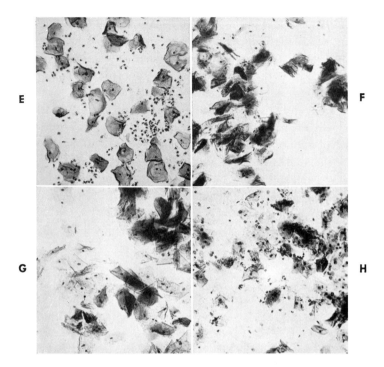

Fig. 1-2, cont'd. E, Ovulatory phase: mature cells with curling and wrinkling. **F,** Postovulatory phase: extensive clumping, marked drop in cornification. **G,** Midprogestational phase: large pale cells, envelope-type folding, and moderate cytolysis. **H,** Premenstrual phase: free nuclei, leukocytes, bacteria, and cellular debris.

the vagina: the pH of the secretions in the vagina and the growth of the Döderlein bacilli. At birth the vagina is sterile and the pH reaction of the secretions is acidic; however, in several days the Döderlein bacilli appear and the degree of acidity is increased to a pH of 4.0 to 5.0 chiefly by lactic acid, most of which is derived from the action of the bacilli on the glycogen in the vaginal epithelial cells. In the first few days of life some of the acidity may be due to contamination of the vagina by amniotic fluid. After the first month the lactobacilli disappear, a mixed flora replaces them, and the pH rises to 7.0. The secretions in the vagina remain neutral or alkaline until puberty, at which time acidity recurs with a pH of 4.0 to 5.0. This acidity is caused by the marked increase in the number of Döderlein bacilli and the changes in the cells. The adult condition of the vagina continues, provided there is normal ovarian function and no infection, until the menopause, after which it returns to the prepuberty state.

The creamy or curded material that normally covers the vaginal walls is a mixture of cervical and endometrial secretions and of desquamated epithelia. Microscopic examination of fluid obtained from the normal vagina of a mature woman during the intermenstrual stage shows a large number of exfoliated vaginal cells, occasional endometrial and cervical cells, and numerous bacteria, leukocytes, and histiocytes. The biosynthesis of lactic acid within the vagina is a matter of some conjecture. It may be that glucose available in blood and tissue fluids is converted into glycogen by the vaginal epithelium. Before storage in the cells the glycogen is evidently reduced to less complex carbohydrates, particularly glucose, by a glycolytic enzyme. The histochemical demonstration of alkaline phosphatase, which is important in glycogenesis, is compatible with this opinion. The role of lactobacilli has already been mentioned, but it is not certain whether they are capable of transforming glycogen into lactic acid without intermediate steps. A low pH serves to inhibit the growth of most pathogenic organisms except fungi. The pH is usually elevated after coitus or in conditions of excessive endocervical secretion or vaginal infection.

Physiology of the vulva and vagina

Response during sexual stimulation and accomodations for parturition are the important considerations.

With sufficient erotic stimulation vascular engorgement to tumescence occurs in the bulbocavernous and ischiocavernous bodies and in the two crura and glans of the clitoris, while vascular engorgement of the vessels of the labia minora causes a twofold or threefold expansion and a change from pink to red. Stimulation originates synergistically through cerebral activity and contact excitation of the numerous sensory nerve endings of the vulva and vagina, as well as tactile response from the lips, breasts, and other readily responding areas. The numerous sweat glands of the vulva are activated, and a copious transudate from the vaginal wall occurs. A small amount of mucus escapes from the Bartholin glands. The smooth muscle of the vaginal wall contracts to dilate the upper vagina. The voluntary muscles of the vulva and around the vagina contract reflexly and frequently at the acme of the orgasmic phase.

The period of time required for maximum response is longer in women than in men. With sufficient stimulation over an adequate period the plateau of response that can be maintained in women is longer than that which occurs for many men.

The distensibility needed for childbirth develops during pregnancy when hypertrophy of the muscles and mucosa occurs, along with increased vascularity due to the continued stimulation of large amounts of estrogens and progestogens.

UTERUS
Anatomy and histology

Situated about the center of the pelvic cavity, the uterus, often compared to an inverted pear, projects upward into the lower part of the peritoneal cavity. In most females the upper part of the corpus uteri is directed forward and the cervix uteri

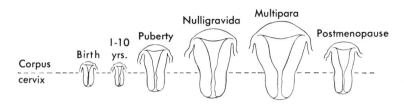

Fig. 1-3. Changes in the relative size of the cervix and corpus of the uterus.

is directed backward and downward into the vagina. The corpus is usually freely movable. That portion above the tubouterine junction is called the fundus.

The uterus has a small central cavity that is lined with mucous membrane and that communicates through the vagina with the external part of the body and through the fallopian tubes with the peritoneal cavity. This is the only continuous opening from the outside of the body into the peritoneal sac; it is because of this direct opening into the peritoneal cavity that peritonitis is so much more common in women than in men.

The size of the uterus is, of course, different in the different periods of life (Fig. 1-3). At birth it is a trifle over 2.5 cm long, and the cervix comprises two thirds of the organ. It is important to keep in mind the peculiarities of the infantile uterus, for occasionally a woman's uterus is somewhat infantile and accompanied by troublesome symptoms due to lack of development. A rather common condition is acute anteflexion of the cervix, the corpus uteri being in practically normal position but the cervix being flexed sharply forward and directed along the vaginal canal toward the opening. In the fetus the uterus lies very high and the cervix is very long. At first the axis of the uterus lies almost in the axis of the vagina. Normally, as development progresses, the corpus uteri gradually comes forward and the cervix becomes directed somewhat backward, across the vaginal axis. In the cases of imperfect development just referred to the corpus uteri comes forward normally, but the cervix fails to assume its backward direction, remaining in practically the fetal position (directed along the axis of the vagina) and causing acute anteflexion of the cervix.

The adult virgin uterus is about 7.6 cm long, with a cavity of 6.3 cm, and the cervix forms one third of the organ. The transverse measurement at the widest part is 3.3 cm, and the average thickness of the wall is 2.5 cm. It weighs 28 to 45 grams. The uterus after childbirth is always larger; the cavity is usually 7.6 cm, and the weight is around 70 grams.

After the menopause there is progressive atrophy of all the genital organs. The extent of the atrophy of the uterus is variable. In the very aged this organ may be reduced to a nodule the size of the end of the thumb; the cervix then no longer projects into the vaginal cavity but is felt simply as an indurated area, usually with a very small central opening, situated in the upper part of the anterior vaginal wall.

The *wall* of the uterus is composed of three layers: peritoneal, muscular, and mucous.

The *peritoneal layer* forms a delicate serous covering for the uterus, with the exception of the lateral portions of the corpus and the front and sides of the cervix. It is continuous with the peritoneum of the posterior surface of the broad ligament on each side and with that of the rectouterine pouch. It covers most of the posterior cervix. The position of the uterus is subject to great variation in different women and in the same woman at different times. If the corpus is anteflexed, the vesical surface of the uterus is separated from the upper surface of the bladder by the vesicouterine pouch.

The *myometrium* is the real wall of the uterus. It is composed of involuntary muscle. At the cornua where the uterine tube traverses the uterine wall there is an interlacing network of uterine muscle fibers. It has been shown that these fibers are responsible for the sphincter mechanism, which may be seen on hysterosalpingography. Most of the uterine *connective tissue* is found in the muscular layer. This also applies to the *blood vessels*. The arteries are distinguished in a microscopic section by their thick walls and folded intima. The outer vessels run in a longitudinal direction, and the inner vessels run perpendicular to the mucous surface, close to which there is a dense capillary network. The veins are very large and have thin walls. The *lymphatics* of the uterus empty into large lymphatic vessels in the external muscular stratum, which drain into the hypogastric, external iliac, obturator, sacral, inguinal, and aortic nodes. The *nerves* of the muscular layer are derived from the sympathetic nervous system. Filaments ramify among the muscle bundles and terminate in the nuclei of the muscle cells.

The *endometrium* is directly on the internal muscular stratum, the usual submucous layer of loose connective tissue being absent. Scattered muscular filaments extend into it, so that the connection between the two strata is relatively firm. The endometrium is 2 to 6 mm thick in the childbearing period and is disposed over the interior of the uterus as a smooth layer. It is soft and velvety to the touch and, when perfectly fresh, is pink. It is thin with but a few glands in infancy, greatly thickened and with many glands in the childbearing period, and thin again in old age. The lining of the cervix is known as the endocervical mucosa.

The basis of the endometrium is a tissue composed almost exclusively of oval cells, each somewhat larger than a leukocyte and having a round or oval nucleus that stains lightly. The nucleus is so large that it occupies most of the cell. When stained it is reticular; i.e., it shows the chromatin bands and does not stain a solid dark color as does the nucleus of a lymphocyte. These oval cells with the large reticular nucleus are known as *stromal cells*. They are packed close together, with nothing separating them except a few cell processes and a small amount of serous or mucoid intercellular substance, referred to as ground substance. The tissue thus formed is known as *cytogenic tissue*. When a specimen of it is stained, the microscopic field seems to be almost entirely occupied by rounded or oval reticular nuclei. The cell protoplasm stains so lightly and is so negligible that it is scarcely noticeable. The stroma probably represents embryonic connective tissue. In the resting endometrium the stromal cells are closely packed and stain very deeply. Under certain conditions, however, they become swollen and stain more lightly. This occurs in the premenstrual stage and especially during pregnancy. During pregnancy they greatly enlarge and become the decidua cells. Under these conditions, also, the intercellular serous or mucoid material becomes noticeable, thus giving the whole an edematous appearance.

The stroma is rich in capillaries that become much increased in size and number in the premenstrual stage. They arise in the basal layer and course upward, forming right-angled loops near the surface.

Embedded in the stroma are the *uterine glands*. These are lined by single layers of epithelial cells, the nucleus of each cell being placed near its center. In the stage of secretion they crowd each other, forming a very irregular line, unlike the regular arrangement of the nuclei in the cervical glands. The glands extend from the depth of the endometrium and open upon the surface. They vary considerably in different parts of their course, especially in the premenstrual stage.

The structure of the cervix differs from that of the body of the uterus in several particulars, as follows:

1. The greater part of the cervix has no peritoneal covering.

2. The muscular layer of the cervix has a much larger proportion of connective tissue and therefore is much firmer. Danforth, in extensive studies of the cervix, has shown that the cervix is composed predominantly of fibrous tissue. The musculature averaged 15% of the total tissue. Except in the peripheral areas of the supravaginal portion of the cervix, where the muscle fibers seem to be concentrated and where they are continuous with the uterus above and the vagina below, the muscle fibers are isolated attenuated strands. He found no evidence of a definite sphincter muscle, although at the internal os there is an abrupt change from the uterine muscle above to the fibrous tissue containing a few muscle cells of the cervix. The contractile ability of the cervix was negligible when compared with that of the uterus.

3. There are no large venous sinuses in the cervix, and the blood vessels have thicker walls and smaller lumina than those of the body of the uterus.

4. The endocervix is disposed in prominent folds, extending more or less obliquely outward from two ridges, one situated near the center of the posterior lip and the other near the center of the anterior lip.

5. The glands of the cervix are of a somewhat racemose variety. They consist of branching ducts with dilated ends. The glands are lined with columnar epithelial cells that are even taller than those on the surface. The nucleus of each cell lies at the base. These cells secrete mucus that does not stain appreciably in ordinary preparations (hematoxylin and eosin); consequently that portion of the cell lying next to the lumen, which is usually filled with mucus, appears clear.

The glands of the cervix secrete a clear viscid tenacious mucus that fills the cervical canal and serves to close it and prevent invasion of the uterine cavity. The ducts of these glands sometimes become obstructed, causing retention cysts. These are sometimes called ovula Nabothi. There may be many of them, in which case the cervix is said to be in a state of "cystic degeneration." Fluhmann, from a study of premature and newborn infants and children from 2 weeks to 14 years of age, concluded that the glands were in reality multiple folds of the cervical lining. In a discussion of this article, however, Hertig stated that in the adult the glands have a tubular or racemose appearance.

The mucus of the cervix shows varying forms of fernlike patterns according to the time of the cycle and the presence or absence of a pregnancy. This is discussed in more detail in Chapter 2.

Atypical changes occur in cells lining the cervical canal during pregnancy, but these usually disappear during or after the puerperium. Howard and co-workers noted certain unusual cells possessing multipotentialities in the cervical mucous membrane, which they named "reserve cells." Pund and Auerbach had previously observed that when these cells were found in other locations in the body they could become malignant. Hellman and associates reported that the cells responded to estrogen stimulation with atypical changes but that these changes were reversible and that there was no evidence that they bore any direct relationship to cervical cancer in the human being.

6. The epithelium covering the outer surface of the cervix is similar to that of the vagina; hence the cyclic changes occurring are included in the discussion of the vagina.

Blood vessels and nerves. The blood supply of the uterus comes from the uterine and ovarian arteries. The *uterine artery* of each side arises from the anterior trunk of the internal iliac and passes inward and downward between the layers of the broad ligament to a point just above the lateral vaginal fornix. It then turns upward and runs in a very tortuous course along the side of the uterus. Near the top of the uterus it joins the descending branch of the ovarian artery.

As it runs along the side or just within the myometrium of the uterus, the uterine artery gives off many branches that run horizontally about the organ and supply various segments. These anastomose with corresponding branches of the opposite artery. The tortuous and spiral arrangement is so marked that these have been called the "curling arteries" of the uterus. A horizontal branch of considerable size at the level of the internal os is known as the circular artery.

The *ovarian artery* of each side supplies the tube, ovary, and upper part of the uterus. The ovarian arteries in the female correspond to the spermatic ones in the male and arise directly from the aorta. The artery of each side passes downward and enters the broad ligament. After giving off the branches that supply the ovary, the artery passes on to the upper part of the uterus where it divides into two branches. The upper branch supplies the fundus uteri and anastomoses with the corresponding branch of the opposite artery. The lower and larger branch descends along the side of the uterus and anastomoses with the uterine artery. Some authorities describe the uterine artery as supplying all the side of the uterus and a part of the tube and anastomosing with the ovarian artery some distance out along the tube. The distribution differs considerably in different individuals.

The *veins* of the uterus are exceedingly numerous. The organ is surrounded by a vast network of these vessels, which receive the blood from the veins and sinuses within its walls. There is free communication of these plexuses with the vaginal and vesical plexus below and with the ovarian (pampiniform) plexus above, the blood ultimately emptying into the internal iliac vein.

An important fact, from a surgical standpoint, is that in the median line the uterus is almost free of blood vessels, so much so that it may be bisected with but little blood loss.

The *lymphatics* of the uterus may be divided into those of the cervix and those of the corpus. The former join with those of the upper part of the vagina and empty into the sacral, hypogastric, and superior iliac glands. The lymphatics from the corpus join with those of the tube and ovary, emptying into the lumbar glands. A few lymphatics from the uterine cornua pass along the round ligaments and drain into the inguinal glands.

The *uterine nerves* are derived from the hypogastric plexus of the sympathetic system and from the third and fourth sacral nerves of the central nervous system passing through the ovarian plexus and the Frankenhäuser ganglion.

Ligaments. The uterus is held in position by the pelvic floor and the *broad* and *uterosacral ligaments*. Ulfelder, as well as others, has emphasized that the role of the uterine ligaments is not to hold the uterus up but to hold it forward in a normal position. This prevents the intra-abdominal pressure from forcing the uterus through the weak sites in the pelvic sling.

The *broad ligament* derives its name from the fact that it has an attachment along the side of the organ from the cervix to the fundus and a corresponding attachment to the pelvic wall. It holds the uterus in its appointed position in the center of the pelvic cavity. Each broad ligament is composed of two layers of peritoneum, and between them there are a number of important structures. This disposition of the peritoneum and consequent formation of the broad ligaments are represented very well by a thin cloth laid over the pelvis and tucked down snugly around the pelvic organs. The peritoneum covering the anterior surface of the uterus, when continued laterally, forms the anterior layer of the broad ligament, and that covering the posterior surface of the uterus, continued laterally, forms the posterior layer of the ligament. Between these two layers of peritoneum is a considerable amount of connective tissue, especially at the lower part. This connective tissue around the uterus is known as the parametrium. Inflammation of this tissue is spoken of as parametritis.

The role of the pelvic sling in preventing uterine prolapse is discussed in Chapter 6.

The *uterosacral ligaments* are flat bands of fibrous tissue, containing some muscle fibers, that can be seen for about 1.5 to 2 cm as they extend dorsally from the posterolateral surface of the cervix and fan out into small strands to be inserted into the anterior surface of the sacrum. These separated strands are not evident as a band but, when made tense, show strong support. Similarly the endopelvic fascia, of which the uterosacral ligaments are a posterior portion, is condensed at its lateral attachments to the cervix and upper vagina (cardinal ligaments) and fans out into strands laterally and anteriorly. This arrangement has been compared to chicken wire, which, when viewed expanded in individual strands, is not nearly so strong as when gathered and pulled taut. Plication of the uterosacral ligaments is employed in uterine replacement operations and in the surgical repair of enterocele.

The *round ligament* of each side is a fibromuscular cord that arises from the top of the uterus just in front of the fallopian tube and extends outward and forward in the upper part of the broad ligament to the internal inguinal ring. It passes through the inguinal canal and at the external inguinal ring divides into fibrous filaments that are lost in the tissues covering the pubic joint. The round ligaments are 10 to 12.5 cm in length and tend to prevent backward displacement of the uterus. Ordinarily they are lax, but, when the uterus is displaced backward by a full bladder, they are made tense and help to bring the uterus back to its accustomed position. It is probable that one of their main functions is to prevent torsion of the uterus.

The *vesicouterine ligament* is simply a fold of peritoneum extending from the uterus to the bladder. It may have some slight stabilizing action.

Physiology

Menstruation and childbearing are the functions of the uterus. The normal nonpregnant uterus serves as a passageway for spermatozoa en route to meet the oocyte, and it undergoes cyclic changes in preparation for gestation. During pregnancy it harbors the products of conception and affords avenues for the exchange of metabolic materials between the mother and the conceptus.

Menstruation is the physiologic uterine bleeding that normally recurs, usually at approximately 4-week intervals, in the absence of pregnancy during the reproductive period of the female of the human species and a few other species of primates. Anovulatory, or anovular, menstruation is the term applied to cyclic uterine bleeding without preceding ovulation. Vicarious menstruation is the name used for a menstrual flow from some part or organ other than the vagina. In the years preceding puberty the endometrium develops slowly, the glands being formed by ingrowth of the surface epithelium. As puberty is approached, more rapid development takes place in preparation for the change from a quiescent structure to an actively functioning membrane that undergoes partial destruction and renewal every few weeks.

Adolescence is the period during which the reproductive organs become functionally active and secondary sex characteristics develop. Formerly it was taught that the onset of the first menstrual period, or the menarche, was the clinical sign denoting the onset of puberty. Changes often referred to as puberty, however, actually precede the menarche by many years. Therefore Stuart suggested dropping the term "puberty" entirely because of its indefinite connotation. In its place he proposed that the changes covered by the term "adolescence" be divided into the prepubescent, pubescent, and postpubescent periods, thus encompassing the process of growing from childhood to womanhood. In the prepubescent period there is little difference between the sexes in build or development. The pubescent period extends from the eighth to the sixteenth year, during which time the secondary sex characteristics develop and the sex organs mature and begin to function, as exemplified by the menarche, which is only one of the signs of sexual development. The postpubescent period usually extends from the sixteenth to the twentieth year, a span within which the girl usually becomes a fully matured woman both physically and psychologically.

Physiologic changes in endocrine glands

The endocrine glands concerned in growth and maturation are the pituitary, the adrenals, the gonads, and the thyroid; their interrelationships are shown in Fig. 1-9. At about the age of 8 years there is an increase in the production of the adrenotropic and the gonadotropic hormones. From the eighth to the tenth year there is an increase of estrogens in the blood, which are responsible for the bodily changes known as the secondary sex characteristics. The estrogens during these years are in part produced by the adrenal glands, as the ovaries have just begun to secrete estrogens. From the tenth to the eleventh year the ovaries have matured enough to respond to follicle-stimulating hormone (FSH), and the ovarian spiral arterioles develop as described under ovulation. When the blood cycle of estrogen reaches a peak high enough that withdrawal causes a breakdown of the endometrium, the menarche appears. This is usually between the ages of 12 and 14 years, but the time varies with climate, race, and socioeconomic conditions. In otherwise healthy girls it may occasionally start as early as 10 or as late as 18 years.

The early cycles are usually anovulatory, and they continue until the ovulatory mechanism becomes established. Mills and Ogle, in a study of a primitive group in which sexual promiscuity among children was frequent, found there was an interval of several years between the menarche and pregnancy.

Changes during adolescence

Along with the changes in the contour of the body and the growth of the sex organs, there are profound changes in the psyche. Interest in the opposite sex, together with the new experience of cyclic bleeding, causes a considerable emotional upheaval, and it is important that those associated with the child understand the problems involved and show a sympathetic interest in them. The changes taking place should be explained, with emphasis on the fact that these are normal and are an important part of the plan of the Creator for survival of the race. General hygienic measures include adequate rest and exercise, balanced diet, and protection from emotional strain whenever possible. Terms such as "the curse," "sick time," and "unwell" should not be used, as they place an erroneous interpretation on a normal process. Pads should be used by younger girls, but tampons may be used when the hymenal opening becomes large enough to permit insertion.

Menstruation

Menstrual discharge consists of blood mixed with the secretion and fragments of the endometrium, secretion of the endocervix, and cells and organisms of the vagina. It also includes many enzymes, hormones, and vitamins, as well as other substances such as proteins, fats, and carbohydrates.

Although normal menstrual blood does not clot, no anticoagulant has been isolated. Glueck and Mirsky decided that the blood clots in the uterine cavity as it leaves the endometrium; it is then acted on by a lytic agent. Such fibrinolytic activity has been demonstrated by other workers. Phillips and associates found a fibrinogenolytic enzyme and a cytofibrinokinase in extracts from the human myometrium, endometrium, decidua, and placenta. Rumbolz and Greene demonstrated that there were heparin granules in mast cells and that there was an increase of mast cells in the endometrium from the time of ovulation up to menstruation. These cells were also increased in certain bleeding states associated with the progestational phase of the cycle.

The amount of bloody discharge lost at each menstruation varies considerably in different women; there is also a variation in the same person at different times. Barer and co-workers, in a careful check on 100 healthy women between the ages of 15 and 43 years, found an actual variation from 6 ml to 178 ml. The average amount was 50 ml. They found that the duration of the period and the number of pads used were not an accurate index of the amount of the flow. They also studied the effect on the hematopoietic system of long-continued loss of iron with excessive menses and concluded that excessive menses were a cause of hypochromic anemia in certain cases.

There is much variation in the duration of the menstrual flow, the average being 3 or 4 days. Some perfectly healthy women menstruate 1 or 2 days, and others have a flow for 5 or 7 days or longer.

Numerous studies have been made on the interval between menstruations, estimated from the first day of the flow. McKeown and associates found that for 819 women with fairly normal periods the mean length of the cycle was 28.4 days. Although the average interval is 28 days, all workers found that in no case did absolute regularity exist and that normal women could expect a variation of 2 days from the mean cycle length in about one third of their menses. Rock stated that variations beyond the limits of 24 to 32 days should be considered abnormal, agreeing with the analysis made by Haman.

Menstruation usually ceases during pregnancy and lactation, but there are exceptions to this rule, and very often the menses return while the woman is still nursing her baby.

Endometrial changes. The relation of cyclic endometrial changes to follicle maturation, ovulation, and corpus luteum formation is shown in Fig. 1-5.

Cyclic glandular and stromal changes. Change in the endometrium during the menstrual cycle may be conveniently divided into five stages: postmenstrual, early growth, later growth, premenstrual, and menstrual. The first stage of the cycle begins immediately after the breaking down of the endometrium in the preceding menstruation and ends with the menstruation, which signifies the breaking down of the endometrium built up in the cycle. It will be of help in mastering terminology to keep in mind that we are dealing with changes in the endometrium itself and that the terms, in the technical meanings used here are not related to the flow, which continues to appear externally some days after the menstrual breaking down of the endometrium is completed. Accordingly the postmenstrual stage begins as soon as the menstrual breaking down of the endometrium is finished, which is in the first part of the menstrual flow. Usually by the time the external flow is over the postmenstrual stage of the endometrium is past and regrowth has begun.

Bartelmez states that the tissue lost with the menses is chiefly stromal ground substance and some of the superficial layer of the endometrium. There is some loss of this substance immediately following ovulation, after which there is an increase until just before the end of the progestational stage. With the death and regression of the corpus luteum there is a marked decrease, resulting in the extravasation of the ground substance and the secretion of the glands, which occurs just prior to actual loss of tissue with the menses. He also points out that the secretion of the endometrial glands is continuous throughout the menstrual cycle, but that the rhythmic contractions of the uterine muscle prevent it from collecting in the lumina of the glands. The reason we see the glands filled with fluid during the last half of the cycle is that the relaxation of the uterine musculature during this part of the cycle allows it to collect there. For this reason he suggests that the use of "secretory phase" be supplanted by the term "progestational phase."

Cyclic arteriolar and venous changes. The vascular events associated with the cyclic changes of the endometrium are of great interest in that, under hormone control, they cause the menstrual flow of blood and are important in the accompanying endometrial disintegration (Fig. 1-5).*

The vessels in the endometrium primarily concerned with menstrual bleeding are the coiled arterioles and the subepithelial capillaries. The coiled arterioles arise from the arcuate branch of the uterine artery in the inner third of the uterine wall. They follow a radial course through the inner fourth of the uterine muscle, in which area there are constricting fibers that Markee called "contraction cones." After leaving the musculature each arteriole extends through the endometrium to its surface as an end arteriole. Immediately after menstruation these arterioles begin to grow into the newly regenerating endometrium. The arterioles grow faster than the other endometrial tissue and thus become coiled or spiral.

The muscle cones surrounding these spiral arterioles are under hormone control, and the terminal portions of the arterioles in the endometrium degenerate when their blood supply is diminished by prolonged contraction of the muscle cones. The interference with the blood supply to the endometrium in the area of the affected terminal arterioles is associated with disintegration of the endometrium in those areas. The basal layer of the endometrium is supplied by another group of arteries, which are not under hormone control and hence do not undergo cyclic changes. Thus the fundal portions of the glands, which lie in the basal layer, are preserved for regeneration of the endometrium.

About 48 hours before the onset of menstruation the endometrium begins to shrink as a result of the withdrawal of estrogen and progestogen caused by the regression of the corpus luteum. The actual shrinkage is due to a loss of stromal ground substance. This shrinkage causes excessive spiraling of the arterioles, with a consequent stasis of the blood circulation in them. Okkels described an anastomosis between the artery and the vein proximal to the superficial portion of the endometrium, and Schlegel believes that the stasis in the superficial portion of the endometrium before necrosis and bleeding is due to the opening of this arteriovenous anastomosis at this stage. For 4 to 24 hours before the onset of menses there is also constriction of the coiled arterioles in the region of the "contraction cones," causing further degeneration of the terminal portions of the arterioles and the adjacent tissue. The actual bleeding results from several factors, including dipedesis (due to increased fragility of the capillary and arteriole walls) and spasmodic flow from intermittent temporary relaxation of the muscle cones.

During menstruation there is a marked loss of stromal ground substance, and the superficial layers of the endometrium are cast off. During the entire menstruation the basal circulation has continued, and it is now accelerated. From the stumps of the coiled arterioles, capillary sprouts develop and the superficial capillary bed is rapidly re-formed.

In contradistinction to the behavior of endometrial glands, these cyclic vascular events preceding and accompanying menstruation appear to be similar whether the bleeding follows an ovulatory or an anovulatory cycle.

Cyclic histochemical changes. As the result of an intensive study of chemical changes occurring in component cells of various tissues, it has been found that in the endometrium, as in other tissues, numerous biochemical reactions occur that are controlled by the hormone-enzyme regulators. Numerous lipids, proteins, and other chemical substances have been isolated, and their location in the various endometrial cells has been determined. The amounts and location of many of these substances vary with different phases of the cycle. In a synopsis such as this the subject cannot be discussed fully, but the brief discussion of acid hydrolases, prostaglandins, and glycogen may help to demonstrate their clinical importnace. It is well known that the general nutrition has a marked effect on menstrual function and in fact on the whole life cycle of a woman. The effect of nutrition in the life cycle of women has been the subject of a study by Macy and Mack.

It has been shown that the glycogen content of the epithelial cells lining the endometrial glands is under both hormone and enzyme (alkaline phosphatase and phosphorylase) control. As the glycogen increases, the alkaline phosphatase in the endometrium decreases. Payne and Latour, using the anthrone method of estimating the quantitative amounts of glycogen in the endometrium, confirmed previous findings that the concentration is greatest on the seventeenth day of the cycle. Then there is a drop; the concentration reaches its lowest point about the twenty-first day and again rises moderately until the twenty-seventh day. Hughes was one of the first to point out the importance of these glycogen deposits in the premenstrual endometrium for the nutrition of the blastula. He found that when they were deficient in the progestational endometrium, sterility and habitual abortion were common.

Electron-microscopic studies have indicated that acid hydrolases elaborated by the Golgi systems are so disruptive of cellular membranes that they must be sequestrated in the lysosomes from which they are liberated at the time of dissolution of the endometrium. These and other changes in the endometrial cells can be correlated with observations using the scanning electron microscope, which beautifully demonstrates the surface changes of the endometrium during the menstrual cycle.

It is thought that prostaglandin may be involved in menstruation. Studies of prostaglandin F_{2a} and prostaglandin E_2 suggest that prostaglandin E_2 levels, which rise near menstruation, may be involved in vascular change and uterine contractility. Clinical use of prostaglandins suggests that premenstrual and menstrual symptoms may, in large part, be due to their presence.

Menopause

In a healthy woman menstruation usually ceases between the ages of 40 and 52. This period of cessation of menstruation is known variously as the menopause, the climacteric, and the "change of life." The changes that take place in the uterus during and after menopause are similar to those occurring in all the genital structures—a gradual atrophy of the functioning part (endometrium and muscular tissue), a general fibrous change, and a gradual diminution in size, particularly of the corpus.

Many of the symptoms that are ordinarily considered as part of the "change of life" are instead due to pathologic conditions and as such require investigation. Such symptoms, for example, are increased menstrual flow, bloody discharge between the menstrual periods, leukorrhea, pelvic pain, and marked nervous disturbances. It seems to be the general impression among women that irregular bloody discharges are natural during the "change of life." Such discharges are not natural, however, and they usually mean either inflammation or cancer. The clinical aspects of the menopause are discussed in a later chapter.

OVARY

The somewhat almond-shaped ovaries are situated on each side of the uterus, near the pelvic brim and close to the outer end of the fallopian tube. Each ovary projects from the posterior wall of the broad ligament on its respective side, and the peritoneal fold thus formed is called the mesovarium (Fig. 1-4). It is through this attachment to the broad ligament that the ovary receives its blood supply, this being the point where the blood vessels enter. In size the ovaries vary greatly in different individuals, and even in the same individual the two ovaries may differ. Ordinarily the ovary is 3.5 to 5 cm in length, about 2.5 cm in width, and about 1.5 cm in thickness. It weighs 5 to 10 grams.

Anatomy

In structure the ovary is a collection of microscopic oocytes, supported and held together by the connective tissue that forms the framework. Each oocyte is inside a minute sac, called the ovisac or graafian follicle. The connective tissue extends

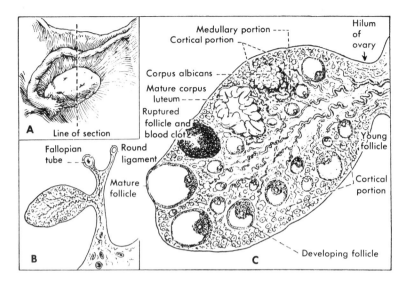

Fig. 1-4. Ovarian structures and relations. **A,** Surface relations of ovary, tube, and round ligament and the line of section for **B. B,** Attachment of the ovary to the broad ligament at the hilus and, incidentally, the relative locations of the tube and round ligament. **C,** Diagrammatic representation of the details of ovarian structure. The blood vessels, lymphatics, and nerves enter at the hilus and, with their connective tissue supports, extend through the center of the ovary, forming the medullary portion. From this central location nutrition, drainage, and nerve control are supplied to the cortical portion, which is the special functioning part of the ovary.

From Crossen, R.J.: Diseases of women, St. Louis, The C.V. Mosby Co.

between the follicles in all directions, and, in addition to supporting and protecting them, it carries the blood vessels that nourish them and also the lymph vessels and nerves. This connective tissue constitutes the ovarian stroma, and it is peculiar in that it is exceedingly rich in cells. These cells are spindle shaped and are packed so closely together that in an ordinary microscopic preparation the tissue seems to be made up exclusively of long, oval nuclei lying close together. Near the periphery of the ovary the connective tissue fibers become more numerous and the nuclei fewer, so that there is a rather dense capsule, known as the tunica albuginea. It is simply a condensation of the ovarian stroma and serves to protect the deeper structures of the ovary. Outside this fibrous layer lies the epithelial covering.

   That portion of the ovary at which the vessels find entrance and exit is called the hilus. Immediately about the hilus and extending some little distance into the ovary is the area known as the medulla or medullary portion. This is occupied by the blood vessels, lymph vessels, nerves and supporting connective tissue. It contains no follicles.

   The remaining part of the ovary contains the graafian follicles and is called the cortex or cortical portion. The free surface of the cortical portion, i.e., the peritoneal surface of the ovary, is covered with cylindric epithelium. The graafian follicles are very numerous and of different sizes. The small, young follicles lie near the surface and are numbered by thousands. They are about 0.25 mm in diameter. The larger, older follicles lie deeper and are not as numerous. The largest of these measure 1 mm in diameter.

The graffian follicle is lined with an epithelial layer serveral cells thick, called the membrana granulosa, and is filled with clear viscid fluid, the liquor folliculi. The oocyte lies within the follicle near one side and is completely surrounded by cells of the membrana granulosa. After full development of the oocyte the follicle ruptures, and the egg is extruded into the abominal cavity; this process is known as ovulation. Most of the follicles never reach maturity but become atretic follicles. Usually only one follicle each month develops to maturity, although occasionally several may develop to allow multiple pregnancy.

After ovulation the remains of the ruptured follicle undergo changes to become the corpus luteum. The yellow color of the corpus luteum is due to the lipid droplets found in the cytoplasm of the hypertrophied granulosa cells, which are now called lutein cells. There is a marked folding of the granulosa wall. The cells of the theca interna also undergo hypertrophy but remain at the bases of the fold of the granulosa. Histochemical studies have shown that both types of cells produce steroid hormones. (This is unlike the situation in the follicle, where granulosa cells are histochemically rather inert.) The principal function of the corpus luteum is to produce progesterone. It also produces large quantities of estrogens. The corpus luteum continues to function for about 13 days, by which time it decreases in size. Blood is extravasated into the central region. The lutein cells undergo lysis and atrophy, and the structure is invaded by connective tissue cells. The corpus luteum persists awhile as a small yellow body but then is eventually reduced in size and becomes hyalinized. At this point it is called a corpus albicans. After a number of corpora albicantia have developed, areas of depression appear on the ovary, giving it an irregular surface.

When pregnancy follows ovulation, the corpus luteum undergoes a similar development but increases in size and persists for several months. The corpus luteum of pregnancy develops because the luteinizing gonadotropic hormone is replaced by chorionic gonadotropin.

Ligaments. The ovary lies in the pelvis obliquely, and its inner end is about 2.5 cm from the uterus. Extending from this end of the ovary to the uterus is a small fibromuscular cord, the utero-ovarian ligament, which joins the uterus just below the fallopian tube. It is the strongest support of the ovary; therefore ovarian position varies with uterine position.

Blood vessels and nerves. The ovary is supplied with blood by several branches of the ovarian artery, which corresponds to the spermatic artery in the male. The ovarian artery arises directly from the abdominal aorta and, passing downward to the side of the pelvis, enters the broad ligament and sends branches to the ovary, uterus, and tube. In the hilus of the ovary the main artery divides into the primary, secondary, and tertiary branches. The first two show some spiraling, but the tertiary branches have a coil-like arrangement, and the diameter of the vessels in this arterial system gradually diminishes until it ends in the capillary bed. The veins form a plexus near the hilus, which is known as the pampiniform or ovarian plexus.

The nerves come from the renal and spermatic ganglia. The fibers pass along in the connective tissue framework to all the graafian follicles and terminate in the follicular epithelium.

The lymphatic spaces surround the graafian follicles and ramify throughout the connective tissue of the ovary. They emerge at the hilus, anastomose with the uterine lymphatics in the broad ligament, and empty into the lumbar glands.

Parovarium. The parovarium is the remaining part of the wolffian body and consists of a triangular group of tubules situated in the part of the broad ligament lying between the ovary and the fallopian tube. When the main tubule becomes distended with fluid, a tiny cyst is formed on the surface of the broad ligament. There are other fetal remnants: The ends of the müllerian ducts occasionally form small cysts called the hydatids of Morgagni. Nearer the uterus there is a smaller group of remnants of the wolffian body called the parovarium and the paroophoron. After a study of the embryologic derivation of these structures, Gardner, Greene, and Peckham proposed a new terminology based on origin rather than on the names of the men who discovered them.

Proposed terminology	Commonly used terminology
Mesonephric body	Wolffian body, organ of Rosenmüller, epoophoron, parovarium
Mesonephric duct	Wolffian duct, longitudinal tubule of epoophoron
Mesonephric tubules	Wolffian tubules, epoophoral tubules, transverse tubules of epoophoron, Kobelt's tubules
Paramesonephric duct	Müllerian duct
Oviduct	Fallopian tube
Accessory oviducts	Accessory fallopian tubes

These structures have no function and are of interest only because they give rise to tumors in the broad ligament.

Physiology

The ovary has closely related and interdependent functions: the formation and discharge of oocytes and endocrine activities.

OOGENESIS

Largely through the studies of Fischel, Politzer, Witschi, and others, ideas on oogenesis have changed. It was formerly thought that oocytes were derived from the surface layer of the gonad, or the so-called germinal epithelium. According to the present concept the development of the ovary and the oocyte is divided into three phases: (1) the undifferentiated or gonadanlage stage, (2) the formation of primary and secondary germinal cords, and (3) the partition of these cords into separate germinal cells and the further development of the future ovarian follicle.

In the earliest stage there is an accumulation of mesenchymal cells on the anterior aspect of the mesonephron. These cells form the future gonad, are specific for this function, and are found nowhere else in the body. The overlying peritoneum gradually loses its characteristics as a serosa and becomes a single layer of epithelial cells. The germinal cells are derived from the dorsal part of the endothelium of the hindgut. They differ from the usual lining cells, for they possess the ability to migrate by ameboid motility. These cells migrate through the dorsal mesenteric epithelium into the epithelium of the genital fold (which later becomes the hilus of the ovary) and then into the central mesenchyme of the ovary. In the first phase of differentiation they arrange themselves in cords called rete ovarii, converging toward the ovarian hilus. In the female these serve no purpose and usually disappear rapidly, although occasionally they persist and remnants are seen in the mature ovary.

The second phase of development is marked by the formation of germinal cords containing the germinal cells and other small round cells that later become granulosa cells. These cords were thought by Waldeyer to be derived from the germinal epithelium but are now known to arise from the ovarian mesenchyme, and they are desginated as the primary sex cords. Secondary sex cords, which fuse with the primary cords and later disappear, are derived from the surface epithelium. Their function is not known, but some investigations indicate that their remnants may be the origin of Brenner tumors and Walthard inclusions cysts.

In the final phase of ovarian development the primary germinal cords are divided into islands of germinal cells by ingrowth of the surrounding ovarian stroma; this process is complete when each germinal cell or egg is surrounded by a single layer of granulosa cells. The final result is the primordial follicle. The development of the follicle to this stage is controlled by the self-contained organizing power of the egg. The proliferating granulosa cells then influence the surrounding stroma cells to form a concentric framework around the follicle. This framework, which is also derived from the ovarian mesenchyme, has a loose inner layer (theca interna) containing the blood vessels and a compact outer layer (theca externa). Between the theca interna and the granulosa cell layer is a clear hyaline membrane called the membrana propria. The granulosa cells proliferate, especially in the region of the egg, and later a cavity filled with a fluid is formed. The mount of cells surrounding the egg on the wall of this cavity is called the cumulus oophorus or discus proligerus. From this point on, development and functioning of the follicle are controlled by the anterior pituitary hormones.

OVULATION

Ovulation is the term applied to discharge of the mature oocyte from the graffian follicle. After the antrum appears, the further maturation of the follicle, ovulation, and development of the corpus luteum are controlled by FSH and the luteinizing hormone (LH), which are in proper balance as to time and concentration. Investigations by Reynolds and by others indicate that the development of the ovarian vasculature is under the control of estrogen. In the early adolescent girl small amounts of gonadotropic hormone reach the ovary through the undeveloped vascular system, but this is sufficient to cause follicular development and secretion. The estrogen acts on the ovarian vascular system, controlling its development and maturation. Over a period of months the ovarian rhythm becomes stronger, with the increased amount of the gonadotropic hormone reaching the ovary through its expanding vasculature, until eventually the amount of gonadotropic hormone is sufficient to stimulate the complete ovulatory cycle. After development of the ovarian vasculature is complete, the distribution of hormones throughout the cortex and the blood pressure within the ovary are controlled by adjustments that the spiral ovarian arterioles undergo during the ovarian cycle.

As the graafian follicle ripens, the theca interna forms a cone pointing toward the surface of the ovary, and the follicle ascends until it reaches and protrudes above the ovarian cortex. An attenuation of the granulosa and theca layers of the follicle wall and of the surface of the ovary develops. This area becomes ischemic and translucent. When sufficient weakening occurs, the oocyte and the follicular fluid can slowly escape through the "rupture" point. The liberated secondary oocyte is then available for the tube to carry it toward the uterus. About 20 follicles develop with each cycle, but only 1 or 2 are involved in ovulation. The remaining secondary follicles are destined to become atretic. Histochemical studies indicate that, contrary to former ideas, the theca interna—not the granulosa—is the principle source of estrogen and progesterone. Sturgis concluded that the extra spurt of estrogen just before ovulation comes from the theca interna of the secondary follicles and that this in turn stimulates the pituitary to secrete LH, which is the factor initiating ovulation (Fig. 1-5).

After the ripened oocyte is discharged, the ruptured follicle fills with bloody serum that clots, forming the corpus hemorrhagicum. The rent in the follicular wall soon heals, and the blood clot becomes partially decolorized. This follicle, now an early corpus luteum, is usually very prominent. When encountered during the course of an operation it should not be mistaken for hematoma of the ovary.

When the secondary oocyte leaves the ovary, it is approximately 100 to 150 μm in diameter. It is surrounded by the corona radiata cells, which are granulosa cells. These cells exhibit tubular processes that extend through the membrane called the zona pellucida. Material passes from these cells through the zona pellucida into the

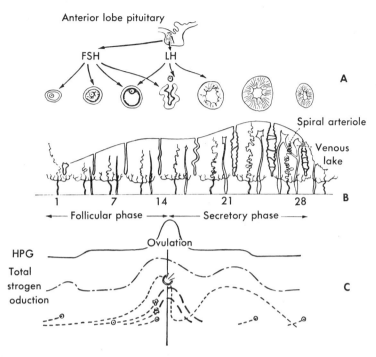

Fig. 1-5. Hormonal relationships in an ovulatory menstrual cycle. **A,** Depicting follicular maturation, ovulation, and corpus luteum formation under the influence of the two fractions of gonadotropins. **B,** Showing endometrial changes. **C,** Showing the relationship of HPG, total estrogens, and estrogenic production by individual follicles. In the lowest portion of the figure secondary follicles, which contribute to the production of estrogens, are illustrated. It is noted that the estrogen production from the follicle that matures to the point of ovulation drops sharply after ovulation.

After Sturgis, S.H.: Fertil. Steril. **1:**40, 1950.

perivitelline space. These specialized granulosal cells, which have been called nurse cells, contribute to the metabolic needs of the oocyte. When the oocyte, surrounded by the corona radiata, enters the tube, the corona cells are dispersed and the oocyte becomes more available for sperm penetration. If fertilization does not occur, the oocyte passes into the uterus and out through the vagina. It is such a small body that it is not seen. In the absence of the uterus this small body disintegrates, and its fragments can be absorbed by the peritoneum.

At the time the oocyte is picked up by the tube the second meiosis has not occurred, and it still contains 46 chromosomes; consequently it cannot properly be called an ovum.

A short review of the chromosomal changes of gametogenesis and fertilization is in order. When sexual differentiation of the gonad occurs during the seventh and eighth weeks after conception the primordial germ cells can be recognized as oogonia. Mitoses of the oogonia continue through the sixth month of fetal life. Meiosis begins at about 8 weeks, and it has been estimated that at 6 months a female fetus has about 7 million germ cells—2 million oogonia and approximately 5 million oocytes. At birth it is estimated that there are roughly 2 million germ cells, the others having been lost by degenerative processes, for which we use the term "atresia." At birth the meiotic process has begun, so that the germ cells are primary oocytes. The meiotic process is arrested in the prophase, and each cell is tetraploid (contains 92 chromosomes). The primary oocytes remain in this resting stage until further influenced by the gonadotropic hormones. When they develop in the secondary follicles, meiosis is complete. During this process the first polar body is removed and the cells become diploid (46 chromosomes). The secondary oocytes do not complete their second meiotic division unless sperm enter them. After the sperm enters, the second meiotic division takes place with a separation of the second polar body. The number of chromosomes of the oocyte is now 23. With the entrance of the 23 chromosomes from the sperm, the zygote is formed with a normal complement of 46 chromosomes. The first polar body can divide, and it is thought that certain tumors (teratomas) originate from polar bodies. An understanding of the mitotic and meiotic processes is essential for comprehension of chromosomal anomalies.

Once the sperm has penetrated the oocyte, the male pronucleus swells to the size of the female pronucleus. It is thought that the two pronuclei fuse and mitotic cleavage begins after about 30 hours. The process continues while the zygote is still in the tube, so that after 4 days a 38-cell blastula has been formed. The zona pellucida does not undergo lysis until cavitation develops. After 4 to 6 days the development is such that implantation in the endometrium can begin. If the blastula has not been transported to the endometrial cavity, implantation in the tube may occur as a tubal pregnancy. With endometrial implantation and development of the cytotrophoblast, the hormones of pregnancy are soon produced.

Certain subjective, objective, and laboratory changes are associated with ovulation. Over a period of 3 or 4 days there is an increase in the quantity and a decrease in the viscosity of the cervical mucus. The patient who is observant may speak of these as her "wet days." Soon after ovulation there may be lower abdominal pain, particularly when there is an appreciable amount of bleeding from the ovary. This is variable and does not always occur. After ovulation there may be slight endometrial bleeding noted vaginally that is thought to be due to the drop in estrogens. If the vaginal cells are studied daily, it will be found that with continuing high estrogen levels the pyknotic cells of the superficial layer are more numerous and more completely developed. After ovulation there is a folding of the cells and a relative decrease in their number so that the maturation index changes. If the basal body temperature is recorded, it is noticed that before ovulation the oral temperature is 98° F or less. After ovulation the temperature increases approximately 0.6° or 0.7° as a result of the influence of progesterone. Determination of an increased amount of progesterone in the blood or pregnanediol in the urine is indicative of the development of the corpus luteum.

The normal human ovary contains about 400,000 eggs at menarche. About 450 eggs are released by ovulation. The others degenerate as atretic follicles. The rate of degeneration is similar with and without ovulation. Menopause will occur when no more follicles are available for ovulation and adequate estrogen production. The stromal cells primarily produce testosterone, androstenedione, and dehydroepiandrosterone; this accounts for slight increases in these substances in some postmenopausal women.

Relation of ovarian, pituitary, and hypothalamic functions (Fig. 1-6)

Follicular development of the ovary is stimulated by FSH of the anterior pituitary, and estrogen secretion occurs with FSH and LH stimulation. Progestogen secretion is stimulated by LH, which is also called ICSH (interstitial cell–stimulating hormone) because of its effects on the testis and on the hilar cells of the ovary. The growth and maturation of the reproductive organs and the development of the secondary sex characteristics depend on the ovarian and gonadotropic hormones.

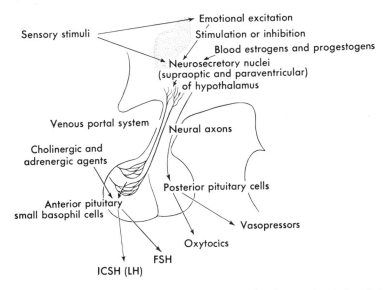

Fig. 1-6. Relation of the hypothalamus and the pituitary. Note that the anterior pituitary is influenced through the portal system and the posterior pituitary by nerve pathways. The principal factors controlling the neurosecretory nuclei of the hypothalamus are indicated.

During adolescence maturation of hypothalamic function allows the releasing factors to be produced and causes gonadotropins to be secreted by the anterior pituitary. The extracts from stalk–median eminence tissue have been shown by in vivo and in vitro methods to cause release of FSH and LH by pituitary tissue. Although originally it was thought that there were separate releasing factors for FSH and LH, recent studies indicate that the gonadotropin-releasing factor (GnRF) exists as a decapeptide that is capable of increasing secretion and release of both FSH and LH. Use of synthetic GnRF has allowed better understanding of relationships of hypothalamic, pituitary, and ovarian functions. These preparations are administered intravenously, intramuscularly, or subcutaneously and are effective. They have a half-life of 4 to 9 minutes and blood levels attained are very low. After intravenous administration the gonadotropin levels increase within 24 minutes.

Clinical investigations have shown that clomiphene increases response to GnRF. The fact that infants aged 3 months and prepubertal children respond suggests that the maturation of the hypothalamus brings on puberty and menarche. Patients with anorexia nervosa and "post pill" amenorrhea respond. Patients who have had a pituitary removed by ablation or injured by pituitary tumors either have a decreased response or fail to respond. It has been shown that small amounts of estrogens increase the pituitary response to GnRF. Larger doses of estrogens and progestogens decrease the degree of response of the pituitary to GnRF

Considerable evidence indicates that neurotransmitters are involved in the regulation of secretions by the pituitary. Dopamine inhibits prolactin and LH secretion. Acetylcholine stimulates and serotonin inhibits the release of GnRF. Norepinephrine neuronal pathways are also involved. The hypothalamus is capable of in situ formation of 2-hydroxyestrone and 2-hydroxyestradiol—catecholestrogens that may serve as biochemical links between estrogens and catecholamines in the modulation of neuronal activity.

According to our present understanding, the inhibition of the hypothalamic and pituitary functions are influenced by three feedback mechanisms—a long, a short, and an ultrashort mechanism. In the long feedback mechanism the estrogens and progestogens (also testosterone) produced by the ovary inhibit the hypothalamus, particularly when these substances exist in higher levels. (There is a positive feedback effect increasing function of the hypothalamus with low levels of estrogens and progestogens.) The short loop feedback mechanism is from the ovary to the pituitary. Estrogens, progestogens, and testosterone inhibit pituitary function. The ultrashort feedback mechanism is from the pituitary to the hypothalamus. Experiments indicate that increased levels of gonadotropins cause some decrease in hypothalamic function.

Experiments in lower animal forms indicate that dopamine is involved in hypothalamic hormonal production. The effect of dopamine can be blocked by estrogens, and it may be increased somewhat under the influence of progesterone.

Whereas the evidence of hypothalamic influence has been ascertained principally by inference, the mechanisms of pituitary influence on the ovaries are better understood because the gonadotropic hormones are produced in sufficient quantity to be extracted from pituitary glands and urine and to be determined in blood and urine by assays. The minute amounts of FSH and LH in blood can be determined by radioimmunoassays; amounts in urine allow bioassay and immunoassay. The multiple antigenic sites of gonadotropic molecules cause heterospecificity of the antibodies produced, so that cross reactions occur. Antisera for human chorionic gonadotropin yield the same results as antisera for human luteinizing hormone. Some cross reactions between FSH and LH antibodies also occur. The accuracy of immunoassay is further limited by the fact that the levels apparently include substances that are biologically inactive as determined by simultaneous assay in animals. The observed effects of purified human FSH and LH extracts administered in known amounts to patients have given more evidence for understanding ovarian hormonal response.

Subunits of FSH and LH have been identified. The α-subunit is common to both FSH and LH. The β-subunit is specific for each gonadotropin and can be used to produce antibodies of good specificity, making accurate immunoassays available.

As indicated in Fig. 1-5, FSH causes an increase in follicular maturation and estrogen production. LH production increases rapidly 2 or 3 days before ovulation so that total urinary gonadotropins are highest at midcycle (Fig. 1-7). For ovulation to occur the rise in LH is essential. As progestogens in the corpus luteum increase, the level of LH decreases so that the corpus luteum, once formed, increases function for about 10 days and then begins to regress.

The estrogen levels, as reflected by urinary excretion, are highest at or just before ovulation. Bioassayable FSH levels in urine are lowest at the time of ovulation. The relationship of FSH and estrogen levels indicates a push-pull mechanism, which appears to be cyclic and perhaps is a major consideration in the control of the menstrual cycle. The regression of the corpus luteum, with decrease in progestogens and estrogens, is correlated with endometrial shedding (menstruation).

If a zygote forms and implantation occurs (Fig. 1-8), the trophoblasts soon produce a gonadotropic hormone that is similar in action to LH of the pituitary. This chorionic gonadotropin maintains the corpus luteum, which enlarges to be recognized as the corpus luteum of pregnancy. This persisting corpus luteum is soon surpassed by the trophoblasts in production of estrogens and progestogens, so that it is not necessary for marked decidual transformation and the continuation of pregnancy as it is in the rabbit. In the rabbit the excision of the corpus luteum will cause abortion. The sustained production of estrogens and progestogens by the placenta inhibits the production of pituitary gonadotropins, FSH in particular, so that ovulation does not take place.

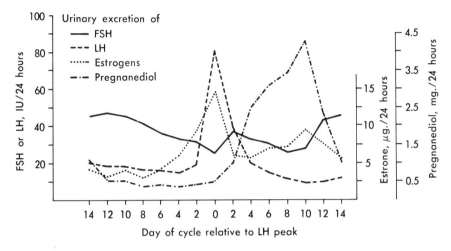

Fig. 1-7. Determinations of urinary excretion during regular ovulatory menstrual cycles indicate the relationship of FSH, LH, estrogens, and pregnanediol. The FSH and LH curves are taken from bioassay studies. Radioimmunoassays are similar for LH but for FSH differ by revealing a peak at the time of the LH peak.

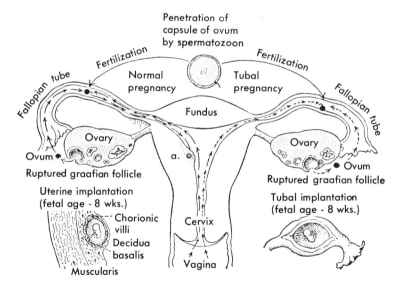

Fig. 1-8. Fertilization of the oocyte (ovum). Note fertilization in the tube and implantation of the fertilized oocyte in the endometrium.

From Falls, F.H., and McLaughlin, J.R.: Obstetric nursing, St. Louis, The C.V. Mosby Co.

OVARIAN HORMONES

The two types of hormones that cause female development and functions are estrogens and progestogens. Estrogens are produced by the maturing follicle. Progestogens are secreted by the mature follicle in small amounts just before ovulation and in larger amounts by the corpus luteum, which continues to produce estrogens.

Estrogens. Since Allen and Doisy in 1923 isolated the female sex hormone estrogen, much knowledge has been accumulated in steroid chemistry regarding molecular structure, synthesis, analysis, enzyme systems, etc. During recent years techniques of chromatographic separation and isotopic labeling have afforded means of investigating the various estrogenic steroids, as well as progestogens and androgens. Smith and Ryan have discussed possible metabolic pathways for the ovarian biogenesis of estrogens, as suggested by their investigations using human follicular linings for incubation in vitro (Fig. 1-9).

From the results of various investigators it is evident that the principal estrogens produced by the ovary are estradiol (the most active form), estrone (which has considerable potency), and estriol (which is relatively inert) and that at least 15 other estrogenic compounds occur in women. Large amounts of estrogens are produced by the chorionic trophoblasts, and small amounts by the adrenal cortex. The normal ovary produces androgens, androstenedione, and testosterone, which exist mainly as intermediate compounds in the synthesis of estrogens. The principal active estrogen produced outside the ovary is estrone, which has androstenedione as its precursor. Androstenedione comes from the adrenal and the ovary and is the main source of estrogen after menopause. Conversion of androstenedione is also a principal source of estrogen in such conditions as chronic anovulation, which occurs with a polycystic ovary syndrome. Estriol is a weak estrogen that occurs in the nonpregnant state as a product of estrone and estradiol metabolism in peripheral tissues. Although it is a relatively weak estrogen when administered orally in large doses over a long period, it can produce estrogenic effects.

The natural estrogens are rapidly metabolized in the liver to various compounds, which are conjugated with glucuronic acid, etc., to be ultimately excreted in the urine (about 65%) and feces (about 10%). Determinations of estrogen levels in blood or urine are time-consuming and expensive and as yet have not been helpful in the management of disorders such as abnormal uterine bleeding and infertility.

The physiologic functions of estrogens are as follows:
1. Stimulation of growth of the upper vagina, uterus, and oviducts
2. Facilitation of development of the primordial follicles and vascular system of the ovary
3. Inhibition of the FSH and LH secretion by the pituitary, due to their effect on the hypothalamus and pituitary

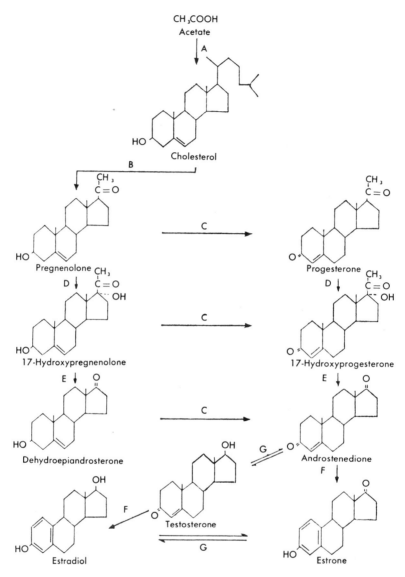

Fig. 1-9. Possible metabolic pathways for the ovarian biogenesis of estrogens. Letters above arrows denote the following metabolic pathways and the enzyme systems involved. **A,** Formation of the sterol nucleus. **B,** Cleavage of cholesterol side chain with formation of C-21 steroid. **C,** Isomerase reaction with changing of double bond from C-5 to C-4 and dehydrogenation at C-3; 3β-ol dehydrogenases. **D,** 17α-hydroxylation, i.e., introduction of hydroxy radical in alpha position on C-17. **E,** Cleavage of side chain converting C-21 to C-19 steroids. **F,** Aromatization, i.e., introduction of double bonds into ring A with conversion of C-19 to C-18 steroids. **G,** 17β-ol dehydrogenase reactions (reversible), i.e., conversion of hydroxy radical in beta position on C-17 to ketone group or vice versa.

From Smith, O.W., and Ryan, K.J.: Am. J. Obstet. Gynecol. **84:**141, 1962.

4. Promotion of growth of the vaginal epithelium to produce cornification of cells and to increase glycogen content
5. Stimulation of the endocervix as evidenced by increased cell height, increased undifferentiated cells beneath the mucosa, and increased clear watery mucus production
6. Stimulation of proliferation of endometrium and increase of myometrial contractility
7. Increase of contractility of oviducts
8. Stimulation of growth of breasts, with ductal proliferation
9. Promotion of growth of bone, closure of epiphyses, and gynecoid shape of pelvis
10. Promotion of female type of body contours and hair
11. Retention of sodium and water
12. Increase in thyroxin-binding and corticosteroid-binding globulin

In addition to the natural occurrence of estrogens, compounds that have estrogenic capabilities have been synthesized. The more commonly used nonsteroid forms are diethylstilbestrol, hexestrol, dienestrol, and chlorotrianisene. Synthetic steroid compounds in which an ethinyl radical has been added at the 17 position of estradiol are called ethinyl estrogens—ethinyl estradiol (Estinyl) and ethinyl estradiol 3-methyl ether (Mestranol). These potent, orally administered compounds can be used to produce the physiologic effects of natural estrogen. In addition they can be used to inhibit the production of pituitary gonadotropins for long periods and to stimulate hyperplasia of the endometrium. When administered immediately after parturition they can prevent engorgement of the breasts, probably by interfering with stimulation of the breasts by prolactin.

Progestogens. The ovary produces small amounts of progesterone before ovulation, although the significant production is by the corpus luteum after ovulation. The liver is the major site for the conversion of progesterone to pregnanediol, which is conjugated to be excreted in the urine as sodium pregnanediol glucuronide. Since only about one fifth of injected progesterone can be accounted for by urinary excretion, this determination is not a complete reflection of total progesterone. As judged by the amount of pregnanediol excreted in the urine, the placenta is capable of producing 8 to 10 times as much progesterone per day as the ovary.

Progesterone causes the following physiologic effects:
1. Secretory changes in an endometrium previously stimulated by estrogen; formation of decidual cells in the stroma with sufficient stimulation
2. Increased growth in myometrium
3. Secretory changes in tubal epithelium and decreased motility
4. Change in the cervical mucus, which becomes viscid with increased leukocytes, and disappearance of ferning

5. Acinar and lobular development of breasts
6. Slight rise in basal body temperature
7. Depression of the response of the ovary to pituitary gonadotropin
8. Reduction of the pyknotic index of vaginal cells by antagonizing the action of estrogens (noted particularly during pregnancy)
9. Increase of the sodium content and reduction of the potassium content of myometrial cells

Synthetic progesterone is readily available and inexpensive. It is administered by injection in oil solution, since it is destroyed for the most part by digestive processes. In recent years synthetic progestogens have been produced by substitution of groups on the progesterone nucleus or by variation of the chemical structure of testosterone. Two esters of hydroxyprogesterone are 17α-hydroxyprogesterone caproate (Delalutin) and 6α-methyl-17α-hydroxyprogesterone acetate (Provera). These preparations have not caused severe acne or hirsutism when administered over long periods in human subjects. When these compounds have been given in large amounts by injection, ovulation has been inhibited. Provera is effective orally or intramuscularly, whereas Delalutin is given only intramuscularly. Chlormadinone is 6-chloro-6-dehydro-17α-acetoxy progesterone and is about 30 times as active as Provera.

Several compounds similar in structure to testosterone have been administered orally to produce progestogenic effects. Ethinyl testosterone (Pranone) has been found to be of relatively low potency. Norethindrone, 17α-ethinyl-19-nortestosterone, acetate (Norlutate) is a potent oral progestogen with androgenic potential that can inhibit the pituitary. Norethynodrel 17α-ethinyl-17β-hydroxy-5 (10)-estren-3-one is combined with ethinyl estradiol 3-methyl ether and marketed as Enovid. It has less androgenic potential than norethindrone and is effective in inhibition of the pituitary. Megestrol acetate, 17α-acetoxy-6-methylpregna-4,6-diene-3,20-dione, is a potent oral progestogen used to treat endometrial adenocarcinoma.

There are potentially many variations in the chemical structure of synthetic progestogens. These variations affect the estrogenic, androgenic, and progestogenic effects of these compounds. All synthetic progestogens are capable of inducing secretory changes in the estrogen-primed endometrium. They also tend to mimic the other physiologic effects of progesterone. Their principal uses have been to promote secretory changes and cause withdrawal bleeding in nonpregnant amenorrheic patients with adequate estrogens; to control hypermenorrhea and polymenorrhea due to dysfunction by opposing the proliferative effects of estrogens; to forestall pregnancy by inhibiting ovulation, by fostering an unphysiologic endometrium, and by producing an unfavorable cervical mucus for migration of sperm; to prevent primary dysmenorrhea by inhibiting ovulation and decreasing the production of prostaglandins by the endometrium; and to assist in the production of the pseudo-pregnancy state with ultimate endometrial atrophy in managing endometriosis.

Among the drawbacks of oral progestogens are nausea with occasional vomiting, variation in individual response regarding uterine bleeding during administration and the occurrence of withdrawal bleeding after cessation, and slight weight gain. Delalutin in oil solution is not likely to result in bleeding for 12 days. Depo-Provera in aqueous suspension may result in amenorrhea for several months. Long-term administration in large doses has not resulted in major structural changes and appears to be safe.

A retroisomer of progesterone, dydrogesterone (Duphaston), is available as a weak oral progestogen that usually does not cause a rise in basal body temperature or inhibit ovulation. It is rapidly eliminated and must be ingested several times daily to have an appreciable effect.

GONADOTROPIC HORMONES

The actions of the two gonadotropic hormones upon the ovary have been described under endocrine function. FSH and LH are water-soluble glycoproteins that have been isolated in electrophoretically pure forms. Levels of these complex proteins are determined in human subjects by bioassay and immunoassay of blood and urine specimens.

FSH is found in the urine and blood of girls in increased amounts just before puberty. After the menopause the amount found rises and remains high for about 10 years. Estrogens and androgens, natural or synthetic, inhibit production of FSH.

LH is found in the urine of mature women and reaches a peak in concentration just before ovulation. Neither FSH nor LH alone is associated with ovulation. They must act in proper combination. Administration of sufficient estrogens, androgens, or synthetic progestogens for 7 days or more before the anticipated time of ovulation can produce an anovulatory cycle in women. Prolonged administration of these preparations has been shown to cause a decrease in total gonadotropin levels.

Human chorionic gonadotropin (HCG) is a glycoprotein produced by the trophoblasts. As previously indicated, there is an immunologic cross reaction with LH. Chorionic gonadotropins are combinations of bioassayable FSH and LH. They are present in the urine in an amount approximately 1000 times that of the pituitary gonadotropins, which are recoverable during the reproductive life of women. The urine of pregnant women serves as a source of gonadotropin, which is extracted and purified for therapy. Methods of extraction depend on adsorption on Kaolin and purification by ion exchange chromatography. Some separation of FSH and LH can be effected by chromatography on cellulose and by gel filtration. The bioassay of total chorionic gonadotropins that has been used in the past is the uterine weight response in rodents, which shows the influence of a joint action of FSH and LH. The bioassay commonly used to determine FSH is the ovarian augmentation assay in rats or mice, whereas LH is determined by the ovarian ascorbic acid depletion assay.

Prolactin, which is secreted by the lactotropes of the pituitary, acts on osmoregulation, metabolism, and reproduction. Mammary gland responses are stimulation of growth, initiation of milk secretion, and stimulation of established milk production. High levels are found in women with galactorrhea and in some women with secondary amenorrhea. Prolactin has been shown to inhibit progesterone formation by granulosal cells. Unlike FSH and ICSH, which appear to be released on stimulation, prolactin is principally controlled by inhibition, that is, through the release of prolactin-inhibiting factor from the hypothalamus. Thyrotropin-releasing factor increases prolactin production by the pituitary. Radioimmunoassay studies of prolactin levels during the menstrual cycle indicate that prolactin usually shows no consistent pattern. In situations with high prolactin levels there is interference with the release of FSH and LH by the pituitary, and ovulation does not occur. This matter will be further discussed in the section dealing with amenorrhea.

OTHER HORMONES CONCERNED IN OVARIAN FUNCTION

The amounts of tetraiodothyronine (T_4) and triiodothyronine (T_3), as well as thyrotropin-releasing hormone (TRH) and thyroid-stimulating hormone (TSH), influence ovarian function. When there is a deficiency of the active thyroid hormones (hypothyroidism), amenorrhea, anovulation, and prolonged or excessive uterine bleeding are more apt to occur. The absence of a feedback mechanism on the hypothalamus and the pituitary results and the secretion of thyrotropin-releasing factor is increased. This, in turn, may cause an increase in the production of prolactin, which may interfere with production of gonadotropins by the pituitary. There is good evidence to suggest that estrogen metabolism is decreased with a deficiency in thyroid function.

With hyperthyroidism the amount and duration of menstrual flow are apt to be decreased. There is some question regarding a central hypothalamic-pituitary mechanism and possibly an effect on estrogen and other steroid metabolism. It is well known that estrogens increase the thyroxin-binding globulin. This usually has little effect on the free thyroxin and is not thought to be of great significance except in interpretation of thyroid tests.

Hormones produced by the adrenal cortex, particularly when in excessive amounts, can affect estrogen production and the ovulatory mechanism, which, in turn, may result in irregular menstruation, amenorrhea, or oligomenorrhea resulting in infertility. Dehydroepiandresterone and androstenedione are mildly androgenic and they are precursors of testosterone, estrone, or estradiol. When these precursors are converted by the adrenal gland and by the liver, kidneys, and blood to testosterone, there is an interference with ovarian function as well as development of symptoms due to excess androgens such as hirsutism, acne, enlarged clitoris, and voice and muscle changes. The glucocorticoids are essential for many

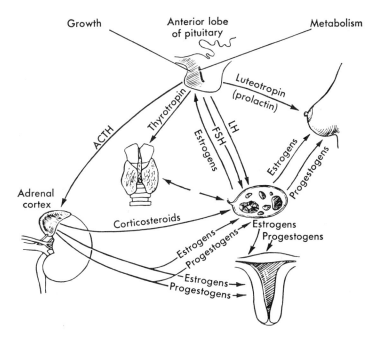

Fig. 1-10. Interrelationship of the various hormones concerned directly or indirectly with pelvic function. Thyroxine arrows not labeled because of lack of space. Ovarian effect on the thyroid is not clear.

metabolic functions, and patients with adrenal failure develop ovarian malfunction.

The adrenal gland and ovary have common capabilities in steroid production. Both organs can sensitize acetate to cholesterol and cholesterol to pregnenolone, as well as change pregnenolone to progesterone. The adrenal gland does not have the capability of producing any large amount of progesterone, whereas the ovary with corpus luteum formation does produce progesterone in large quantities. The adrenal gland can produce only small amounts of estrogens. The adrenal gland and the ovary can produce androgens. Under normal circumstances the androgenic substance produced in largest quantity by the adrenal gland is dehydroepiandrosterone, whereas the androgenic substance produced in largest quantity by the ovary is androstenedione. The ovary cannot provide the hydroxylation that is necessary for the formation of the glucocorticoids (cortisone and cortisol). If the adrenal glands are removed or effectively destroyed by disease, administration of glucocorticoids is essential for ovulation and normal ovarian function. In diseased states in which there is excessive secretion of adrenal steroids, some degree of disturbance in ovarian function is anticipated, as will be discussed under functional disturbances of the ovary.

Fig. 1-10 shows the interrelationship between the various hormones.

FALLOPIAN TUBES

The fallopian tubes, or oviducts, are two small muscular tubes, one on either side, that extend from the fundus uteri outward into the upper part of the broad ligament toward the pelvic wall (Fig. 1-11). Each tube has a small central cavity extending its whole length. The inner end of this cavity communicates with the uterine cavity, and the outer end opens into the peritoneal cavity. Thus there is a direct opening from the outside of the body into the great peritoneal sac, through the vagina, uterus, and fallopian tubes. This is why infection of the genital tract in women so frequently causes peritonitis.

The tubes vary considerably in size and somewhat in shape in different individuals. The length of each tube is 7.5 to 12.5 cm, and the direction is outward, backward, downward, and inward. The tube somewhat resembles a shepherd's crook and partly surrounds the ovary.

That portion of the tube lying in the uterine wall is known as the *intramural portion* or uterine portion. It has a very narrow lumen. That part of the tube extending from the margin of the uterus to the beginning of the curve is called the *isthmus*. It has about the diameter of a slate pencil and is firm. The lumen is small but becomes gradually larger toward the outer end. The outer curve, dilated portion of the tube is known as the *ampulla*. It is about the size of a lead pencil, and its lumen also is much larger than that of the isthmus. The outer end of the tube is called the *fimbriated extremity* or the infundibulum. This consists of a funnel-shaped expansion surrounded by a fringe of slender, fingerlike processes called fimbriae.

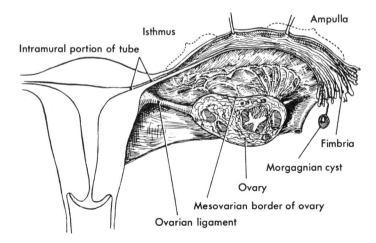

Fig. 1-11. Diagrammatic lateral section through the uterus and tube.

Anatomy and histology

The wall of the tube is largely muscular. It is derived from the same fetal organ as the uterus. The tube lies beneath the peritoneum of the upper margin of the broad ligament and its wall presents three layers: peritoneal, muscular, and mucous.

The *peritoneal layer* does not differ materially from peritoneum elsewhere. It is composed of flat endothelial cells lying on a base of firm connective tissue. Immediately beneath the peritoneum is a layer of connective tissue, sometimes called the subperitoneal layer. In this run blood vessels and lymphatics. The intramural portion of the tube has, of course, no peritoneal layer, as the muscular tissue of the tube is in immediate contact with the muscular tissue of the wall of the uterus.

The *muscular layer* of the tube is composed of involuntary muscular tissue disposed in two strata, an outer longitudinal and an inner circular one.

The *mucous layer* of the tube, like the uterine mucosa, is placed directly upon the muscular layer; there is no intervening submucosa. The surface of the mucous membrane is composed of a layer of ciliated cylindric cells. The cells are somewhat taller than those lining the body of the uterus but not as tall as those lining the cervix uteri. Beneath the epithelial layer the mucosa is composed of stroma cells, which are very much like those found in the uterus, except slightly smaller.

The mucous membrane is folded longitudinally. In the intramural portion and in the isthmus the folds are few and simply longitudinal, but in the outer portion of the tube (the ampulla) they become very complex and fill the tube with folds extending in every direction, so much so that it is sometimes difficult to decide which is the main canal of the tube. The cilia of the epithelium project into the lumen of the tube and, by their movement toward the uterus, aid the passage of the oocyte in that direction. In the presence of this delicate and much-folded mucous membrane, inflammation in the tube quickly causes serious changes. The cilia are lost, the folds become adherent, pockets of serum or pus form, and the tube is blocked and disorganized.

The *blood supply* of the tube comes from the ovarian artery through several small branches. The uterine artery helps to supply the tube in some cases. The veins open into the pampiniform or ovarian plexus and pass into the broad ligament. The lymphatics join with those from the ovary. The nerve supply comes from the pelvic plexus of each side.

Physiology

The primary function of the fallopian tube of each side is to convey oocytes from the corresponding ovary to the uterus. It is supposed to require several days for the oocyte to pass down the length of the tube. In addition to this, spermatozoa traverse the tube in the opposite direction, and it is usually in the tube that the union of the oocyte and the spermatozoon takes place.

The mechanism by which the oocyte is carried from the ovary into the tube is complicated. After the graafian follicle in the ovary opens, the liquor folliculi causes the oocyte to adhere slightly to the surface of the ovary. Some of the fimbriae are in contact with the surface of the ovary, and when an oocyte comes into contact with one of them, the cilia carry it toward the entrance of the tube. Besides this action of the cilia directly on the oocyte, the constant movement of all the cilia causes a slight current of peritoneal fluid toward the interior of the tube from all directions. This helps to carry the oocyte or any other particles into the tube. The fact that there is such a current toward the interior of the tube has been demonstrated in animals by the injection into the pelvic peritoneal cavity of numerous small insoluble particles, which were found later in the tubes.

Cyclic variations in the intratubal pressure, interpreted as peristaltic contractions, have been shown experimentally in the sow's oviduct. These variations are controlled by estrogen and progestogen in the blood.

Kymographic records of Rubin tests made on human beings show similar variations, which were interpreted by Rubin as evidence of peristaltic contractions of the tube. The rate of contraction varies at different times in the cycle, contractions being frequent just before and after ovulation and least frequent about the time of menstruation.

Doyle observed during a laparotomy in a patient on the twelfth day of the cycle that the fimbriated end of the tube was firmly attached to the ovary by suction. He also observed peristaltic movement in the tubal wall.

NORMAL CHANGES IN TUBES

Just as the uterus, particularly the uterine mucosa, is subject to normal changes under three conditions—menstruation, pregnancy, and menopause—so, too, is the fallopian tube. Generally the changes that occur in the fallopian tube are like those occurring in the uterus but less marked.

During *menstruation* there is congestion of the tube and possibly a slight effusion of blood into the interior of the tube. If this does take place, however, it is slight and is of no importance when considering the source of the menstrual blood. Practically all the menstrual blood comes from the uterus. In a case of removal of the uterus by operation and the fastening of one of the tubes in the vaginal incision, a slight bloody flow is noticed at the menstrual periods for a few months. Such tubes, though, are pathologic, and it is an open question as to whether bloody flow would take place from a normal tube.

The tubal epithelium contains two types of cells: the ciliated or nonsecretory and the nonciliated or secretory.

The epithelium of the tubes also goes through cyclic changes during the menstrual cycle. The following stages have been described by Novak and Everett:

1. In the postmenstrual stage the epithelium is low at first but rapidly increases in height, so that by the third or fourth day after menstruation it is almost as tall as during the interval. The cells are narrow, closely packed, and, after the first day or so, of uniform height.

2. In the growth phase the epithelium is uniformly tall, and the ciliated cells are broad, with rounded nuclei near the free margin. The nonciliated cells are narrower, and the nuclei are deeply placed. There is a progressive increase in the nucleotides and the polysaccharides during this phase.

3. In the premenstrual phase the ciliated cells become lower, so that the secretory cells project beyond them, giving the margin a ragged appearance. The secretory cells show a bulbous herniation into the lumen of the tube, often carrying the nucleus with it. Mitoses are rarely seen. In the latter part of the progestational stage the epithelial cells expel chemical substances into the tubal lumen; one of these substances has been identified by Green as α-amylase.

4. During the stage of menstruation the epithelium becomes quite low. The secretory cells, having emptied into the lumen, are very low, and frequently the nucleus is quite bare of cytoplasm.

During *pregnancy* the epithelium becomes flat and no secretory changes are seen. There is, however, a congestion of the tube, and the vessels and lymphatics are dilated.

In the *menopause* the ciliated and nonciliated cells disappear and the tube becomes smaller and firmer.

PELVIC PERITONEUM

The pelvic peritoneum is that portion of the wall of the peritoneal sac that lies in the pelvis. It is attached more or less closely to the pelvic organs, and its free surface comes in contact with the peritoneal surface of the intestines as they move about in the lower abdomen. To get an idea of the distribution of the peritoneum in the pelvis, imagine a piece of thin cloth laid over the pelvic organs and tucked down firmly around them.

Starting from the abdominal wall, the peritoneum passes onto the bladder and from the posterior surface of the bladder to the uterus. The height of the abdominovesical fold of peritoneum varies much with the varying size of the bladder, a fact that is of much importance in surgical work. The distance to which the peritoneum extends down the anterior surface of the uterus varies considerably in different persons. Usually it extends to the level of the internal os and is about an inch above the anterior vaginal fornix. When the bladder is distended, the peritoneum is drawn upward somewhat. The vesicouterine fold of peritoneum forms the two so-called vesicouterine ligaments.

The peritoneum then folds over the uterus, the tubes, and the round ligaments, covering these structures and forming the broad ligament of each side. All the posterior surface of the uterus above the vagina is covered with peritoneum. The fold of peritoneum extends a considerable distance below the point of attachment to the uterus before being reflected on to the rectum. The deep pouch of peritoneum thus formed is called the cul-de-sac of Douglas. This posterior cul-de-sac is very important surgically. A collection of exudate or a tumor in this situation can be easily felt from the posterior vaginal fornix, and this is the point of incision in posterior or vaginal drainage.

The peritoneum, as it is reflected from the uterus to the rectum, helps to form the uterosacral ligaments. The uterosacral ligaments, one on each side, extend backward from the lower part of the uterus and around the rectum to the sacrum. They are composed of connective tissue, a few muscle fibers, and peritoneum. The cul-de-sac of Douglas dips down between them for a considerable distance. The expanse of peritoneum extending from the uterosacral ligament to the broad ligament of each side forms a kind of shelf. The two together are sometimes called the rectouterine shelves. There is also a fold or shallow pouch of peritoneum on each side between the fallopian tube and the round ligament. A small portion of the uterus at the sides and in front is not covered with peritoneum.

The structure of the pelvic peritoneum is much the same as that of peritoneum elsewhere. It is a very thin and smooth membrane, formed of a basis of delicate fibrous and elastic tissue, supporting large endothelial cells.

PELVIC CONNECTIVE TISSUE

Between the pelvic peritoneum and the pelvic diaphragm there is connective tissue. This is distributed to fill all the spaces. When it is necessary for organs to change their relation to each other in physiologic activity, the connection is open and loose to permit free movement and much stretching. The principal collections of connective tissue are at the sides of and in front of the cervix uteri and at the base of each broad ligament. The areas of connective tissue are exceedingly rich in lymphatics and veins. Inflammation taking place in the connective tissue is called pelvic cellulitis.

The connective tissue about the uterus is often spoken of collectively as the parametrium or parametrial tissue, and inflammation of it is accordingly called parametritis, a very convenient term.

It was formerly supposed that nearly all inflammation in the pelvis outside the uterus was inflammation of the connective tissue (i.e., pelvic cellulitis), but it has been found that in the majority of individuals the inflammation invades first the tube and later the peritoneum and that usually the involvement of the connective tissue, if present at all, is a late development and of only secondary importance. There are exceptions to this rule, for example, those inflammatory conditions resulting from tears of the cervix. Also in puerperal infections, particularly streptococcic, the inflammation usually extends directly through the wall of the uterus into the pelvic connective tissue.

SELECTED REFERENCES

Arrata, W.S.M., and Iffy, L.: Normal and delayed ovulation in the human, Obstet. Gynecol. Surv. **26:**675, 1971.

Barer, A.P., Fowler, W.M., and Baldridge, C.W.: Blood loss during normal menstruation, Proc. Soc. Exp. Biol. Med. **32:**1458, 1935.

Bartelmez, G.W.: The phases of the menstrual cycle and their interpretation in terms of the pregnancy cycle, Am. J. Obstet. Gynecol. **74:**931, 1957.

Brown, J.B., and Beischer, N.A.: Current status of estrogen assay in gynecology and obstetrics, Obstet. Gynecol. Surv. **27:**205, 1972.

Carey, H.M.: Modern trends in human reproductive physiology, Washington, D.C., 1963, Butterworth & Co.

Cohen, V.J.B., and Gibor, Y.: Anemia and menstrual blood loss, Obstet. Gynecol. Surv. **35:**597, 1980.

Corner, G.W. In Engle, E.T., editor: Menstruation and its disorders, Springfield, Ill., 1950, Charles C Thomas, Publisher.

Danforth, D.N.: Distribution and functional activity of the cervical musculature, Am. J. Obstet. Gynecol. **68:**1261, 1954.

Downie, J., Poyser, N.L., and Wunderlich, M.: Levels of prostaglandins in human endometrium during the normal menstrual cycle, J. Physiol. **236:**465, 1974.

Doyle, J.B.: Tubo-ovarian mechanism, Obstet. Gynecol. **8:**686, 1956.

Faiman, C., and Ryan, R.J.: Radioimmunoassay for human follicle stimulating hormone, J. Clin. Endocrinol. **27:**444, 1967.

Fischer, R.H.: Progesterone metabolism. III. Basal body temperature as an index of progesterone production and its relationship to urinary pregnanediol, Obstet. Gynecol. **3:**615, 1954.

Fluhmann, C.F.: The nature and development of the so-called glands of the cervix uteri, Am. J. Obstet. Gynecol. **74:**753, 1957.

Franchi, L.L., and Baker, T.G.: Oogenesis and follicular growth. In Hafez, E.S.E., and Evans, T.N., editors: Human reproduction, New York, 1973, Harper & Row, Publishers Inc.

Fukushima, M., Stevens, V., Gantt, C., and Vorys, N.: Urinary FSH and LH excretion during the normal menstrual cycle. J. Clin. Endocrinol. **24:**205, 1964.

Gardner, G.H., Greene, R.R., and Peckham, B.M.: Normal and cystic structures of the broad ligament, Am. J. Obstet. Gynecol. **55:**917, 1948.

Glueck, H.I., and Mirsky, I.A.: Clotting mechanism of menstrual fluid, Am. J. Obstet. Gynecol. **42:**267, 1941.

Grant's atlas of anatomy, Baltimore, 1978, The Williams & Wilkins Co.

Green, C.L.: Identification of alpha-amylase as a secretion of the human fallopian tube and "tubelike" epithelium of Müllerian and mesonephric duct origin, Am. J. Obstet. Gynecol. **73:**402, 1957.

Haman, J.O.: Length of the menstrual cycle, Am. J. Obstet. Gynecol. **43:**870, 1942.

Hellman, L.M., Rosenthal, A.H., Kistner, R.W., and Gordon, R.: Some factors influencing the proliferation of the reserve cells in the human cervix, Am. J. Obstet. Gynecol. **67:**899, 1954.

Henzal, M.R., Smith, R.E., Boost, G., and Tyler, E.T.: Lysosomal concept of menstrual bleeding in humans, J. Clin. Endocrinol. Metab. **34:**860, 1972.

Homburg, R., Potashnik, G., Lunenfeld, B., and Insler, V.: The hypothalamus as a regulator of reproductive function, Obstet. Gynecol. Surv. **31:**455, 1976.

Howard, L., Jr., Erickson, C.C., and Stoddard, L.D.: Study of incidence and histogenesis of endocervical metaplasia and intraepithelial carcinoma; observations on 400 uteri removed for noncervical disease, Cancer **4:**1210, 1951.

Huffman, J.W.: Gynecology and obstetrics, Philadelphia, 1962, W.B. Saunders Co.

Hughes, E.C., Van Ness, A.W., and Lloyd, C.W.: The nutritional value of the endometrium for implantation and in habitual abortion, Am. J. Obstet. Gynecol. **59:**1292, 1950.

Hunter, R.G., Henry, G.W., and Civin, W.H.: The cornual sphincter of the uterus, Surg. Gynecol. Obstet. **103:**475, 1956.

Klopper, A.I.: The excretion of pregnanediol during the normal menstrual cycle, J. Obstet. Gynaecol. Br. Emp. **64:**504, 1957.

Lang, W.R., Rakoff, A.E., and Gross, M.: Alkaline phosphatase in vaginal biopsies, Am. J. Obstet. Gynecol. **68:**815, 1954.

Leckie, F.H.: Study of histochemistry of human foetal ovary, J. Obstet. Gynaecol. Br. Emp. **62:**542, 1955.

Macy, I.G., and Mack, H.C.: Implications of nutrition in the life cycle of woman, Am. J. Obstet. Gynecol. **68:**131, 1954.

McKay, D.G., Hertig, A.T., Bardawil, W., and Velardo, J.T.: Histochemical observations on the endometrium. I. Normal endometrium, Obstet. Gynecol. **8:**140, 1956.

McKay, D.G., Hertig, A.T., Bardawil, W., and Velardo, J.T.: Histochemical observations on the endometrium. II. Abnormal endometrium, Obstet. Gynecol. **8:**140, 1956.

McKeown, T., Gibson, J.R., and Dougray, T.: Study of variation in length of menstrual cycle, J. Obstet. Gynaecol. Br. Emp. **61:**678, 1954.

Mills, C.A., and Ogle, C.: Physiologic sterility of adolescence, Hum. Biol. **8:**607, 1936.

Novak, E., and Everett, H.S.: Cyclical and other variations in tubal epithelium, Am. J. Obstet. Gynecol. **16:**499, 1928.

Okkels, H.: The histophysiology of the human endometrium. In Engle, E.T., editor: Menstruation and its disorders, Springfield, Ill., 1950, Charles C Thomas, Publishers.

Payne, H.W., and Latour, J.P.: Quantitative estimations of endometrial glycogen, using anthrone method, J. Clin. Endocrinol. **15:**1106, 1955.

Philipp, E.E., Barnes, J., and Newton, M.: Scientific foundation of obstetrics and gynecology, Philadelphia, 1970, F.A. Davis Co.

Phillips, L.L., Butler, B.C., and Taylor, H.C., Jr.: Study of cytofibrinokinase and fibrinolysin in extracts of tissue from human myometrium, endometrium, decidua, and placenta, Am. J. Obstet. Gynecol. **71:**342, 1956.

Pozo, E.D., Goldstein, M., Friesen, H., et al.: Lack of action of prolactin suppression on the regulation of the human menstrual cycle, Am. J. Obstet. Gynecol. **123:**719, 1975.

Reynolds, S.R.M.: The vasculature of the ovary and ovarian function. In Pincus, G., editor: Recent progress in hormone research, vol. 5, New York, 1950, Academic Press, Inc., p. 65.

Rumbolz, W.L., and Greene, E.G.: Observations on metachromic granules in human endometrium, Am. J. Obstet. Gynecol. **73:**992, 1957.

Ryan, K.J.: Hormones of the placenta, Am. J. Obstet. Gynecol. **84:**1695, 1962.

Schlegel, J.U.: Arteriovenous anastomoses in endometrium in man, Acta Anat. **1:**284, 1945.

Shettles, L.B.: Further observations on living human oocytes and ova, Am. J. Obstet. Gynecol. **69:**365, 1955.

Shettles, L.B.: Parthogenetic cleavage of the human ovum, Bull. Sloane Hosp. **3:**59, 1957.

Shettles, L.B.: The living human ovum, Obstet. Gynecol. **10:**359, 1957.

Smith, O.W., and Ryan, K.J.: Estrogen in the human ovary, Am. J. Obstet. Gynecol. **84:**141, 1962.

Stevens, V.C., and Vorys, N.: Gonadotropin secretion in the normal cycle. In Greenblatt, R.B., editor: Ovulation, Philadelphia, 1966, J.B. Lippincott Co.

Stuart, H.C.: Medical progress; normal growth and development during adolescence, N. Engl. J. Med. **234:**666, 1946.

Sturgis, S.H.: Mechanism and control of primate ovulation, Fertil. Steril. **1:**40, 1950.

Tanner, J.M.: The development of the female reproductive system during adolescence, Clin. Obstet. Gynecol. **3:**135, 1960.

Ulfelder, H.: Mechanism of pelvic support in women: deductions from a study of the comparative anatomy and physiology of the structures involved, Am. J. Obstet. Gynecol. **72:**856, 1956.

Venning, E.M., and Browne, J.S.L.: Urinary excretion of sodium pregnanediol glucuronidase in the menstrual cycle, Am. J. Physiol. **119:**47, 1937.

Verhage, H.G., Bareither, M.L., Jaffe, R.B., et al.: Cyclic changes in ciliation, secretion and cell height of the oviductal epithelium in women, Am. J. Anat. **156:**505, 1979.

Waldeyer, W.: Eierstock und Ei, Leipzig, 1870.

Yen, S.S.C., and Jaffee, R.B.: Reproductive endocrinology, Philadephia, 1978, W.B. Saunders Co.

Chapter 2

GYNECOLOGIC EXAMINATION AND DIAGNOSIS

The physician who wishes to be accurate in the diagnosis and treatment of diseases of women must possess certain information: (1) knowledge of the anatomy and physiology of the organs involved, (2) reliable history and examination of the patient, and (3) knowledge of the organic and functional disturbances to which the parts are liable and of the differential diagnosis and treatment of them, along with coordinating knowledge that will enable the understanding of the situation as a whole as well as of the local disturbance. Problems are recognized in diagnosis and/ or therapy, and plans for resolution are made. The problem-oriented medical record is a means of organizing the subjective and objective findings, assessing those findings, and developing plans to be followed. Flow sheets allow for correlation of diagnostic data with therapeutic agents and procedures over periods of time.

Diagnosis is based upon the symptoms given by the patient, the signs found on examination, and objective evidence from special examinations, reports of specimens examined in the laboratory, and response to therapy. It should, as far as possible, be both an anatomic and a pathologic diagnosis; i.e., it should state the structures involved and the character of the pathologic process, whether organic or functional. The fact that a diagnosis must eventuate from the history and examination requires that the diagnostic significance of symptoms and signs be kept in mind and utilized as the examination proceeds. Diagnosis improves with experience. When on previous occasions a diagnosis has been made, it is later made with less conscious correlation of findings, much as a person well known by previous contacts is easily and quickly recognized.

IMPORTANCE OF KEEPING A RECORD

A short record, showing in a systematic way the principal facts of a case, can be made quickly and more than repays one for the time consumed. The major advantage is not the permanent record it gives for reference after some years, although that is important, especially to the teacher, but the fact that it systematizes, steadies, and improves the physician's work day by day. Such an account of the case in black and white, referred to frequently as the patient returns for treatment, is a constant stimulus to accurate diagnosis and a constant help in the treatment, particularly if the case is a long-continued one. The importance of legible, accurate, and complete notes on the history, findings, and treatment for future statistical reporting can be fully appreciated only by one who has done this type of work. Furthermore in court a physician is expected to have a record of his work. He may at any time be called upon to testify as to the exact findings in the case of some patient whom he saw several years previously.

PSYCHOSOMATIC ASPECTS OF GYNECOLOGY

Because of the importance of the emotional and environmental background as a factor in gynecologic problems, this information is needed, along with the patient's complete medical history, to evaluate properly the influence of such factors.

In the following paragraph Miller succinctly states in an understandable way the importance of finding out something about the patient's life:

> One must always remember that there is an organ above the neck called the brain and that it has been active since early childhood. In fact, in childhood it probably received its most vivid and important impressions, which will determine the attitude of its owner for life. Is there any reason why it is less important to learn that Mary Smith acquired a lasting hate for men because she was treated cruelly by a drunken father than to learn that she had measles, mumps, and chickenpox before the age of ten? For the gynecologist it is a much better clue to the understanding of her frigidity in marriage than any other item in the examination. It is well to remember that sexual function is more closely related to the powerful emotion of love than any other and, as far as I know, love still seems to have a universal appeal. When it is interfered with and the woman is unhappy, depressed, worried, and frustrated, it is more than likely that the physiologic counterpart will reflect most of the disturbance.*

The fallacy of limiting our inquiry to diseases of a physical nature while obtaining a history is evidenced by numerous reports of cures by psychotherapy in patients who have had many ineffective medical and surgical treatments. In a group of 150 psychiatric patients Bennett found that 121 had had a total of 205 surgical operations and had received a total of 368 medical treatments of various types before the psychogenic origin of the trouble was recognized. Lock and Donnelly analyzed the histories of patients in the gynecologic practices of several colleagues and concluded that 33% of the patients had psychosomatic disturbances.

The importance of considering the patient as a whole person, who is subject to internal and environmental stresses with their resulting emotional reactions, should

---

*From Miller, W.R.: J.A.M.A. **134**:938, 1947.

be obvious to the gynecologist, for pelvic function is concerned with the most compelling of human emotions—love. According to some authorities this elemental emotion begins in intrauterine life and continues in its various phases through infancy, adolescence, marriage, motherhood, and menopause. Its interplay with other emotions can result in deep-seated complexes. These complexes are expressed, consciously or unconsciously, as symptoms such as pain, frigidity, infertility, or menstrual disturbances. Many of the functional diseases have a background of psychosomatic disturbances. As Mandy and associates suggested: "Many women seeking aid for female trouble are, instead, troubled females."

The knowledge that the hypothalamus controls the release of the gonadotropins from the pituitary has helped us to understand how the psyche, acting through the higher centers, can cause endocrine disturbances.

A point stressed by all psychiatrists is that one needs to be a good listener to obtain an adequate history. A sincere, sympathetic, leisurely attitude on the part of the physician does much to establish the rapport needed for a free discussion of the patient's intimate thoughts and actions. It would be very time-consuming and impossible to obtain a complete life history for every gynecologic patient. However, by starting the history in this way instead of by the usual rapid "check-off" method, one quickly gains insight into the patient's problem and can tell whether the trouble is chiefly organic, psychosomatic, or a combination of both.

In the history there arise a number of symptoms and actions that enable one to suspect a psychosomatic element. Alvarez states: "The harder it is to get a clear history out of the person, the less likely he or she is to have organic disease." These patients bring in many irrelevant facts that they have written down. Instead of answering the questions put to them, they interrupt the physician to give their own interpretation of the symptoms and their diagnosis. Hart emphasized the "resistance symptoms" characteristic of these patients, such as procrastination in seeking medical advice, self-treatment, vagueness and evasion, broken appointments, medical shopping, misleading explanations, fear of personality study, numerous ineffective operations, and many others.

When an extensive, detailed history seems indicated, it is important to learn of the environmental forces present throughout the life of the individual and her responses to them, both expressed and repressed. When episodes of stress or emotional conflicts are mentioned further details are sought concerning the chronology of the events and the patient's reaction to them. By tactful inquiry the physician can usually get the necessary social and psychologic data in a systematic way.

Table 2-1 shows the factors involved in psychosomatic disorders that express themselves in gynecologic complaints.

In addition to information about the patient's psychologic background, the history should include a review of the various systems with symptoms referable to

Table 2-1   PSYCHODYNAMICS OF FUNCTIONAL PELVIC DISORDERS*

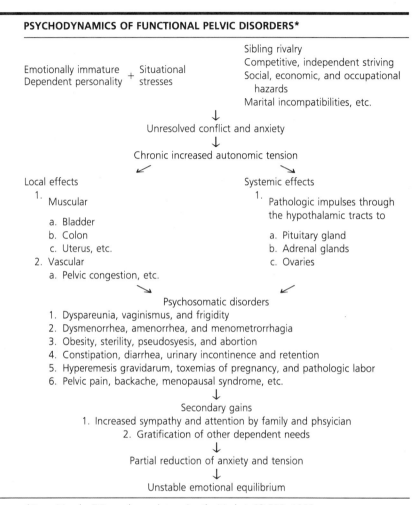

Emotionally immature   +   Situational
Dependent personality   stresses

Sibling rivalry
Competitive, independent striving
Social, economic, and occupational
   hazards
Marital incompatibilities, etc.

↓
Unresolved conflict and anxiety
↓
Chronic increased autonomic tension
↙   ↘

Local effects
1. Muscular
  a. Bladder
  b. Colon
  c. Uterus, etc.
2. Vascular
  a. Pelvic congestion, etc.

Systemic effects
1. Pathologic impulses through
   the hypothalamic tracts to
  a. Pituitary gland
  b. Adrenal glands
  c. Ovaries

↘   ↙
Psychosomatic disorders
1. Dyspareunia, vaginismus, and frigidity
2. Dysmenorrhea, amenorrhea, and menometrorrhagia
3. Obesity, sterility, pseudosyesis, and abortion
4. Constipation, diarrhea, urinary incontinence and retention
5. Hyperemesis gravidarum, toxemias of pregnancy, and pathologic labor
6. Pelvic pain, backache, menopausal syndrome, etc.
↓
Secondary gains
1. Increased sympathy and attention by family and phsyician
2. Gratification of other dependent needs
↓
Partial reduction of anxiety and tension
↓
Unstable emotional equilibrium

*From Mandy, T.E., and associates: South. Med. J. **48**:533, 1955.

them: social status of the patient, family history, past history (especially regarding operations, about which the physician should obtain the patient's signature on an authorization-request form addressed to the hospital at which the surgery was performed, so that accurate data can be obtained concerning the findings, the procedure, and the reports of the pathologist, radiologist, etc.), and marital history, including pregnancies with their outcomes, conflicts and their causes, etc. The present illness should be investigated in detail, allowing the patient to tell her story with guidance as needed. Details as to time of onset, duration, disability, and previous treatment are important. Any adverse reactions to medications and benefits from therapeutic regimens are essential. All present physicians and all medications should be known. In the menstrual history the significant facts are age of onset, regularity, duration, amount, and pain or associated symptoms.

A summary of the chief symptoms is helpful in fixing these facts in mind before passing on to the examination.

Although this chapter is concerned with diagnosis, a few remarks on treatment of psychosomatic problems are indicated. All too frequently when the physician finds that the physical examination and various tests are negative, he concludes that the patient is not really sick. As Ashenburg stated:

> In a way, it is not too different from telling the patient who comes in because of symptoms of diabetes to go home and stop worrying about his polyuria and polydipsia. Both patients come to the doctor for help because of disturbing symptoms. Both may be helped to a better adjustment and to regain their functional stability. To dismiss either patient without help or support places the entire burden back on the patient's shoulders. This adds to his anxiety and fears, and he leaves the doctor's office in a dilemma with the unsatisfying reassurance that he is well.*

If a little more time is taken to listen to the story, to explain the physical or psychologic reasons for the symptoms, and to offer reassurance and support, it may make the difference between a sick, frustrated, and discouraged patient and an appreciative person who is well on the way to recovery.

The gynecologist will probably refer his more disturbed patients to a psychiatrist, but others can frequently be benefited by his understanding and sympathetic advice. In an exhaustive study of anxiety neurosis, for instance, Cohen and White concluded:

> As judged by published therapeutic results, patients with this dsiorder do as well with simple reassurance and the passage of time as do apparently similar cases managed by prolonged psychotherapy, psychoanalysis, electric convulsion procedures, ergotamine tartrate, and adrenal denervation.†

The physician should not minimize the symptoms that, of course, are very real to the patient, but he should attempt to find the etiologic factors. Pain is one of the most difficult symptoms to fathom, since the only interpretation of it is that given by the patient. Frigidity is seldom a primary complaint, although it is present to some degree in most patients with functional disorders.

PHYSICAL EXAMINATION

The general examination should be pursued far enough to give a reliable idea of the general physical condition and to discover any serious disturbance that may

---

*From Ashenburg, N.J.: GP **12**:111, 1955.
†From Cohen, M.E., and White, P.D.: A. Res. Nerv. Ment. Dis., Proc. **29**:832, 1950.

indicate whether the patient's disability is probably caused by pelvic disease or some extrapelvic trouble. It is important that the *breasts* be checked carefully for any abnormalities. Some patients who attempt to examine their breasts worry because of the possibility of cancer, some think they feel a tumor that is not present, others fail to detect an abnormality that does exist, and some substitute the "self-examination" for an examination every 6 months by a competent physician. Such a substitution may prove to be disastrous.

The regular steps in the examination are as follows:
1. Abdominal examination
2. Inspection of external genitals; inspection of introitus, vagina, and cervix; smears for cytologic and any other indicated examinations
3. Instrumental examination
4. Vaginal examination (digital)
5. Vaginoabdominal examination (bimanual)
6. Rectoabdominal palpation

In most cases the history and regular examination give all the information needed for diagnosis and treatment, but in some cases further special examination is necessary to establish a diagnosis.

Abdominal examination

Have the patient lie near the edge of the bed or table in a comfortable position, with the head slightly raised on a pillow and the knees drawn up sufficiently to relax the abdominal muscles. The abdomen is examined as follows:
1. Inspection for contour, colors, scars, eruption, hair
2. Palpation for tension, tenderness, mass (occasionally fluid wave, fat wave, fetal movement, uterine contraction, friction rub)
3. Percussion for area of dullness (stationary, shifting)
4. Auscultation for fetal heart sound, placental souffle, aneurysmal murmur
5. Mensuration for accurate comparison of changes in the abdominal circumference caused by ascites or intestinal distention (The distance that a pelvic mass extends above the symphysis pubis should be recorded for future comparison.)

INSPECTION

The contour is the principal thing to determine by inspection of the abdomen. Has the patient the smooth, moderately full contour of the normal abdomen; the flat, sunken abdomen of wasting disease; or a swollen, prominent abdomen?

PALPATION

The best way to begin palpation is to place the palmar surface of the whole hand flat on the abdominal wall. Hold it still for a moment so that the patient may see that you are not going to cause pain. Then, as the muscular tension relaxes, depress the wall carefully with the fingers in various directions as the hand is moved slowly over the surface. Avoid the use of sudden movements and force, particularly digging movements with the fingertips, as these stir up muscular resistance that makes deep palpation impossible. In the palpation, distinction should be made between tension, tenderness, and a mass, for each has its particular diagnostic significance.

When *tension* of the abdominal wall is found, it may be caused by voluntary contraction caused by fear of pain or by the involuntary muscle guard of inflammation, a mass (solid or cystic) under the wall, or hysteric contraction. Voluntary contraction usually disappears as the examination progresses and the patient becomes convinced there will be no pain.

Definite *tenderness* has diagnostic significance according to its location (organ probably involved) and severity (grade and extent of inflammation or other process).

In the case of an apparent *mass* or of prominence of the abdomen the first point to decide is whether the enlargement is because of something in the abdominal wall or something under the wall. Either a thick layer of fat in the wall or a relaxed wall with some distention is quite misleading at times and has caused mistaken diagnoses of tumor. For this reason it is important to test the thickness of the abdominal wall to see whether that accounts for the prominence, either wholly or partially. The thickness of the wall is determined by picking it up, as shown in Fig. 2-1. The fingers are thus brought close together under the wall, showing definitely how much of the prominence is due to the wall and how much to something underneath.

If a mass is found, decide whether it comes from the pelvis (free margin upward and fixed part below) or from one of the upper abdominal organs (free margin below and fixed part above). If it comes from the pelvis, the anatomic and pathologic diagnosis is made by determining as far as possible its position, size, shape, consistency, tenderness, mobility, and attachments.

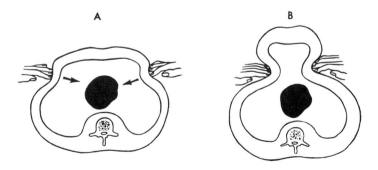

Fig. 2-1. A, First step, testing thickness of abdominal wall. **B,** Second step, fingers carried beneath the wall.

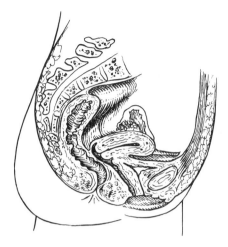

Fig. 2-2. Anteroposterior section of pelvis showing left half of body with intestines removed.

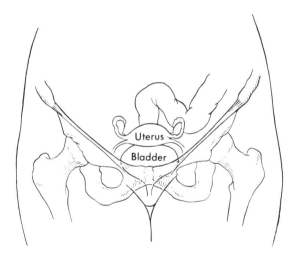

Fig. 2-3. Diagrammatic anterior view of major pelvic organs.

Sketches of the pelvic organs in sagittal and anterior views are shown in Figs. 2-2 and 2-3.

For recording the location of a mass or of tenderness the abdomen is divided into regions that are conveniently designated as follows: right lower quadrant, left lower quadrant, central lower abdomen, right upper quadrant, left upper quadrant, central upper abdomen, umbilical area, and lumbar regions (right and left). Within

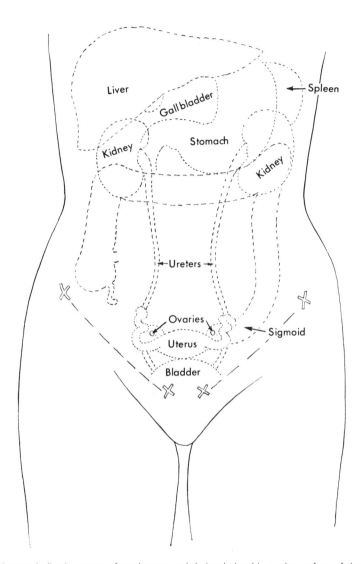

Fig. 2-4. Diagram indicating areas of tenderness and their relationship to the surface of the abdomen.

each of these regions there are certain points where tenderness or a mass takes on special diagnostic significance because of the organs normally situated underneath, as shown in Fig. 2-4.

PERCUSSION

The distinctive information obtained by percussion relates to the presence or absence of an *area of dullness* and, if such an area is present, its location and

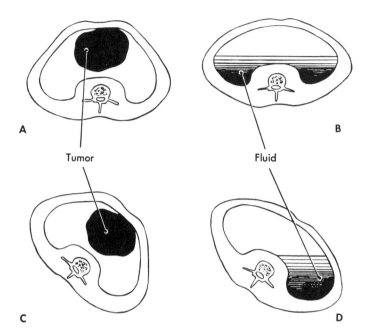

Fig. 2-5. Cross sections of the abdominal cavity. **A,** Encysted fluid or tumor with resonance in the flanks. **B,** Free fluid in the cavity with dullness in the flanks and resonance above the fluid. **C,** The effect of changing the position of the patient on the encysted fluid or tumor, no shifting area of dullness. **D,** On shifting the position of the patient when there is free fluid in the abdomen, the fluid gravitates to the lower flank and dullness is found in the flank with resonance above the fluid.

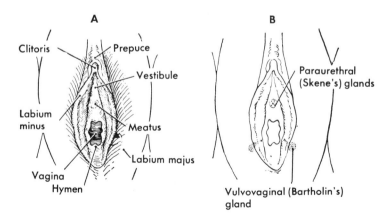

Fig. 2-6. A, External genitals. **B,** Areas most likely to harbor persistent infection.

outline and whether it shifts with change of the patient's position. The change of outline of dullness according to gravity is the definite and certain sign of free fluid (ascites). The differential percussion signs between ascites and a tumor are shown in Fig. 2-5.

Inspection of external genitals, meatus, perineum, and anus

The various structures comprising the external genitals are shown in Fig. 2-6, *A*, and the special areas most likely to harbor persistent inflammation are indicated in Fig. 2-6, *B*. The physician should determine if any of the following conditions are present:

1. Discharge (mucoepithelial, mucopurulent, purulent, bloody, watery, malodorous)
2. Inflammation (gonorrheal or otherwise)
3. Ulcer (simple, chancroidal, syphilitic, tuberculous, malignant)
4. Swelling (inflammation, stasis infiltration, edema, hematoma, hernia, cyst)
5. New growth (condyloma, urethral caruncle, lipoma, fibroma, malignant growth)
6. Malformation (imperforate hymen, adhesion of labia, pseudohermaphroditism)

Notice also the following:

1. Condition of hymen (intact, lacerated, destroyed)
2. Condition of urethral meatus (pus, polyp, inflammation)
3. Condition of vulvovaginal glands (red spots, discharge, induration, tenderness)
4. Condition of perineum (normal, relaxed, lacerated)

If pus is found, determine just where it comes from, i.e., whether from the urethra or vulvovaginal gland, from inflamed surfaces on the external genitals, or from the vagina.

Dip the tip of a cotton-wrapped applicator in this purulent discharge and spread some on a microscopic slide. If possible, secure some discharge from the urethra or vulvovaginal gland, for the pus from these areas is much more satisfactory for microscopic examination than the mixed vulvar or vaginal discharge.

To secure urethral pus, separate the labia, cleanse the meatus, and compress the internal end of the urethra by pressure against the anterior vaginal wall with the tip of the index finger. Then, still maintaining the pressure, draw the tip of the finger along the urethra toward the meatus. This brings the urethral pus to the meatus.

Chronic inflammation in the urethra is likely to be situated in Skene's glands, and in such a case some pus may be expressed from these small glands by compressing the urethra (by pressure through anterior vaginal wall) just back to the meatus. In some patients, particularly in multiparas, the urethral mucosa pouts, so that by careful examination the orifice of one or both of Skene's glands may be seen (Fig. 2-6, *B*).

The vulvovaginal glands, Bartholin's glands (Fig. 2-6, *B*), are situated symmetrically on each side of the vaginal opening. The opening of the duct of the gland on each side is situated laterally, just in front of the remnants of the hymen and a little below the middle of the lateral margin of the vaginal opening. Draw aside the labia, look for the opening of the gland, and determine whether the opening is reddened and if there is any discharge from it. To determine if there is any thickening or tenderness from inflammation or if pus can be squeezed from it, palpate either vulvovaginal gland by grasping the region of the gland between the index finger in the vagina and the thumb outside.

Instrumental examination

Instrumental examination includes the following:
1. Inspection of the vagina and cervix through the speculum
   a. Vaginal walls (color, discharge, redundancy)
   b. Cervix uteri (position, color, size and shape, lacerations, deviation of axis, eversion, erosion, hypertrophy, cystic change, ulcer)
   c. External os (size and shape, color of edges, discharge, polyps)
2. Excision of tissue from cervix for microscopic examination
3. Exploration of interior of uterus with a sound
4. Exploration of interior of uterus with a small curet when indicated

By means of certain instruments the vaginal walls may be spread apart so that they and the cervix uteri may be seen. Information of much value may be obtained in this way. Usually instrumental examination should be done before palpation to obtain better material for cellular or organism study.

The instruments needed for this examination are shown in Fig. 2-7. They are as follows:
1. Speculum for separating the vaginal walls
2. Long dressing forceps for sponging out the vagina, usually called uterine dressing forceps
3. Tenaculum forceps, vulsella, for catching the cervix and bringing it into better view

The *bivalve speculum* (Fig. 2-7, *B*) is used most frequently in ordinary office work. It consists of two blades, which are introduced closed and then are opened by a mechanism at the handle. The vaginal walls are thus held apart (Fig. 2-8), and a very good view of both the vaginal walls and the cervix may be obtained.

There are many different modifications of the blades and also of the mechanism for separating the blades. The most satisfactory type that we have found is shown

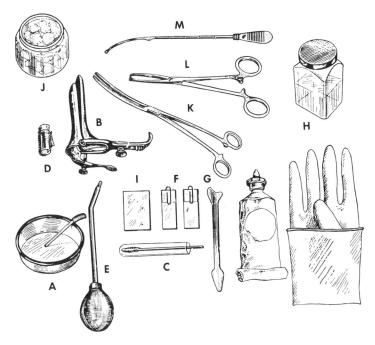

Fig. 2-7. Equipment used for vaginal examination. **A,** Catheter to empty bladder if necessary. **B,** The Graves speculum. **C,** Vaginal applicator, cotton-tipped. **D,** Culture medium. **E,** Vaginal pipette. **F,** Slides for Papanicolaou smears (paper clips hold slides apart and also facilitate their removal from the fixing solution). **G,** Ayre's cervical scraper. **H,** Fixing solution, 50% ether and 50% alcohol. (A rapidly drying protective coating may be used.) **I,** Slide for wet smear. **J,** Sterile cotton balls. **K,** Uterine dressing forceps. **L,** Vulsella or long Allis forceps. **M,** Uterine sound. (Gloves and lubricant are shown but not lettered.)

in the illustration. It is called the Graves speculum and has the advantage of being easily and quickly transformed into a fairly satisfactory Sims speculum, which is a decided convenience for office work. Three sizes are useful—small (virgin), medium, and large. Narrower-bladed specula, such as the Pederson, are used advantageously in some patients. As a rule, the bivalve speculum is used with the patient in the dorsal posture and the Sims speculum with the patient in a knee-chest position.

The *uterine dressing forceps* (Fig. 2-7, *K*) is a long, strong forceps for sponging out the vagina and for making vaginal applications. It may be straight or curved as preferred. A vaginal depressor for pushing the vaginal wall out of the way is usually included in an examining set, but it is generally not necessary because the vaginal wall may be pushed aside sufficiently with the dressing forceps.

The *uterine tenaculum forceps* (Fig. 2-7, *L*) is needed for catching the cervix

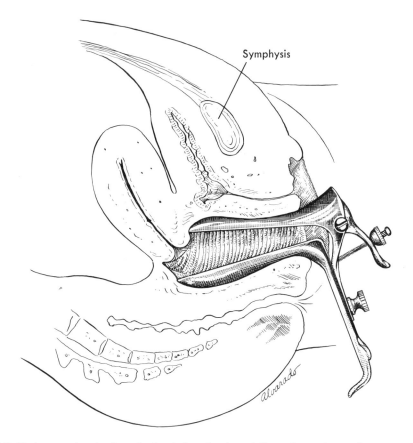

Symphysis

Fig. 2-8. Bivalve speculum in place. Sectional view showing relations of speculum and exposure of the cervix and vaginal vault by opening the blades.

and bringing all parts of it into view. It should be light but strong, especially about the lock, where it is likely to work loose. The 19 cm Allis forceps with a box lock is excellent.

STEPS IN SPECULUM EXAMINATION

Introducing speculum. The blades of the speculum are closed, the outer surfaces are moistened or lubricated, and the speculum is held in the right hand; with the other hand the labia are separated and the perineum depressed somewhat with one finger. The speculum is introduced and carried all the way to the upper part of the vagina without being opened. In most patients the speculum passes the vaginal entrance most easily when held with its width almost vertical. The edge should be held just far enough to one side to miss the urethra. When well within the vagina, it is turned transversely and carried in as far as it will go (Fig. 2-8).

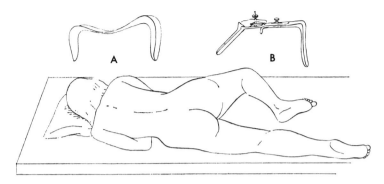

Fig. 2-9. Patient in the Sims position. **A,** Sims speculum. **B,** Graves bivalve speculum changed to the Sims type.

Care is necessary that painful pressure not be made on the urethra or other structures beneath the pubic arch. Remeber that when more room is required the pressure must always be directed *against the perineum*, which will gradually yield.

Another common mistake of the inexperienced examiner is to open the blades too soon before the speculum has been introduced all the way. If the blades are not in far enough to expose the cervix satisfactorily, pain is likely to be produced by pinching the vaginal wall, since the blades are closed for further introduction.

Exposing cervix. After the blades have been introduced deeply in the vagina, they are opened and the cervix and vaginal walls are exposed (Fig. 2-8). If the speculum is turned in various directions, all parts of the cervix and the upper end of the vagina may be seen.

Cleansing vagina. If there is secretion obscuring any part of the vaginal wall or cervix, it should be wiped away with cotton held in the dressing forceps.

Exposing vaginal walls. For inspection of the vaginal walls the speculum is turned to bring various portions of the walls within the opening between the blades. Another way is to inspect the various portions of the walls just beyond the end of the speculum as it is gradually withdrawn.

Examination with the Sims speculum. The Sims speculum is a perineal retractor and for use requires that the patient be put in the Sims posture or the knee-chest position. Like any other retractor, it must be held in place by an assistant.

As it is usually made, two blades are placed on one handle, a large blade at one end and a small blade at the other (Fig. 2-9). The Graves bivalve speculum mentioned previously is easily and quickly changed into a satisfactory Sims speculum.

The principal points about the Sims posture, called also the left lateral posture and the semiprone posture, are shown in Fig. 2-9.

For introduction of the speculum the right labia are raised, thus exposing the vaginal opening; then the speculum, well lubricated, is carefully inserted into the opening. At the same time the perineum is pulled somewhat backward with the speculum point to give more room for the instrument to slip in. The blade is then carried all the way in. The speculum is grasped firmly and pulled backward, thus retracting the perineum and exposing the interior of the vagina.

As the speculum is introduced, the vagina becomes distended with air, and, when the perineum is retracted, the cervix and anterior vaginal wall may be seen. To bring the cervix into still better view, catch it with the tenaculum forceps and bring it slightly toward the opening.

The Sims speculum with the Sims posture is of decided advantage when the bivalve speculum fails to expose the cervix satisfactorily either because the vaginal walls are so lax that they fall about the blades and obscure the cervix or because the vaginal opening is so small that the blades cannot be sufficiently separated. Use of the Sims speculum and position is also very helpful in exposing the opening of a vesicovaginal fistula on the anterior wall of the vagina. The *genupectoral position*, also called the knee-chest position, is very valuable in many cases (Fig. 6-4). After the assumption of this position a Sims speculum is introduced into the vagina, which balloons, so that it and the cervix are easily inspected. We consider the genupectoral position so much better than the Sims position that we use the latter only to examine those patients in bed for whom the kee-chest position is contraindicated.

Vaginal examination (digital examination)

With one or two fingers in the vagina, palpate the following structures:
1. Vaginal walls (roughness, tenderness, discharge, induration, swelling, stricture)
2. Base of bladder (tenderness, induration)
3. Urethra (tenderness, induration, discharge)
4. Pelvic floor (size of opening, resistance to backward pressure, protrusion of vaginal walls, scars and distortion, thickness of perineum)
5. Rectum, as palpated through posterior vaginal wall (tenderness, induration)
6. Cervix uteri (position, size, shape, consistency, tenderness, mobility, direction of canal, grooves of lacerations, infiltration and eversion of lips, cyst formation)
7. Pericervical tissue (tenderness, induration, mass)

At the beginning of the examination, as the examining fingers are being introduced, there is frequently a tendency on the part of the patient, who is nervous for fear of pain, to contract the muscles of the pelvic floor and thus interfere with the vaginal examination. In such a case, if one finger is introduced a short distance and steady *pressure backward* is made against the muscle, it slowly relaxes and the second finger may be introduced beside the first. Remember that to obtain more space at the vaginal orifice, either in digital examination or in introducing a speculum, always press downward against the pelvic sling. About and to the sides of the opening is the bony arch, and, if an attempt is made to overcome the resistance by direct forward pressure, without depressing the perineum, the soft tissues above are pinched between the finger or instrument and the bony arch, causing the patient pain and increasing the muscular resistance.

Determine if there is definite tenderness of the vaginal wall, which indicates inflammation either in the wall or in adjacent tissues. The diagnostic significance of tenderness or induration or a distinctly outlined mass depends largely on its location. In making the vaginal palpation, keep in mind the location of the various structures adjacent to the vagina, and you will have the key to the interpretation of any perivaginal tenderness or induration.

The amount or grade of relaxation of the *pelvic floor* is to be definitely tested and noted, for that information, together with the symptoms, determines whether repair of the floor is necessary.

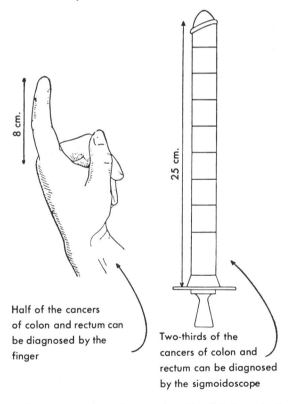

Half of the cancers of colon and rectum can be diagnosed by the finger

Two-thirds of the cancers of colon and rectum can be diagnosed by the sigmoidoscope

Fig. 2-10. Comparison of percentage of rectal cancers found by digital examination and by sigmoidoscope.

From Welch, C.E., and Giddings, W.P.: N. Engl. J. Med. **244**:859, 1951.

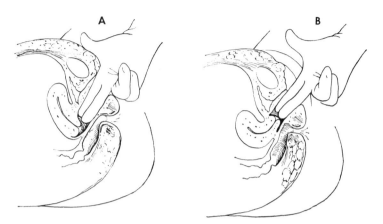

Fig. 2-11. Digital examination to determine position of cervix. **A,** Normal position. **B,** Cervix is low.

Tenderness or induration back of the *posterior vaginal wall* is to be further investigated by rectal palpation. Conditions just within the anal canal—such as fussure, ulcer, or hemorrhoid—can usually be brought into view through eversion of the anal area by pressure from within the vagina.

The *cervix uteri* is felt at the upper end of the vagina as a firm conical body projecting through the upper portion of the anterior wall (Fig. 2-2). It is distinguished from the surrounding vaginal wall by its hardness. The normal position of the cervix is 7.5 to 9 cm from the vaginal orifice. If it takes nearly the full length of the examining fingers to reach the cervix, it is in normal position (Fig. 2-11, *A*). If the cervix is encountered when the fingers are just inserted or only a short distance within the vagina, the cervix is low (Fig. 2-11, *B*).

Determine whether the cervical canal, i.e., axis of the cervix, points *across* the vaginal canal and toward the coccyx as it should (Fig. 2-12, *A*) or *along* the canal (Fig. 2-12, *B* and *C*). Direction of the cervix forward along the vaginal canal is usually caused by backward displacement of the uterus (Fig. 2-12, *B*). However, sometimes it is simply caused by anteflexion of the cervix (Fig. 2-12, *C*).

The size and shape of the cervix vary greatly in different individuals and in the same individual at different periods of life. In women who have never been pregnant the normal cervix has the shape of a rounded cone. The external os is small and round and is at the flattened apex of the cone.

In certain abnormal cases the cervix is very long and pointed. This condition is known as conical cervix.

In women who have borne children the cervix is larger and broader and comparatively shorter. The os is a transverse slit or may be somewhat irregular in

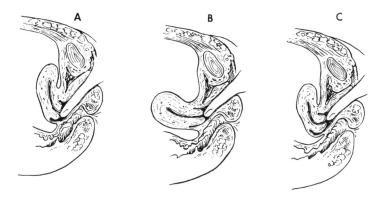

Fig. 2-12. Digital examination to determine relation of cervix to the examining finger. **A,** Uterus in normal position with cervix pointing across canal. **B,** Retroplacement of uterus with cervix pointing along canal. **C,** Anteflexion of uterus with cervix pointing along canal.

shape. When the cervix has been severely lacerated, there may be two or three distinct lips. Again, with chronic inflammation it may become enlarged two or three times and be felt as an irregular ball at the top of the vagina.

In consistency the cervix is firm, like hard connective tissue, almost as hard as tendon. Its consistency is closely approached by that of the end of the nose when firmly pressed. During pregnancy the cervix softens, the *softening* beginning at the lower end and gradually involving more and more as pregnancy advances. The softening is so marked that the softened portion is sometimes missed entirely, the cervix apparently being simply shortened. This is what gave rise to the former idea that the cervix became gradually shortened as pregnancy advanced. The softened portion feels like thick velvet or a fold of vaginal wall as it slips back and forth beneath the examining finger. A partial idea of it may be secured by the following experiment: Cover a finger with a piece of velvet with a very thick nap, the nap side out. Then shut the eyes and with the other hand, with the fingers usually used in vaginal examination, endeavor to make out exactly the thickness of the nap by passing the fingers over it with varying pressure and in different directions. First press firmly to appreciate the fingers beneath, and then press lightly to estimate the thickness of the nap. These same maneuvers are carried out in appreciating the presence and extent of marked softening of the cervix.

This softened, velvety condition of the cervix is very characteristic, and its presence should always arouse suspicion of pregnancy. Slight softening of the cervix is found in some patients with inflammation of the cervix and also in some whose circulation is interfered with, as when the pelvis is filled with a tumor or with a mass of inflammatory exudate or when there is marked displacement of the uterus.

Abnormal *hardening* of a portion of the cervix may be caused by scar tissue, cystic disease, a myomatous nodule, or malignant infiltration.

In regard to *tenderness*, the cervix is much less sensitive than the vaginal wall and rarely becomes very sensitive even when diseased. Complaints of pain when the cervix is pressed upon are usually because of inflammation in the connective tissue about the cervix (parametrium).

As to *mobility*, the cervix is freely and painlessly movable for a short distance in all directions. Its range of mobility may be diminished by scar tissue or by malignant infiltration in the upper part of the vagina, by an inflammatory exudate in the pelvis, by a uterine tumor, or by any pelvic tumor that fixes the uterus. Its range of mobility may be increased by laceration or overstretching of the supports posteriorly, anteriorly, or laterally, a common accompaniment of pelvic floor injuries.

Vaginoabdominal examination (bimanual examination)

With one or two fingers in the vagina and the fingers of the other hand pressing into the pelvis from above, palpate the following:

1. Body of uterus (position, size, shape, consistency, tenderness, mobility, attachments by adhesion or infiltration)
2. Tubo-ovarian regions (mass, induration, tenderness)
3. Posterior part of pelvic cavity (mass, induration, tenderness)
4. Anterior part of pelvic cavity (mass, induration, tenderness)
5. Ureteral regions (mass, induration, tenderness)
6. Pelvic nerve trunks (tenderness)

The vaginoabdominal examination is, as its name implies, an examination from the vagina and the abdomen at the same time. The pelvic structures are caught between the fingers in the vagina and the fingers over the abdomen and carefully examined by touch. By this means the body of the uterus may be located and outlined, the region to each side of the uterus and also the space back of the uterus palpated, and the presence or absence of any mass or tenderness determined.

To the beginner in clinical work this important bimanual examination is often unsatisfactory. He has heard a great deal about tubal and ovarian diseases and he expects to feel the tube and ovary at once. After examining several patients and failing in each to distinguish definitely either tube or ovary (as is likely if those organs are normal), he is discouraged and thinks he has learned nothing from the examinations. Probably he has not learned much for the simple reason that he was feeling for something that he could not feel and he did not appreciate the significance of what he did feel. Close attention to details of the examination will keep the experience from being unprofitable.

STEPS IN PALPATION OF THE CORPUS UTERI

If a catheterized specimen is not needed, have the patient empty the bladder just before the examination. A partially filled bladder pushes the uterus back and interferes generally with the palpation in the pelvis, as indicated in Fig. 2-13, *A*. It has happened on several occasions that a supposed ovarian cyst has disappeared when the bladder was emptied.

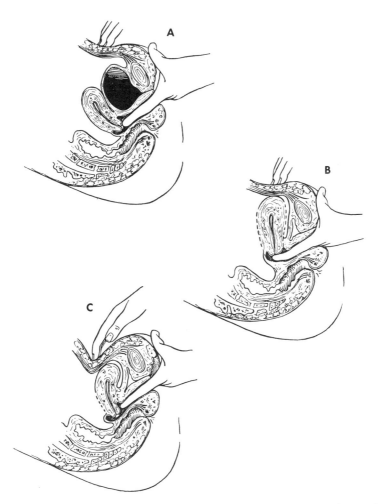

Fig. 2-13. Bimanual examination. **A,** Uterus displaced backward by a full bladder. This interferes with deep palpation. **B,** Difficult case in which the uterus cannot be adequately outlined. Dotted line shows area about which the examiner cannot be certain. **C,** Uterus foward and easily outlined.

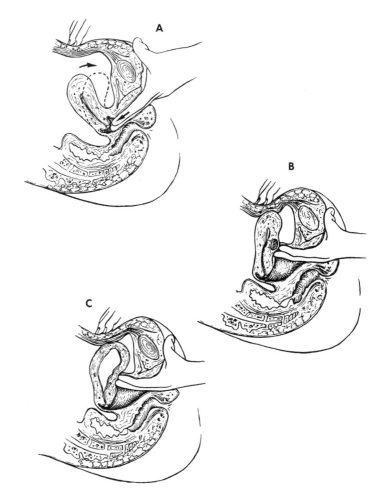

Fig. 2-14. A, The cervix uteri is pushed back to bring the corpus uteri forward. **B,** Palpating a nodule on the anterior surface of the corpus uteri. **C,** Softening of the uterus present with pregnancy of fluid in the cavity.

The distinctness with which the corpus uteri can be palpated and the extent of surface within reach of the examining fingers vary much in different individuals, even with the organ in normal position. In some patients interfering conditions prevent the corpus uteri from being felt. In others the corpus uteri can just barely be identified by catching it between the vaginal fingers on the cervix and the abdominal fingers creating counterpressure (Fig. 2-13, *B*). In other patients deep bimanual palpation is possible and a considerable part of the outline of the uterus can be definitely identified (Fig. 2-13, *C*).

In beginning palpation to locate the corpus uteri it is well to push the cervix back and upward (Fig. 2-14, *A*). This tends to tip the fundus slightly forward into better position for bimanual palpation. Then, with the abdominal fingers making counterpressure, feel (with the vaginal fingers) for the body, tracing up the front of the cervix into it. If the corpus uteri is not felt in front, examine back of the cervix in the center and laterally. In a patient with no undue tension of the abdominal wall and no mass obstructing the pelvis, the body of the uterus should be distinctly outlined (Fig. 2-14, *B* and *C*).

The uterus is more distinctly felt when it is moved up and down between the vaginal and abdominal hands and laterally by a finger placed on each side of the cervix (in the lateral fornices). Apply gentle pressure first on one side and then on the other in a rocking manner.

When the corpus uteri has been found, fix in your mind the following facts concerning it:

1. *Position*. Is it in anterior position as it usually is or is it turned backward or drawn to one side?
2. *Size*. Is it apparently normal, i.e., about 7.5 cm, or is it as large as the fist, as large as a child's head, or as large as the pregnant uterus in the sixth month?
3. *Shape*. Is it approximately pear shaped and regular in outline or does it present irregularities?
4. *Consistency*. Is it apparently a firm, solid body? Does it contain fluid or are there hard nodules in it?
5. *Tenderness*. Does pressure on the uterus or the attempt to move it cause pain?
6. *Mobility*. Can the uterus be moved easily, up and down and laterally, or is it fixed and stationary in the pelvis?
7. *Attachments*. Is the uterus attached to any other organ or to the pelvic wall by adhesions or infiltration?

After these facts regarding the uterus are determined, explore the pelvis at each side or the uterus (tubo-ovarian regions) and behind it. If all the tissues are soft and yielding and no pain is caused by the manipulation, you may be certain the tubes and ovaries are not seriously diseased although you have not felt them.

If a mass is found at either side of the uterus or behind or in front of it, you must determine the same facts concerning it that you did concerning the uterus— its *position, size, shape, consistency, tenderness, mobility,* and *attachments*. If a mass is fastened to the uterus, determine, if possible, whether it is fastened by a broad attachment or a narrow one.

Common errors. The following errors are made so often by students and practitioners during examination that it is advisable to call particular attention to them.

Error 1—Depression of abdominal wall too close to pubis. If the uterus happens to be rather high, as it frequently is, the depression of the wall close to the pubis tends to push the uterus backward. Consequently the corpus uteri is not felt between the examining fingers, although there is no real displacement.

To *avoid this error* start the depression of the abdominal wall about midway between the pubis and the umbilicus so that the depression is made into the posterior part of the pelvis. After the abdominal wall is thus depressed into the pelvic cavity, the examining fingers are brought gradually forward until the body of the uterus is felt or until the vaginal and abdominal fingers are so closely approximated that the absence of the uterus from that part of the pelvis is demonstrated.

Error 2—Frequent shifting of position of abdominal fingers. Some students gouge about roughly in the lower abdomen in various directions in an effort to feel the fundus uteri with the abdominal fingers. This is likely to make the examination a failure in a healthy patient, and it is almost certain to do so in a difficult one. Remember that tension of the abdominal wall interferes with the examination and may defeat it entirely. Remember also that the tension is increased by frequent movements of the abdominal fingers, such as placing them in one position after another in rapid succession, and particularly by gouging rapidly and forcibly in various parts of the pelvis in an endeavor to overcome the resistance of the wall.

To *avoid this error* place the abdominal fingers so that the depression of the wall will be into the back part of the pelvis, and then carry the fingers by steady and continuous pressure toward the desired region. When you have advanced the fingers as far as possible, hold them there steadily and direct the patient to take a deep breath and then to let the breath all out. As expiration takes place, the fingers may be carried deeper into the pelvis, not by any sudden forcing movement but by strong steady pressure that does not excite muscular contraction and resistance. If the fingers still are not deep enough in the pelvis, the same movements may be repeated several times. Because the uterus is not felt at once, do not cease the pressure there and begin to depress the wall at some other place. Start the fingers in the right direction at first and then keep them going in that direction steadily, firmly, persistently, and without relaxing the pressure, until the depth of the pelvis is reached and the corpus uteri is brought within reach of the vaginal fingers palpating from below.

In the subsequent steps of the palpation of the uterus the slight movement of the abdominal fingers that is necessary to bring them into position for good counterpressure at the various parts of the uterus may usually be made without relaxing the pressure, since the skin is loose enough to be slipped about over the underlying structures.

Error 3—Depending on abdominal fingers to feel uterus. The principal function of the abdominal fingers is to press the pelvic structures down within reach of the vaginal fingers. The particular work of the vaginal fingers is to outline the deep structures in the pelvis and determine the various points about them. A moment's thought will make this clear, for the vaginal fingers palpate through the soft and comparatively thin vaginal tissues, whereas the abdominal fingers must palpate through the thick and resistant abdominal wall. The average student, though, will waste much time and effort trying to feel the uterus or other deep-seated structure with the fingers of the abdominal hand instead of using that hand simply to press the structures down within reach of the vaginal fingers and to furnish counterpressure for accurate palpation from within.

STEPS IN PALPATION OF LATERAL REGIONS

In the lateral region, on each side, lies the large area of connective tissue beside the cervix and lower part of the corpus uteri. Here induration from inflammation or other cause is felt at once low about the cervix, just under the vaginal wall. Higher, beside the uterus, lie the fallopian tube and the ovary. They are near the upper part of the broad ligament and so close together that ordinarily it is impossible to say, simply from the position of a mass there, whether it springs from the tube or from the ovary. Hence the region is spoken of as the tubo-ovarian region. It is also called the adnexal region, the tube and ovary of each side being considered the appendages of the uterus. The tubo-ovarian region lies high. To palpate it satisfactorily requires special care. In endeavoring to palpate this region proceed as follows:

1. Place the tips of the vaginal fingers to that side of the cervix and push them backward, outward, and upward as far as possible. In order to carry the fingertips sufficiently far into the posterior lateral area of the pelvis, it is sometimes necessary to push the perineum for some distance into the pelvis.

2. With the abdominal fingers, locate the anterosuperior spine of the ilium on that side and then bring the fingers directly inward (not downward toward the pubes, but directly inward or slightly upward) toward the median line or about 5 cm (Fig. 2-15, *A*).

3. At that point, depress the abdominal wall into the posterior part of the side of the pelvis until the tips of the abdominal fingers come close to the tips of the vaginal fingers. This brings the fingers near to each other *back* of, or at least in the region of, the tube and ovary (Fig. 2-15, *B*).

4. If the adnexa are not felt in the back part of the pelvis, bring the fingers of the two hands held in the same relation to each other slowly downward toward the pubis. In this way the tube and the ovary are made to pass between the examining fingertips, and they may be felt if decidedly enlarged.

By proceeding gently, so as not to excite contraction of the abdominal muscles, and at the same time by steadily pressing the two sets of fingers toward each other a little with each expiration, the fingertips may be brought almost together in the various parts of the pelvis. The ovary is best felt as it slips from the palpating

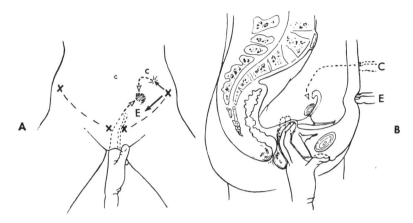

Fig. 2-15. A, Diagram illustrating a common error in efforts to palpate the adnexa—placing the abdominal fingers too low on the abdominal wall. In attempting to depress an area of abdominal wall into the pelvis above and back of the adnexa so as to catch the ovary and tube between the abdominal and vaginal fingertips, allowance must be made for a sufficient length of movable wall to reach from the fixed pubic end into the back of the pelvic cavity. This is secured by placing the fingers on an area inward and upward from the iliac spine, as indicated by *C* (correct). When the necessity of this allowance is overlooked, the fingers are likely to be placed on an area inward and downward from the iliac spine, as indicated by *E* (error) and in **B** by the solid-line fingertips. The correct area to be depressed is indicated in **B** by the abdominal fingertips in dotted outline. **B,** The points emphasized in **A** are used in conjunction with this diagram. A point of importance in difficult cases is to push the vaginal fingers as far back as possible, as is indicated by the dotted outline, before turning them outward and upward. If this precaution is neglected, as indicated by the solid-line vaginal fingers, the ovary and tube are likely to be missed in the examination.

vaginal fingertips, having been gently pushed downward by the abdominal fingers.

In these manipulations the palpation proper is made principally with the vaginal fingers, the abdominal fingers serving simply to push the structures down within reach of the fingers below.

A *common error* is to bring the tips of the examining fingers together too close to the pubis; hence the palpation is of the tissue in front of the tube and ovary. It must be kept in mind also that the tube and the ovary are likely to be displaced, especially if diseased, and the displacement is nearly always backward. Hence it is important to get far back in the side of the pelvis when endeavoring to palpate these structures accurately.

To *avoid this error* be certain that the point of depression of the abdominal wall is well above the tubo-ovarian region (Fig. 2-15, *A*).

GENERAL OBSERVATIONS ON BIMANUAL EXAMINATION

It may seem hardly worthwhile to take the trouble to locate all these points in regard to the uterus or a mass beside the uterus; however, it is, and the further one advances in diagnosis the more he appreciates this fact. The ability to make a correct diagnosis of deep-seated pelvic disease depends largely on the ability to answer the questions listed on p. 69 correctly, and until one can determine the facts just indicated in regard to the uterus or other pelvic mass, one's diagnosis is simply a guess and not a diagnosis at all.

Importance of educated touch. It is necessary to emphasize the importance of *training the hands*—of acquiring the "tactus eruditus." The multiplicity of instruments for diagnostic purposes has to some extent obscured the importance of the educated touch. The beginner in gynecologic work is bewildered by the great variety of specula, tenacula, and other instruments for diagnosis, and he is accordingly impressed with the idea that the principal thing is to learn how to use instruments and then to use them on every occasion. One of the first duties of a teacher in gynecology is to displace this erroneous idea by showing the importance of the use of the hands. Most of the serious diseases of women affect structures that lie beyond the reach of sight. To the teacher falls the duty of directing the student's efforts in such a way that he will acquire the ability to distinguish these intrapelvic conditions in the only way that such conditions can be distinguished—by touch. This is not a matter of a few days. It takes weeks and months of patient work and many careful examinations to be able to recognize normal conditions. The abdominal wall and the vaginal wall intervene between the examining fingers and the important organs. These intervening structures vary so much in thickness, in consistency, in tension, and in sensitivity that there is infinite variety in the facility with which the organs may be outlined. Again, the organs themselves vary much within normal limits, both in different patients and in the same patient at different times.

The beginner must learn to read the conditions by first learning the separate letters, so to speak, and then learning what certain groupings of letters mean. The separate items that must be recognized in this examination should be memorized. They are the *position, size, shape, consistency, tenderness, mobility,* and *attachments* of the organs. Mastery takes much time, patience, and well-directed efforts through many examinations. It cannot be learned from lectures. It cannot be learned by seeing someone make examinations and applications. It can be learned only through repeated bimanual examinations by the student himself under competent instruction; hence the clinical portion of a gynecologic course is important. Although it takes considerable time to learn to recognize normal conditions, the time is well spent, for no real progress is possible without this knowledge. The *normal must be known* before the abnormal can be appreciated.

In the recognition of pathologic conditions the same points must be considered (position, size, shape, consistency, tenderness, mobility, and attachments), and this information supplemented by the history determines the diagnosis. This determination of the particular pathologic conditions present is accomplished almost totally by the hands, either in the ordinary bimanual examination or in the examination under anesthesia.

We do not wish to minimize the value of diagnostic instruments (specula, sounds, curets, etc.). They are often helpful and in some cases indispensable to a positive diagnosis, and their use should not be neglected; however, we do wish to emphasize the fact that in gynecologic examinations generally, instruments are of secondary importance and only supplemental to the trained hand.

Take every opportunity to educate the fingers to appreciate as accurately as possible the various conditions found in the pelvis. When examining a suitable patient, outline the uterus and all the pelvic structures as clearly as you can, even if it is not necessary to the diagnosis in that particular case. Each careful examination made serves to educate the fingers, or rather serves to educate the mind to appreciate what is between the fingers, and better prepares you to determine the exact conditions in difficult cases.

Observe the intra-abdominal findings during surgery of the patients you have examined, for correlation of palpatory findings with operative inspection is essential in maximum development of interpretation.

Train one hand. In the bimanual examination it is well to train one hand for the vaginal manipulations. For this purpose either the right or the left hand may be selected, as the examiner finds more convenient. The advantage of using the same hand in vaginal manipulations in practically all cases is that the *power of discrimination* by the fingers of that hand increases as more and more examinations are made. At the same time the abdominal hand becomes accustomed to the abdominal manipulations, and, as the examining hands are in practically the same relation in every case, deviations from the normal are more readily recognized and more accurately defined than if the two hands were used indiscriminately and hence in different relations. This is especially true when the examiner has had the opportunity of only a limited number of examinations.

In exceptional cases it is an advantage to use first one hand and then the other for vaginal palpation. In some situations the right side of the pelvis can be explored better with the fingers of the right hand and the left side with the fingers of the left hand.

Use two fingers. Use two fingers in the vagina when the vaginal opening is large enough to permit their use without pain. A *deeper* and *more accurate* examination can be made with two fingers (index and middle finger) than with the index finger alone. The upper part of the vagina is capacious; the only difficulty is at the vaginal entrance. By lubricating the fingers well, depressing the perineum, and working carefully, the two fingers may be used without discomfort in practically all parous women and in most sexually active women. In most cases water can be used as the lubricant.

Examine deeply in pelvis. In many patients, to palpate the posterior part of the pelvis and particularly to palpate the tubo-ovarian regions satisfactorily, the vaginal fingers must reach farther than their length will permit. The extra reach is secured by *pushing the perineum into the pelvis* (invagination of the pelvic floor) by strong steady pressure inward. The soft structures closing the pelvic outlet can be pushed for a considerable distance inward without particular discomfort to the patient provided all the muscles are relaxed. In parous women 2.5 to 5 cm may usually be thus added to the effective length of the examining fingers.

If exerted by the arm muscles alone, the required force, although not great, is likely to interfere with delicate palpation by the examining fingers. It adds much to the effectiveness of the examination to exert this pressure by the body muscles, leaving the arm muscles free for the internal palpation movements. This may be accomplished either by placing the left foot (when examining with the left hand) on a stool or chair and resting the elbow on the knee or by letting the elbow rest against the hip.

Preferable position for examiner. For the vaginal and the vaginoabdominal or bimanual examination it is decidedly advantageous for the examiner to stand directly *in front* of the vaginal opening. This is especially important when very deep pelvic palpation is necessary. This is the usual position when the patient is examined on the table with footrests so that the hips may be brought entirely to the end of the table.

When a patient is examined in bed, however, the examiner should sit on the bed so that the examining arm passes between the thighs.

Diminish tenderness. In many patients satisfactory pelvic exploration is prevented by tenderness, particularly in those with a pelvic inflammation that is a primary or complicating lesion. In some of these patients the symptoms are so urgent that an examination under anesthesia is advisable at once. In most instances, however, the symptoms are not so threatening as to necessitate immediate examination under anesthesia. In these patients a few days of treatment for the inflammation with hot douches and antibiotics, if needed, will reduce the tenderness so that an adequate examination can be done. A sedative given a half hour before the examination will help to relax the muscles and reduce the pain.

Rectoabdominal palpation. In every patient it is of decided advantage to follow the vaginoabdominal and speculum examinations by a rectoabdominal examination. The index finger, gloved and lubricated, is introduced into the rectum, and the anal and rectal tissues are palpated. Search is made for evidences of hemorrhoids (with or without thrombosis or inflammation), stricture, malignant disease, ulceration, proctitis, fistula, and fissure. The examining finger is then passed upward between the uterosacral ligaments, as far as possible up the posterior surface of the uterus. With the fingers of the other hand pressing down the organs from above,

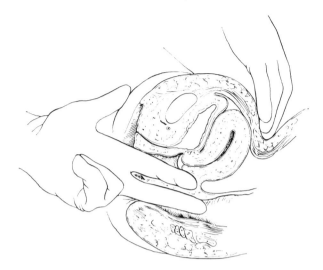

Fig. 2-16. Rectovaginoabdominal examination.

all the structures within reach are palpated with the palmar surface of the rectal finger. With one finger in the rectum and the thumb over the coccyx it can be determined whether the coccyx is normal and whether movement of the coccyx causes pain.

This rectal palpation is especially helpful in cases of suspected cul-de-sac abscess and in cases of carcinomatous infiltration of the parametrium. In an inflammatory mass in the posterior cul-de-sac, fluctuation can sometimes be detected by rectal palpation while still not detectable by vaginal palpation. In cancer of the cervix uteri, rectal palpation aids greatly in outlining the extent of the parametrial infiltration. Rectovaginal examination is also very helpful in determining the involvement of the rectovaginal tissues (Fig. 2-16).

When palpation of the interior of the pelvis is necessary in a girl, sufficient information may sometimes be obtained by rectoabdominal palpation, thus avoiding vaginal examination. If the patient complains of unexplained tenderness of transvaginal palpation, transrectal movement of the uterus and adnexa may reveal no tenderness of these areas, suggesting a psychic cause.

SPECIAL EXAMINATIONS AND TESTS

1. Vaginal and cervical smears
2. Colposcopic magnification of cervical lesions
3. Schiller's test
4. Cervical biopsy

5. Endometrial biopsy
6. Hysteroscopy
7. Cervical mucus arborization test
8. Culdocentesis
9. Pregnancy tests
10. Endocrine investigations
    a. Pituitary hormone determinations
    b. Estrogen and progestogen determinations
    c. Thyroid function tests
    d. Adrenal function tests
11. Chromatin examinations
    a. Sex chromatin bodies
    b. Chromosomal counts
12. Tubal tests
13. X-ray examinations
14. Ultrasonography
15. Pelvic examination under anesthesia
16. Intra-abdominal inspection with culdoscope or peritoneoscope
17. Urinary tract investigation
18. Premarital examination and counsel
19. Pediatric or adolescent examination

Vaginal smears

In 1928 Papanicolaou suggested the use of the vaginal smear as an aid in the diagnosis of early genital cancer in women. In 1943 he introduced a special stain for clear differentiation between basophilic and acidophilic cells. His method has proved to be a boon to an untold number of women, and it rightfully should be a part of every woman's initial examination and annual checkups thereafter. Its use has been extended to determine cellular changes relating to estrogen and progestogen effects that have been observed on the maturation index (% parabasal cells/% intermediate cells/% superficial cells).

To obtain the secretion the speculum is introduced without any lubricating jelly, but it is moistened with warm water (Fig. 2-8). A pipet or spatula can be used to obtain mucoid material from the posterior vaginal pool. An Ayre wooden spatula is excellent for removing a specimen from the surface of the external cervical os by rotating it 360 degrees. It is important to include endocervical mucus, when present, to improve chances of finding abnormal cells. A cotton-tipped applicator can be used inside the cervical canal and either a spatula or cotton-tipped applicator for obtaining a specimen from the lateral vaginal wall, which is the best area to study endocrine effects in cells. Immediately after smears are spread they should be fixed by dropping them in a solution of one-half alcohol (95%) and one-half ether or by applying a rapidly drying fixative such as Cyto Dri Fix Paragon.

Material from the vaginal pool can be viewed in a wet, unstained fresh preparation to identify trichomonads, mycelia, and spores; to evaluate the number of leukocytes; and to estimate the hormonal status by observation of squamous cells. Wet preparations may be rapidly stained. They can be observed under a coverslip while wet. The nuclear and cytoplasmic features then become more apparent. Two drops of 20% potassium hydroxide solution added to a wet slide preparation will cause rapid dissolution of cellular material and allow more definitie identification of hyphae and conidia of *Candida*.

The accurate reading in the search for malignant cells requires permanent staining with Papanicolaou or hematoxylineosin stains. Permanently stained single smears should allow detection of malignant cells in more than 90% of patients with squamous cell carcinoma of the cervix. False-negative smears in cervical intraepithelia neoplasia (CIN) occur more frequently. From 50% to 75% of patients with adenocarcinomas of the endometrium will have positive cytosmears.

The Papanicolaou classification formerly used for reporting is as follows:

Class I—negative

Class II—atypical cells, not suspicious of tumor

Class III—atypical cells, suspicious of tumor

Class IV—probable tumor cells

Class V—tumor cells

The following classification is presently used:

1. Inadequate for diagnosis
2. Essentially normal findings
3. Atypical cells present suggestive of (specify)
4. Findings consistent with:
   a. CIN grade I (mild dysplasia)
   b. CIN grade II (moderate dysplasia)
   c. CIN grade III (severe dysplasia to cancer in situ)
   d. Invasive squamous cell carcinoma
   e. Endometrial carcinoma
   f. Other cancer (specify)

All patients with smears consistent with CIN, invasive squamous cell carcinoma, or other cancer require biopsy. If no gross lesion is seen, colposcopically directed biopsy is often required. When no area requiring biopsy is seen with the coloposcope or when the upper portion of the transitional zone can not be seen, repeated smears and endocervical curettage should be done. If adenocarcinoma is suspected, endometrial biopsy is indicated.

Trichomoniasis and reaction to podophyllin may cause nuclear changes that result in false-positive smears. Negative smears do not rule out cervical cancer completely, and endometrial cancer cells are frequently not found. Patients should very rarely undergo surgical treatment based only on repeatedly positive smears, biopsy may be necessary based on clinical inspection and palpation and knowledge of symptoms and treatment.

When women have had negative annual smears for several years, the first abnormal smears are usually interpreted as atypical cells suggestive of inflammation or possible dysplasia. The inflammatory process should be treated and the smears repeated. With persistent atypical cells colposcopy is indicated. When the first abnormal cellular changes are consistent with CIN, biopsy is best performed with colposcopic direction. Therapy for mild or moderate dysplasia is commonly cryo-conization, an outpatient procedure. Severe dysplasia or carcinoma in situ requires accurate diagnosis, which may be colposcopic biopsy, but when the entire transitional zone cannot be seen, surgical conization is needed to allow accurate histologic diagnosis.

When the transitional zone is completely accessible, routine cytologic screening allows diagnosis of precancerous lesions that often exist for 6 or 8 years before invasive squamous cell cancers develop. The accessibility of the cervix and the relatively long period from dysplasia to invasion in the transitional zone of the cervix are the factors allowing prevention of invasive cervical squamous cell cancer.

Acridine-orange fluorescence microscopy has been advocated as a routine method for more rapid screening of vaginal smears. It appears to offer some advantage in reading smears when adenocarcinoma of the endometrium is suspected and when the material is bloody, but cytologic centers have not generally adopted this method as it has not improved their function.

Special tampons and irrigation-aspiration kits have been tried in large groups of women to obtain specimens on a do-it-yourself basis. These methods have allowed recognition of previously unknown cancers but cannot replace the examination by a physician and the physician-prepared smears.

Colposcopic examination

The colposcope provides magnification and control of intensity and color of illumination, so that changes can be recognized in surface contours, color patterns, and vascularity, which are associated with dysplasia, carcinoma in situ, and invasive cancer. The exocervix and lowest portion of the endocervix are usually well visualized. The transitional zone is the area of greatest concern. The vaginal surface, particularly in the upper vagina, can be searched for evidence of adenosis or malignant change.

Use of colposcopy is limited to the area that is visualized. All or only a portion of the transitional zone may be obscured by changes due to previous cauterization, cryoconization, or conization. Retraction of the transition zone occurs after menopause. Cyst formation may distort the cervix. Vaginal stenosis may limit illumination and proper visualization.

When the expert uses the colposcope, the accuracy of the diagnosis of dysplasia and cervical neoplasia is comparable to that attained in cytologic study. Cervical smears can be obtained by the less expert and examined in numbers in cytologic diagnostic centers. Routine cytologic screening is more feasible than routine colposcopic screening. Colposcopy is essential to select areas for biopsy and often allows avoidance of in-hospital conization for diagnosis.

Schiller's test

When the cervix is painted with Gram's iodine solution, normal squamous epithelial cells take a uniform brown stain because these cells contain glycogen. Areas of eversion, erosion, and cancer, however, fail to stain because the cells in these areas do not contain glycogen. This test is not diagnostic, but it enables one to know the area in which a biopsy should be done.

Daro and associates recommend using a solution of 0.3% to 1% iodine. This is squirted vigorously against the cervix by means of a 10 ml syringe and a 25-gauge needle. This cleanses the cervix, stains it, and avoids the disadvantages of rubbing the surface with cotton.

Cervical biopsy

Histologic diagnosis of excised tissue is essential for accurate diagnosis of CIN, invasive cancer, and endometriosis of the cervix. When a lesion has gross characteristics of neoplasia (including all endocervical polyps), biopsy is essential. Most biopsies are performed as a result of abnormal cytology. The extent of biopsy may be a very small area obtained with a special small biopsy forceps, or it may be a conization specimen that includes the transitional zone and adjacent squamous epithelium of the cervix as well as adequate endocervical tissue.

When the entire transitional zone can be adequately inspected with the colposcope, biopsy is directed to the areas of change. In such cases, with adequate visualization and properly directed biopsies, the accuracy of diagnosis is excellent and conization for diagnosis can be avoided. When visualization of the transitional zone is incomplete, endocervical curettage is indicated. However, material obtained on endocervical curettage, which is a blind procedure, may miss the area of neoplasia. When moderate dysplasia, carcinoma in situ, or invasive cancer is suspected because of cytologic findings and the transitional zone cannot be completely seen, diagnostic conization should be performed.

When visualization is incomplete and dysplasia or carcinoma in situ has been diagnosed by biopsy, outpatient therapy should not be instituted, since the extent of neoplasia has not been accurately determined.

Despite negative cytologic reports, bloody mucoid endocervical drainage, irregular spotty bleeding, and mucopurulent material from the endocervix that have not responded to therapy are an indication for endocervical curettage and possible diagnostic conization.

The extent of diagnostic conization should be determined by iodine stain of the cervix, knowledge of the colposcopic findings (mapping), and the degree of distortion of the cervix. The importance of recognizing the extent of conization needed is examplified by studies showing that up to 30% of specimens removed at hysterectomy after conization contained residual neoplastic tissue. Other studies, however, have shown that residual neoplastic tissue is rarely found after conization.

Endometrial biopsy

Invasion of the uterine cavity with a sound or an endometrial biopsy instrument should be done so as to avoid perforation and spread of infection. The internal os is dilated, and the biopsy instrument is introduced to the top of the uterus and withdrawn while scraping the endometrial surface. Suction should be used during scraping to remove more tissue. The specimen is then placed in 10% formalin and sent to the laboratory. For determining ovulation this procedure is done in the late premenstrual phase or on the first day of menstruation. It is recommended for patients in whom endometrial carcinoma is suspected, for evaluation of functional bleeding problems and infertility, and when tuberculosis of the endometrium is suspected. When a complete search of the endometrial cavity is desired, curettage under anesthesia is necessary. Similarly endometrial biopsy is usually not successful for the removal of endometrial polyps and the retained products of pregnancy.

Various methods have been employed for obtaining material from the endometrial cavity for cytologic study. These methods have included brushes that are introduced and equipment for lavage of the cavity. The Gravlee jet washer properly used affords material that, when properly examined, reveals adenocarcinoma of the endometrium as often as endometrial biopsy. Although these methods can obtain cells and fragments of tissue, more information can be obtained by endometrial biopsy.

Hysteroscopy

The contact hysteroscope (Hysteroser), designed by Institut d'Optitue de le Paris, has recently become available for improved inspection of the endometrial cavity. The optical glass stem surrounded by metal allows for the transport of light and permits a magnifying optical system. This instrument uses the ambient light of the examining room, which is collected and concentrated in a special sleeve. Only the area in contact can be visualized; however, any blood is pressed away so that blood in the cavity offers no problem. Similarly, since distention of the cavity is not required, there is no danger of intravascular or transtubal excape of liquids or gases that have been used for panoramic hysteroscopy. Attemtps at visualization in the endometrial cavity have allowed improved diagnoses of submucous myomas, endometrial cancer, endometrial polyps, endometrial hyperplasia, uterine septa, and uterine synechiae. Use of the contact scope will allow visualization of all or part of an intrauterine device (IUD) within the cavity as well as residual portions of hydatidiform moles. This instrument has been used as an amnioscope during pregnancy.

Cervical mucus arborization (fern) test

In 1945 Papanicolaou discovered that cervical mucus, when spread on a slice and rapidly dried by heating, crystallizes with "arborization," giving a fern or palm leaf–like reaction. Abou-Shabanah and Plotz proved that this fern reaction depends solely on electrolyte concentration. The presence of the fern pattern occurs from the seventh to the twenty-second day of the cycle because of the secretion of estrogen. After ovulation the fern pattern disappears, as a result of the action of progesterone (Fig. 2-17). Roland recommended that this test be used for determining estrogen activity, ovulation, and the early diagnosis of pregnancy.

In utilizing the ferning phenomenon as a diagnosis for pregnancy it should be emphasized that some ferning will be noted in the mucus during early pregnancy. Consequently the test indicates that pregnancy could not be present only when the ferning is marked and the mucus is acellular. The test is particularly useful during the climacteric, when it can readily exclude the presence of pregnancy, which would be very distressful to the patient.

Culdocentesis (cul-de-sac puncture)

Culdocentesis as a diagnostic procedure has proved to be of great value in the recognition of hemoperitoneum or of the purulence of pelvic peritonitis. It has been found especially valuable in proving the presence of hemoperitoneum in cases of suspected ectopic pregnancy. A discussion of the technique will be given in Chapter 13. The conditions in which blood may be aspirated from the cul-de-sac are corpus hemorrhagicum, ectopic pregnancy, and bleeding from an ovarian tumor or other abdominal organ, such as massive bleeding from a ruptured ulcer, spleen, or liver. Small amounts of blood may be found with incomplete abortion because of retrograde tubal flow. Aspiration of purulent fluid usually indicates peritonilis or a pelvic abscess, and stained smears will frequently point to the organisms involved. Final identification is made by culture. If fluid from an adherent ovarian cyst is aspirated, cytologic study of the cells present will aid in the identification of its type

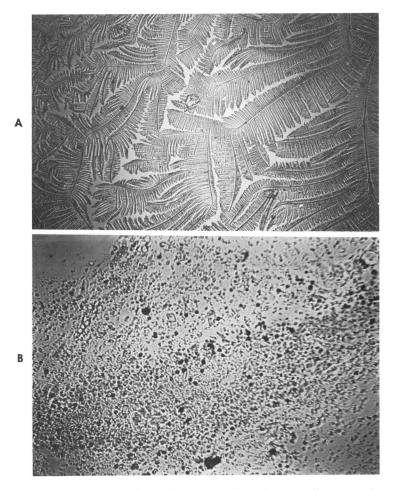

Fig. 2-17. A, Typical arborization of cervical mucus at midcycle in a normally menstruating patient. **B,** Cervical mucus showing effect of progesterone. Note absence of "ferning."

Courtesy Dr. J.C. Ullery, Ohio State University School of Medicine, Columbus, Ohio.

and may show whether or not it is malignant. Fluid from the cul-de-sac may contain malignant cells cast off from malignant growths of abdominal organs.

Culdocentesis can be performed with minimal pain after infiltration of the vaginal wall with a local anesthetic. Analgesics may be given intramuscularly or intravenously if desired. Complications are rarely encountered, and aspiration of the bowel in the absence of intestinal obstruction causes no sequelae in the work mentioned (Fig. 13-5).

In our experience, when hemoperitoneum was present, aspiration of blood was recorded in 95% of the cases. When checked by laparotomy, bloody fluid caused by needling has rarely been misinterpreted as indicating hemoperitoneum.

Pregnancy tests

When the diagnosis of pregnancy is entertained, examination of the cervical mucus may be done to aid in establishing the absence of pregnancy by finding clear acellular mucus, which is productive of typical ferning. These findings indicate estrogen stimulation without progesterone stimulation.

The most accurate means of determining the presence of a normal pregnancy is to observe the patient for the expected increase in the size of the uterus, which can be determined by examinations every 2 to 4 weeks. The fetal circulation will give ultrasound changes with Doppler equipment at 11 to 12 weeks. Real-time ultrasound may be utilized to determine fetal movement at 6 weeks. When urgency indicates early diagnosis, assays of chorionic gonadotropin are used.

Formerly bioassays were done using the effect of chorionic gonadotropins on the reproductive organs of laboratory animals. More rapid, sensitive, and reliable assays can now be determined with immunologic tests for pregnancy. Antiserums for HCG are produced in an animal. Urine to be tested is mixed with the antiserum. If chorionic gonadotropin is present it combines with the antiserum. The neutralized serums then will not cause clumping and precipitation of latex particles coated with HCG. Red blood cells are used instead of latex particles for hemagglutination-type tests.

Like all glycoprotein hormones (LH, FSH, TSH) HCG is composed of an α-subunit and a β-subunit. With minor modifications the α-subunit is common to all glycoprotein hormones, and the β-subunit confers unique specificity to the hormone. Although neither of these subunits is active alone and only the intact molecule exerts hormonal effect, subunits can be separated and used to produce antibodies. These specific antibodies then allow more specific immunoassay and particularly allow for the elimination of LH, which otherwise would participate in the assay of HCG. β-Subunit antiserums are now available for slide and test tube tests as well as for radioimmunoassays.

Pregnancy tests should be considered as qualitative tests for the presence of certain levels of HCG. Quantitative radioimmunoassays can be performed and are essential for the proper management of trophoblastic neoplasms. Pregnancy tests should not be used in an effort to follow cases of hydatidiform mole, much less patients being treated for trophoblastic neoplasms. Table 2-2 indicates the varying sensitivity of pregnancy tests and allows one to select the more sensitive pregnancy tests for the earlier pregnancies. Since the majority of tubal pregnancies do not

Table 2-2	SELECTION OF PREGNANCY TEST			
	Amenorrhea days	Specimen	Type test*	Sensitivity I.U. HCG/ml
	None	Serum	RI-βHCG	.015-.030
	7	Serum	RRA-HCG	.2
		Urine	βHCG tube	.2-.25
	7-14	Urine	βHCG slide	.5-1.0
	14	Urine	βHCG slide	1.0-2.0

RI, radioimmune; *RRA*, radioreceptor assay. For a suspected tubal pregnancy use *RRA*-HCG or *RI*-βHCG on serum or βHCG tube test on urine. Slide tests require less than 5 minutes, tube tests require 60 to 90 minutes, and radioimmune and radioreceptor tests require 12 or more hours for reports by large laboratories.

produce normal amounts of chorionic gonadotropin, it is essential that the more sensitive pregnancy tests be utilized in the management of eccyesis.

It is important to realize that chorionic gonadotropins are not rapidly cleared from the blood and can be found in the urine for several days. Studies done on patients having first trimester terminations by aspiration and curettage have shown that the slide test for pregnancy remains positive for 5 to 6 days. The tube pregnancy test remains positive for 6 to 8 days, and radioreceptor assays remain positive for 10 to 15 days. It then becomes evident if one is seeking to determine the completeness of abortion that some time must elapse before the test is performed. Similarly, use of chorionic gonadotropin assay as a pregnancy test is of little or no value in determining the inevitability of spontaneous abortion. In such considerations one must realize that the syncytiotrophoblast can continue hormonal production without significant fetal development.

Endocrine investigations

The clinical suspicion of major endocrine disturbances is usually not difficult. Minor changes are more likely to be unsuspected. As indicated in the discussion of ovarian endocrine function, the pituitary, adrenal, and thyroid glands influence ovarian function; disturbances in them therefore result in reproductive malfunction. The liver is an important organ for chemical conjugation of steroid compounds and is essential to their proper excretion. Marked hepatic disease over a period of months can result in endocrine changes. The excretion of steroids by way of the kidneys can be decreased by marked renal impairment. Severe malnutrition results in abnormal hormonal balance. From the foregoing statements it is evident that diagnosis of endocrine disturbances must be made with consideration of the function of various organs. The importance of mental function as related to emotional disturbances is particularly appreciated when evaluating hypothalamic-pituitary-ovarian balance and when the effects of stress on adrenal function are well-established.

PITUITARY HORMONE DETERMINATIONS

The hormones of the anterior portion of the pituitary are proteins that do not lend themselves to chemical analysis. Formerly bioassays were used; however, radioimmunoassays now allow less expensive tests on smaller amounts of hormone. When a bioassay is utilized, an aliquot of a 24-hour specimen of urine must be provided. This is then extracted and injected into immature rats or mice. Increased levels of gonadotropin cause an increase in the size of the ovaries and uterus or the prostate gland as compared with control animals. High levels of FSH and LH can be assayed in this manner; however, these tests do not lend themselves to determination of absent or low levels. Total gonadotropin bioassays are considered principally assays of FSH.

The radioimmunoassays can be performed on small amounts of plasma or on aliquots of 24-hour specimens of urine. FSH determinations are specific; LH determinations cross-react with chorionic gonadotropins that exhibit a combination of LH- and FSH-type activities. Isolation of the immunospecific β-subunits of LH and HCG have allowed for elimination of most of the cross reactions that existed with antibodies produced against the combined α- and β-subunits. Because radioimmunoassays of FSH and LH are easily performed and are inexpensive, they can be used more often.

FSH levels are particularly increased with ovarian failure and can be used to aid in the diagnosis of premature menopause. With ovarian dysgenesis the FSH levels are higher in children. When ovaries are removed surgically or destroyed by radiation, it is anticipated that the FSH levels will increase. FSH levels are frequently decreased by the administration of estrogens, particularly those used in oral contraceptives. Similarly there is often a decrease in FSH levels with larger doses of drugs that affect catecholamines, such as the tranquilizers and antidepressants. When excess estrogens or androgens are secreted by tumors of the ovary or adrenal gland, a decrease in FSH is anticipated. Pituitary function is decreased with marked malnutrition, as occurs with anorexia nervosa, and also when the adenohypophysis is injured by shock (Sheehan's syndrome) or when there are pituitary tumors or cysts or tumors adjacent to the pituitary gland. Pituitary tumors rarely excrete increased amounts of FSH and LH; however, they do secrete increased amounts of prolactin, growth hormone, or adrenocorticotropic hormone (ACTH) on occasion. When a pituitary tumor is suspected, determinations of the levels of these hormones may be of value. (The determination of ACTH is not yet feasible as a radioimmunoassay; thus the ACTH must be determined indirectly.)

When FSH and LH are at low levels and the ovaries should be producing estrogens but there is no evidence that they are, pituitary failure must be suspected and tumors of the pituitary or the adjacent area sought. In instances when the FSH and LH are low the responsiveness of the ovary can be determined by the administration of menopausal gonadotropins. With chronic anovulation associated with the polycystic ovary syndrome LH levels remain higher than FSH levels and the LH surge required for ovulation is not seen.

In patients with galactorrhea syndromes the determination of prolactin is important. Increased prolactin may be found without galactorrhea in some patients during lack of ovulation. It has been recognized that high prolactin levels are associated with decreased LH and FSH levels and particularly with the absence of the LH surge, which is essential for ovulation. With treatment to lower the prolactin levels there is an increase in gonadotropins and ovulation may occur.

GnRF from the hypothalamus has been sensitized and its use has allowed research investigation of certain patients to determine whether failure in FSH and LH production is predominantly hypothalamic or pituitary. Similarly in certain laboratories radioimmunoassays for the levels of hypothalamic-releasing factor are now available and aid in study of certain hormone disturbances.

Roentgenograms of the sella turcica may reveal the erosion of expanding neoplasms. Recognition of small adenomas requires polytomography. Changes in the visual fields may occur because of pressure on the optic nerves. Pneumoencephalography is required for diagnosis of the empty sella syndrome.

The changes in general caused by hyperpituitarism are indicated in the discussion of amenorrhea (see Chapter 14).

ESTROGEN AND PROGESTOGEN DETERMINATIONS

The total 24-hour output of estrogen in urine can be measured along with the free fractions of estrogens, estrone, estradiol, and estriol in urine. It should be remembered that estrogen levels vary during the menstrual cycle and are low in postmenopausal women (usually less than 10 μg per 24 hours). During pregnancy large amounts of estrogen are produced and urinary estrogen may rise to 45 mg per 24 hours. Estriol is the estrogen produced in greatest quantity by the placenta and during pregnancy is measured as an indicator of fetal welfare. The rise in urinary estrogens after the administration of human menopausal gonadotropins is the best indicator of the ovarian response to administration of this source of FSH and LH.

Determination of picograms per milliliter of estrogen (usually Estradiol-17 β) in serum is made by competitive binding radioimmune assay. This serum assay may be used to determine ovarian response to stimulation.

In clinical gynecologic practice the changes in cervical mucus and vaginal cells are commonly used as estimates of estrogen production. Withdrawal bleeding after progestogen administration indicates that endometrial proliferation induced by estrogens has occurred.

Progesterone is excreted in the urine as pregnanediol. Plasma progesterone assay is replacing pregnanediol assay in evaluating clinical conditions. Progestogen determinations are limited in clinical value because progestogen influence can be determined by a change in basal temperature and biopsy of the endometrium. In the few patients who have deficient corpus luteum function these tests are of particular value.

THYROID FUNCTION TESTS

In general, hypothyroidism is associated with amenorrhea, anovulatory cycles, and excessive or prolonged uterine bleeding, whereas hyperthyroidism is associated with a decrease in the amount and duration of the menstrual flow. At times hyperthyroidism causes anovulation and amenorrhea to occur. Although reproductive dysfunction is more apt to occur with marked degrees of disturbance in thyroid function, which are readily suspected by clinical observation, lesser degrees of disturbance may cause irregularities in ovarian function.

The two active compounds produced by the thyroid gland are T_4 and T_3. Of these two substances T_4 is produced in much greater amounts. These two substances are bound to thyroxin-binding proteins that act as carriers. To be effective at the cellular level on all tissues, as well as in the feedback mechanism on the hypothalamus and the pituitary, T_4 and/or T_3 must be in a free state. Since thyroxin exists in a reversible equilibrium between the free and protein-bound states, estimations of free thyroxin must take into consideration the total amount of thyroxin, i.e., free and bound, as well as the amount of thyroxin-binding proteins. Although tests are available to give a direct reading of free thyroxin, they are subject to considerable technical error and are expensive. Currently T_4 and tests indicative of thyroxin-binding protein are used in combination to estimate free thyroxin.

Since intrinsic estrogens such as those present during pregnancy and extrinsic estrogens such as those used in oral contraceptives or those used during the climacteric will increase the amount of thyroxin-binding protein, it is particularly important that free thyroxin be estimated when estrogen levels are known to be high.

The protein-bound iodine (PBI) test was the first blood serum test to be utilized, and it continues to be of value in screening patients. It is particularly sensitive to increased amounts of thyroxin-binding protein and has the disadvantage of being susceptible to interference when iodine compounds have been used for diagnostic tests. The accuracy of the test is lost for as long as 6 months after the administration of iodine-containing, aqueous contrast media such as those used for hysterograms, urograms, cholangiograms, and arteriograms. Oil-based media containing iodine may cause false high readings for years. If inorganic iron is ingested or applied to the skin, discontinuation should result in its excretion in 2 or 3 days. Iodized salt does not cause significant elevations.

The T_4 tests are based on the specific binding properties of thyroxin-binding globulin. Exogenous organic iodine contaminants do not interfere with these determinations. A radioimmunoassay for T_4 is available as a direct method of estimation. The most commonly used method is the competitive protein-binding method. This technique involves the interaction of the patient's T_4 (extracted from serum with ethanol) with a reagent containing human thyroxin-binding globulin saturated with radioactive T_4. The radioactive T_4 is displaced from the reagent in an amount proportional to that in the patient's serum. It can be separated from the bound T_4 through use of a Sephadex column or resin. With appropriate radioassay of the separated fraction the value can be compared to a standard curve that permits direct expression of the thyroxin level in the patient's serum. With an increase in the patient's thyroxin-binding protein the value will be higher. Since this test involves radioactive measurements, when the patient has been given a radioactive material, sufficient time should elapse before employing this test; otherwise abnormal high readings will occur.

T_3 can be determined directly by radioimmunoassay. This test is not commonly needed. It is important only in special hyperthyroid states.

The T_3 uptake test is a very important test that gives an index of the unsaturated thyroxin-binding protein in the serum. Since ordinarily the patient's T_3 level is very low, it is not involved in this test. The principal substances involved in the test are radioactive T_3, the patient's thyroxin-binding protein (both the part that is saturated with the patient's T_4 and the part that is unsaturated), and a special resin reagent. When these substances are placed together an equilibrium results. The resin is separated, and the radioactivity of the T_3 bound to the resin is determined. If the patient has an increased amount of unsaturated thyroxin-binding protein, it binds with the radioactive T_3 and causes less to remain bound to the resin, so that the value will be lower. If the unsaturated portion of the thyroxin-binding protein is less, less radioactive T_3 will be bound to the protein, more will remain bound to the resin, and the value will be higher. The amount of radioactivity determined in the separated resin is then inversely proportional to the amount of unsaturated thyroxin-binding protein. If the thyroid produces more thyroxin, then more of the binding protein is saturated, so that the radioactive activity of the resin is higher and the reading is higher. This explains why in hyperthyroidism the T_4 results and T_3 uptake readings are both increased. When the thyroxin-binding protein is increased by high estrogen levels, the T_4 results are higher and the T_3 uptake reading is lower. It then becomes evident that when these two tests are considered together they will give a reliable index of the free thyroxin in the serum. To reiterate, it is evident that during pregnancy and with the administration of extrinsic estrogens these two tests should be done simultaneously. Otherwise an increased T_4 might erroneously lead to the suspicion of hyperthyroidism.

The TSH from the pituitary can be determined by radioimmunoassy. It has its principal use in determining whether hypothyroidism is caused by thyroid gland failure or lack of pituitary stimulation. With inadequate production of thyroid hormone the TSH levels of a functional normal pituitary gland will increase. Conversely with excessive amounts of free thyroxin the TSH levels will decrease. The determination of TSH may be of particular value in managing primary amenorrhea and rare cases of precocious puberty.

Determination of iodine 131 uptake by the thyroid gland reflects the ability of the gland to retain iodine but does not determine the rate of formation of the thyroid hormones and is not a substitute for thyroid hormone blood level tests. The iodine 131 uptake is influenced by TSH, T_4, T_3, and the presence of inorganic iodides. It is of particular value in determining the nature of the pathologic states of the thyroid gland and is essential in accurate diagnosis of thyroid diseases, neoplasms, and cysts.

When patients have hypothyroidism and are given thyroid supplements, the clinical response is generally used as the best means of determining whether the replacement dose is adequate. When PBI and T_4 tests are used while thyroid preparations are being administered, it is important to understand the effects of extrinsic thyroid compounds on blood levels as determined by these tests. If the ratio of T_4 and T_3 in the preparations is similar to that which exists in normal individuals, the test results will be indicative of proper replacement therapy. If T_3 is used alone or in a high ratio, since it is more active than T_4, contains less iodine, and has a greater influence on the feedback mechanism, the PBI and T_4 tests will yield low results and should not be used as indications for determining T_3 dosage.

The TRH increases in amount when insufficient amounts of T_4 and T_3 are present to provide a feedback control. High TRH values lead to increased prolactin production; it is thought that correction of hypothyroidism may thus improve hyperprolactemia.

ADRENAL FUNCTION TESTS

The three principal types of adrenal cortical hormones are the androgens, the glucocorticoids (cortisone and hydrocortisone), and the mineralocorticoids (aldosterone). Small amounts of estrogen and progesterone are also produced. When an excess of androgens is suspected, the possibilities of adrenal neoplasm or hyperplasia or of excessive pituitary stimulation are considered. Masculinizing tumors of the ovary may produce androgens. If primary adrenal failure as in Addison's disease is

Table 2-3   **PRECURSORS OF EXCRETED 17-KS**

Urinary metabolite	Principal precursors	Androgenicity of precursor
Androsterone	Androstenedione	+
	Testosterone	+ + +
	Dehydroepiandrosterone	+
	Adrenosterone	+
Etiocholanolone	Androstenedione	+
	17-OH-progesterone	+ or −
	Testosterone	+ + +
	Dehydroepiandrosterone	+
	Compound S	−
11β-OH-androsterone ⎫ 11-ketoandrosterone ⎭	11β-OH-androstenedione	+
	Adrenosterone	+
11β-OH-etiocholanolone ⎫ 11-ketoetiocholanolone ⎭	Cortisone, cortisol	+ or −

suspected, ACTH stimulation will not elevate the low hormone levels. The effect of cortisone administration on adrenal function is discussed later.

The chemical determination of the 17-ketosteroids (17-KS) excreted in the urine as sulfates and gluconates is a principal test to measure androgenic hormones in women. In the normal female practically all the 17-KS that can be determined as urinary metabolites is produced by the adrenal cortex, with just a trace coming from the ovary. Table 2-3 indicates the hormonal precursors of the various 17-KS excreted.

It is evident from Table 2-3 that total urinary 17-KS is derived from precursors of varying androgenicity; the clinical evidence of masculinization may not correlate unless the amounts of the various fractions are determined by column (partition) or paper chromatography.

The normal adult female excretes 6 to 15 mg 17-KS per 24 hours, with considerable variation from day to day. Increased excretion occurs in patients with adrenal hyperplasia, some adrenal tumors (malignant and benign), some arrhenoblastomas or lutein cell tumors of the ovary, severe stress, treatment with ACTH, and treatment with testosterone. Decreased excretion occurs in Addison's disease, panhypopituitarism, myxedema, and nephrosis. When adrenal cortical hyperplasia or carcinoma is suspected, the 17-KS should be determined. Administration of dexamethasone will decrease the 17-KS caused by hyperplasia but will not effect the 17-KS caused by carcinoma. Compared with the α-fractions the β-fractions of 17-KS when increased indicate carcinoma. Some patients with Stein-Leventhal syndrome will have slightly elevated 17-KS. Hirsutism as the only indication of virilization is seldom associated with increased total 17-KS.

At times the diagnosis of adrenal cortical hyperplasia is suspected but the 17-KS are not elevated. The diagnosis then can be made by finding high urinary pregnanetriol levels, which occur only with adrenal hyperplasia. In Cushing's syndrome the 17-OH-corticosteroids, which are urinary cortisone and hydrocortisone, are elevated and can be determined along with the 17-KS in clarifying the diagnosis. The 11-hydroxycorticosteroids can be determined in plasma as an estimation of cortisol (hydroxycortisone) and corticosterone, since hydroxylation at this position occurs only in the adrenal cortex.

Blood cortisol is a very practical test and has become somewhat less expensive. In considering the findings of cortisol estimations, diurnal variation, suppression of levels with dexamethasone given in varying amounts, and the effect of ACTH stimulation are important in determining whether the syndrome is caused by adrenal tumor, ectopic production of ACTH, or excess pituitary production of ACTH. The term "Cushing's disease" is reserved for that variety of Cushing's syndrome that is caused by abnormal pituitary function. Usually no pituitary tumor is found. The characteristic feature of the disease is that ACTH secretion is inappropriately excessive and that there is a relative resistance to glucocorticoid negative feedback, so that it takes a greater than normal plasma cortisol level to suppress ACTH release.

Recently radioimmunoassay techniques have been the most commonly utilized methods for determining testosterone in plasma or serum. Androstenedione and dehydroepiandrosterone can also be determined by radioimmunoassay methods. With clinical evidence of defeminization and marked virilization (recent onset of clitoromegaly, marked hirsutism, etc.), high levels of testosterone are expected and a search for ovarian and adrenal tumors is indicated. When the polycystic ovary syndrome is studied or when minor degrees of adrenal hyperfunction are suspected, the determination of the more mildly androgenic substances, androstenedione and dehydroepiandrosterone, along with the evaluation of levels after stimulation or suppression of the ovary and adrenal gland, may afford a better understanding of the hormonal abnormality and perhaps allow a more rational therapeutic plan.

Chromatin examinations
SEX CHROMATIN BODIES

Buccal or vaginal smears stained by Papanicolaou's method can be searched for chromocenters, which have been described by Barr as sex chromatin masses located at the periphery of the nucleus. These masses are apparently the inactive X chromosomes. Genetic females have 50% to 85% of cell nuclei containing chromocenters. Genetic males have less than 15% of nuclei with chromocenters. Cells can be stained with quinacrine and examined in ultraviolet light to allow demonstration of the fluorescent Y chromosomes, the F bodies of male cells.

CHROMOSOMAL COUNTS

In recent years technical improvements have allowed culture of human cells with addition of colchicine to arrest mitosis in the metaphase. "Squashed," stained cell preparations then allow individual identification of chromosomes. When photomicrographs are cut to remove images of individual chromosomes, they can be arranged in proper order for the autosomes and sex chromosomes. This array is an ideogram, a display of the karyotype. Normal females have 22 pairs of autosomes and 1 pair of sex chromosomes (XX). The XX pair is associated with sex chromatin bodies. The normal male has 22 pairs of autosomes and 1 X and 1 Y sex chromosome, and few or no chromocenters are associated.

For specific recognition and pairing of chromosomes, staining to display bands in chromosomes is essential. The demonstration of G-bands by Giemsa staining is most commonly used. The Q-bands are elicited by staining with quinacrine and are helpful in identification of Y chromosomes and autosomes 21 and 22. Banding techniques allow more precise recognition of translocations, inversions, and deletions. Knowledge of such changes is necessary for counseling, prognosis, and specific diagnosis. Recent studies have indicated that cytogenic studies of couples reveal chromosomal abnormalities in about 10% when habitual abortion has occurred. About 5% of infertile men have chromosomal anomalies.

Abnormal ideograms are presently explained by nondisjunction and translocation of chromosomes during meiosis or early mitosis. Patients with ovarian dysplasia (Turner's syndrome) typically have 45 chromosomes (XO) and usually are chromatin body–negative or genetic males. Testicular dysgenesis (Klinefelter's syndrome) is associated with 47 chromosomes (44 autosomes and XXY sex chromosomes) in chromatin body–positive or genetic females. Mongolism (Down's syndrome) is associated with 47 chromosomes with an extra autosome (trisomy). The chromatin findings given in this brief discussion are those most commonly found with the respective clinical abnormalities. Variations are found at times among patients with similar anomalies and in cells of the same patient. When the ideograms from a single patient vary, the pattern is termed "mosaic." Nuclei of malignant cells usually reveal chromosomes of bizarre shapes and numbers.

Since each chromosome contains genetic material controlling the development of many individual characteristics, changes in chromosomes associated with anomalies are found in patients with multiple morphologic changes such as Down's or

Turner's syndrome. In many genetic cnnditions such as congenital adrenal hyperplasia the karyotypes are normal and the abnormality may be caused by genetic material controlling the development of one or more important enzymes.

Chromatin examinations now afford a means of yielding additional information in the diagnosis of genital anomalies and mongolism. The genital anomalies of genetic origin usually preclude childbearing, and the probability of their occurrence in future siblings cannot be predicted by present-day chromatin study of parents of the afflicted person.

Tubal tests

Tubal insufflation by introduction of carbon dioxide in measured amount and measured pressure is performed to determine tubal patency. If one or both tubes are open, the gas passes through into the peritoneal cavity. The pressure rises to a height of about 120 mm Hg, and then as it passes into the peritoneal cavity the pressure drops rapidly to around 40 mm Hg. If both tubes are closed, the passage of gas is blocked. One negative test does not necessarily mean that the tubes are permanently closed since tubal spasm may sometimes resist passage of the gas even at 200 mm Hg. Consequently, if the tubes seem closed, a subsequent test is advisable.

This test is a step in the systematic examination in cases of sterility that do not yield to minor measures. It is also occasionally a therapeutic aid in opening closed tubes.

Careful technique is required to avoid erroneous interpretation. With occlusion the site is not determined and with patency the extent of tubal distortion and adhesion is not known. However, the limited equipment required, the ease of performance, the safety, the low cost to the patient, and the percentage of pregnancy occuring after performance lead to continued employment of this test.

Laparoscopy allows the visualization of colored aqueous solutions passing through and from the tubes for a more complete assessment of tubal patency and normalcy.

Hysterosalpingography is discussed under x-ray examinations.

X-ray examinations

X-ray examination has proved very valuable in the diagnosis of certain conditions in the genital tract and also in the differential diagnosis of certain conditions of adjacent organs.

The *plain film* (KUB) may reveal the following:
1. A pelvic mass (normal as the pregnant uterus or the full bladder; abnormal as a myoma or adnexal tumor)

2. Calcifications (for example myomas that have undergone calcification; bones of the fetal skeleton noted at 12 to 16 weeks' gestation; or teeth seen in a dermoid cyst along with the radiolucence of the sebaceous material)
3. Renal, ureteral, or vesical calculi
4. Erosive areas of pelvic or vertebral bones, indicating metastatic cancer

The *pyelogram* (usually intravenous) allows recognition of the following:

1. Ureteral displacement by pelvic tumors or evidence of ureteral obstruction by large pelvic masses or infiltrating cancer (most commonly cervical)
2. Anomalies that are more commonly found if genital anomalies are present

The *barium enema study* is of interest in determining whether diverticula or sigmoid cancer is present to account for the pelvic changes. Endometriosis or genital cancer may infiltrate the sigmoid to cause distortion or partial obstruction. The colon may be displaced by pelvic masses.

With *hysterosalpingography* the tubal lumina and uterine cavity can be visualized after injection of radiopaque iodized aqueous or oily solutions. Congenital malformations of the uterus or distortion by uterine myomas or polyps can be noted. The site of obstruction or change in tubal contours can be determined if present. With proper technique the incompetent internal os of the cervix can be demonstrated.

Gynecography by pelvic pneumoperitoneum is infrequently used to outline the uterus, ovaries, and abnormal pelvic masses when palpation is inadequate.

Lymphography, arteriography, and *venography* are further diagnostic aids. The lymph vessels and glands of the inguinal, femoral, iliac, and aortic areas can be demonstrated by injection of an oil medium such as Eithiodol into a lymphatic of each ankle. This procedure may indicate the likelihood of metastatic tumors in lymph glands. Arteriography by retrograde catheterization of the aorta through the femoral artery allows visualization of the uterine blood supply and the intervillous spaces of the placenta. Pelvic phlebograms can be obtained by infiltration of an aqueous contrast medium into the corpus of the uterus. The iliac veins and inferior vena cava can be visualized by the rapid injection of the medium into the common iliac veins. Although the value of these specialized procedures is limited, their use in recognizing the areas of lymph node metastasis preoperatively may be justified in selected cases. Large pelvic tumors or abdominal pregnancies may at times be better detailed by arteriography.

Ultrasonography

Sound waves of supra-audible frequency in a continuous form can be used to measure fetal heart rate and blood flow because of the Doppler principle. Equipment presently available allows for recognition of the fetal pulse at 11 or 12 weeks.

Employment of this principle also allows for blood flow studies, which may be important in recognition and management of thromboses and thrombophlebitis of the lower extremities associated with gynecologic problems.

When the pulse-echo sonar range–finding technique is employed, one can delineate structures of varying densities. Equipment allowing for a gray-scale visualization improves the ability to discern borders of masses and to attempt to delineate intramass structure. Real time equipment allows for the observation of motion. Sonography has been a great aid in obstetrics and is ideal for the diagnosis of hydatidiform mole and placental localization and the determination of fetal head size as a growth measurement. Multiple gestation is easily recognized, and anomalies and external genitalia may be recognized during advanced pregnancy.

The employment of ultrasound in gynecology is of limited value, since the majority of uterine and adnexal masses can be palpated. In some patients who are obese, in pain, or have intestinal distention, delineation of the pregnant uterus, myoma, ovarian cyst or tumor, or pelvic abcess may be done. Essentially a mass is identified. On occasion one may get good evidence as to whether a mass is solid or cystic. IUDs can be localized accurately. The pregnancy ring can be seen after 5 or 6 weeks' gestation to diagnose early pregnancy in the uterus. (Pregnancy rings are seldom seen in tubal pregnancies.)

Sonographic visualization does not provide complete and sharp borders of many pelvic masses. Fluid and feces in bowel may cause confusion. Gases within intervening bowel prevent adequate transmission of sound waves. These factors limit the information obtained. To properly interpret sonograms all diagnostic findings (historical, physical, and laboratory) must be known. Sonographic written reports should be objectively descriptive, and diagnoses should be included only when adequate criteria are met.

To use real time equipment for gynecologic diagnosis, the transducer is held on the abdomen with one hand and the other hand is used vaginally to manipulate the uterus and pelvic structures. This maneuver can at times provide more accurate determinations.

Pelvic examination under anesthesia

The advantage of anesthesia is that it eliminates *pain* and *muscular tension,* the two factors that make the ordinary pelvic examination of certain patients incomplete and unsatisfactory.

PREPARATIONS

In preparation for this examination the patient's rectum should be cleansed with an enema an hour or two before the examination. The same preparatory examination of the heart, lungs, and urine should be made as though anesthesia were for an operation. Catheter evacuation of the bladder should be done. Have ready a light, strong tenaculum forceps, so that the cervix may be caught and the uterus pulled down as desired. If the interior of the uterus is to be explored, the antiseptic preparation for curettage must be carried out and the instruments prepared.

EXAMINATION METHODS

The various manipulations employed in examination under anesthesia are as follows:

1. Bimanual palpation of pelvic interior
   a. Vaginoabdominal palpation
   b. Rectoabdominal palpation
   c. Rectovaginoabdominal palpation
   d. Rectovesical palpation
2. Uterine investigation
   a. Curettage
   b. Exploration of interior of uterus by digital examination in postpartum cases
   c. Conization or biopsy of cervix for examination

All specimens obtained should be preserved in 10% formalin for microscopic examination.

Intra-abdominal inspection

When the usual pelvic examination fails to furnish sufficient information for diagnosis in a difficult case, intra-abdominal inspection is sometimes indicated. Such inspection may be accomplished by culdoscopy or peritoneoscopy through a puncture in the abdominal wall or by an incision, either in the cul-de-sac or in the abdominal wall, large enough to permit adequate inspection.

CULDOSCOPY

Ruddock developed an instrument for peritoneoscopy that Decker later adapted for use in culdoscopy. Doyle developed an instrument that he calls a pelviscope, which is also used for visualization of the pelvic organs through a culdotomy opening.

Decker uses local anesthesia for the procedure. Josey and associates state that the procedure was valuable in the diagnosis of ectopic pregnancy in which other methods were inconclusive. In addition it was found to be useful in some cases of endometriosis, pelvic masses of uncertain origin, pelvic tuberculosis, sterility, and certain endocrine disorders. In most of their cases intravenous thiopental (Pentothal) sodium was used as the anesthetic, and they stress the importance of using a tracheal catheter in all patients having a general anesthetic. For technique, to-

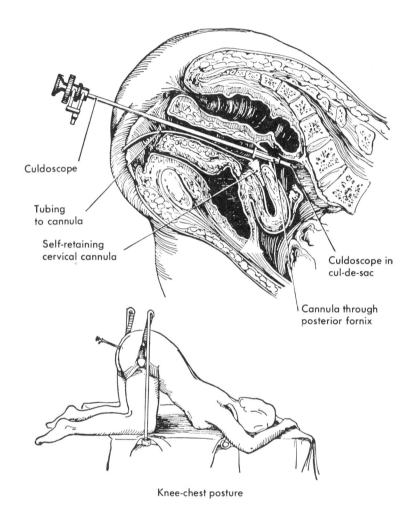

Culdoscope

Tubing to cannula

Self-retaining cervical cannula

Culdoscope in cul-de-sac

Cannula through posterior fornix

Knee-chest posture

Fig. 2-18. Culdoscope is shown in the cul-de-sac, and the screw-tip cervical cannula is in the cervical canal. The lower figure illustrates a method to maintain the knee-chest posture.

From Decker, A., and Cherry, T.H.: Am. J. Surg. **64**:40, 1944.

gether with indications and dangers, the reader is referred to the original article. Failure by experts to successfully introduce the culdoscope in 5% of the cases reduces enthusiasm for use of this method for the limited number of patients in whom an adequate diagnosis cannot be made by other methods.

LAPAROSCOPY

Modern laparoscopes utilizing fiberoptic illumination allow excellent visualization of the pelvic viscera. Instillation of measured amount of carbon dioxide under controlled pressures creates a space within the peritoneal cavity so that instruments can be introduced. Introduction is done through the umbilicus where the peritoneum is usually adherent. The principal uses of laparoscopy have been (1) for tubal sterilization by fulguration, ligation with a small band, or obstruction with a small clip and (2) inspection of the adnexa when there is a question about the cause of infertility and when the possibility of laparotomy is being considered. Adhesions of the bowel and the omentum to the anterior abdominal wall interfere with visualization of the pelvis, and perforation of the bowel is a likely complication under such circumstances. Preperitoneal fatty tissues may interfere with the introduction of the instrument and with proper pelvic visualization. Pelvic adhesions limit movement of the uterus and adnexa and may prevent adequate visualization. In properly selected patients under ideal conditions the rate of complication is very low, and the majority of patients can have the procedure performed and leave the facility after they have recovered from the general anesthesia.

EXPLORATORY LAPAROTOMY

When culdoscopy or peritoneoscopy is indecisive, abdominal incision is usually indicated, and with large masses that need removal anyway it should supplant the other procedures. Abdominal incision permits thorough inspection of different sides of a growth. In addition it allows palpation of the lesion, lysis of adhesions, detailed exploration to determine definitely whether it is removable, and removal if such is found feasible. When finished the surgeon knows definitely the character of the mass and whether it was removable, and, if so, whether it has been removed. If not removed, the family knows beyond a doubt that it is irremovable and that no further operative work is advisable. The decisive factor in choosing between culdoscopy or peritoneoscopy and regular incision is not simply how much can be seen through a tube in a puncture wound but which procedure will be most beneficial to the patient when everything is considered.

Urinary tract investigation

The close association of the urinary tract with the genital tract may cause misinterpretation of symptoms, the symptoms of one being attributed to the other. For example, the common complaint of pressure or fullness about the vagina or uterus is often due to a mild cystitis, urethritis, or trigonitis. This fact must be kept in mind, particularly in those cases where the patient insists that there is real discomfort in this region even though examination shows no genital lesion to account for it.

Inquiry as to urinary function will often reveal some symptom indicating that the location of the trouble is in the urinary tract. Symptoms such as urgency, frequency, pain after urination, or occasional leakage on coughing or sudden exertion would indicate trouble in the bladder or urethra.

Pelvic pains supposedly from the genital tract are occasionally caused by ureteral stricture or stone. Sears has emphasized the frequent association of intractable dysmenorrhea with ureteral stricture. A stone in the lower third of the ureter may cause a tender area simulating parametritis or salpingo-oophoritis.

When upper urinary tract involvement is suspected, intravenous pyelograms (especially of infusion type) may reveal the lesion, or it may be necessary to obtain retrograde pyelograms after ureteral catheterization. A cystogram helps in the diagnosis of stone, foreign body, or diverticulum. Urethral diverticula are diagnosed by noting a discharge of urine or pus from the meatus, after the bladder has been emptied and when pressure is made along the urethra with the examining finger. Exact location of the pocket is made by use of a probe, urethroscopy, or urethrography. Cystoscopy is essential to diagnosis of bladder neoplasms, location of fistula, identification of diverticula, recognition of neurogenic distortion, and description of bladder injury. Measurement of bladder capacity and intravesical and intraurethral pressures are required to recognize dysfunction mechanisms.

Premarital examination

The premarital examinations required by law are primarily to exclude syphilis and gonorrhea. The exact requirements vary somewhat in different states. Detailed information and the forms to be filled out may be obtained from the state health department.

In addition to the designated legal requirements the patient wishes to know, of course, if there is anything that would interfere with marital life. In such a conference one practical point is to avoid disturbing the patient's happy mood by attaching undue importance to certain findings—such as uterine retroplacement without symptoms, erosion of cervix, small fibroid, cystic ovary, or other local variation from the usual that may not cause trouble. It is usually best to tell the patient that there is a slight variation from the usual findings, which may need observation or possible local treatment later, but to assure her that it will in no way interfere with successful marriage or childbearing. If the hymenal opening is so small as to preclude coitus except with severe trauma, it is advisable to enlarge the opening. This can normally be accomplished by having the patient use graduated dilators, but if the hymen is very thick, incision after anesthesia is preferable.

The premarital conference is now recognized as an important means of aiding the young couple toward a successful married life by helping them avoid the marital tragedies that often have their origins in small misunderstandings, lack of knowledge, or initial physical or psychic trauma. We advocate aptitude tests for our young people to determine their fitness for various occupations, and yet we have been slow to recognize the importance of a similar examination for the most vital occupations in life—marriage and parenthood. The need for it has been forcibly impressed upon us by the end results of its omission—marital maladjustment, frustration, divorce, and psychosomatic problems. Formerly many of our young people came to marriage handicapped by all sorts of taboos, inhibitions, fears, and anxieties, but in recent years many of our high schools and colleges have offered courses on preparation for marriage. Numerous books dealing with marriage are on the market, so that general information on the subject is available.

The physician should be prepared to give wise premarital counsel that will help the couple to start their marriage with a sense of security that they would not otherwise have. This confidential contact with the young couple will usually make them feel free to return promptly for intelligent advice if new problems or conflicts arise, rather than to delay until irreparable damage has occurred.

Contraceptive advice should be routinely offered. Time to allow for marital adjustments, completion of education, and accumulation of home furnishings and financial resources before pregnancy is desired by many couples. The knowledge gained can be used for child spacing during future family planning. The matter of contraception is presented in a separate chapter in this book.

During premarital examination abnormalities may be found that deserve correction before pregnancy. On the other hand, if evidence of minimal endometriosis is found, pregnancy should not be deferred for more than a few months, since conception may become more difficult after a considerable period of contraception. Similarly a patient with small myomas might be encouraged to conceive as soon as practical.

Pediatric or adolescent examination

In certain cases it becomes necessary to examine an infant or an older child as in the case of persistent discharge, foreign body, or developmental abnormality. Examination of wet smears and stained smears and cultures may be needed. Examination with a sound in the vagina and the finger in the rectum will reveal a metallic foreign body. Rectoabdominal palpation will often allow palpation of ovarian tumors, of which benign teratomas comprise about one half. Less common are malignant teratomas and granulosa cell tumors. In searching for the origin of persistent discharge or a soft foreign body the use of a small vaginoscope is indicated. General anesthesia may be necessary for adequate inspection of the vagina and avoidance of psychic trauma.

PELVIC PAIN

Pain is a difficult complaint to evaluate because of its subjective nature. For instance, pelvic pain may be caused by trouble in the pelvis, back, or other organs, may be referred pain, or may be caused by psychosomatic problems.

Pain in the back is a prominent symptom in many pelvic diseases and in numerous extrapelvic diseases. Its diagnostic significance depends on its location, i.e., on the structure involved. Consequently a careful localization of the backache should be made in each case, exactly as pain or tenderness in the abdomen is accurately located. If the backache is a prominent symptom or of doubtful origin, the patient is directed to sit up, the back is bared and inspected, and the different areas of the lumbar and sacral regions are palpated systematically. The area in which the patient had noticed aching and also any area in which there is tenderness should be located accurately.

DIFFERENTIAL DIAGNOSIS

The ultimate purpose of an accurate history and a careful examination is to establish a diagnosis. All too frequently authors spend a great deal of time on the methods of acquiring the necessary facts and then completely neglect to explain the method by which these facts should be utilized in the important process of making a diagnosis. Eventually through years of experience one acquires a particular system of ferreting out and assembling the pertinent facts needed to reach a conclusion. A brief summary of some of the general principles we have found useful in the fascinating art of diagnosis will, we hope, be helpful to others.

Method in diagnosis

Accurate and prompt diagnosis is much facilitated by a *grouping of diseases under certain prominent symptoms*. This is the natural method, the one that is followed unconsciously. The prominent sign or symptom in the case brings to mind a group of diseases, and then by the consideration of other ascertained facts the diagnosis is narrowed down to one or two of these. This differentiation should be made as one proceeds with the examination. For example, suppose during an examination an ulcer is found on the external genitals. Immediately arises the question, "Is this a chancroidal, a syphilitic, a tuberculous, a malignant, or a simple ulcer?" Endeavor to settle the question then and there. Recall the facts in the history bearing on the differential diagnosis. Notice the characteristics of the lesion. Is there lymphatic involvement and, if so, of what type? Are there in other parts of the body evidences of syphilis or tuberculosis?

Each important sign must be thus critically considered, and the habit of so considering them should be cultivated. In a few cases the diagnosis is apparent from a few prominent facts, but in most cases, particularly in deep-seated and serious diseases, the diagnosis must be established by a *critical analysis* of the mass of information obtained in the history and examination. It is this critical analysis— this testing, with elimination of diseases that do not stand the test—that makes the difference between the careful diagnosis and the snap diagnosis, between a reliable diagnostician and an unreliable one.

This effective application of the signs to the diagnosis should, as far as practicable, be *made promptly and rapidly* as they are encountered in the examination. In a systematic history and examination all the important facts are supposed to be obtained. Yet, if the application of the symptoms to the diagnosis is made as one proceeds, certain points in the history of particular importance in the diagnosis in that case will be given the special attention that they require, hence the importance of having in mind for immediate use the diagnostic significance of the common signs encountered.

Consideration of extragenital conditions

Disturbing symptoms in the lower abdomen or back do not necessarily mean genital disease. The trouble may be in some other structure in that vicinity or elsewhere. In this connection we must consider the following structures:

1. Digestive system—Gastroenteritis, appendicitis, regional ileitis, cecal tuberculosis or tumor, colitis, diverticulitis, proctitis, hemorrhoids, tumor of rectum or colon
2. Urinary system—Urethritis, cystitis, bladder stone or tumor, pyelitis, ureteral stone or stricture, kidney stone or tumor
3. Skeletal system—Arthritis of sacroiliac, sacrococcygeal, lumbar, or lumbosacral joints; vertebral tuberculosis, tumor, or injury; postural backache or occupational strain
4. Nervous system—Tabetic crises, transverse myelitis, neutritis and neuralgia, hysteria or other psychosomatic disturbances

It is not necessary to go into detail regarding these conditions; to name them is sufficient to call attention to them for differential diagnosis. Most of the serious mistakes in diagnosis come not from ignorance of the symptoms of various diseases but from the fact that the missed disease *was simply not thought of* when deciding on the cause of the patient's symptoms.

Grouping of pelvic symptoms

After one concludes from the brief preliminary questioning that the trouble is probably in the genital tract, the next step is to determine to what general group of pelvic disturbances this belongs. It is interesting to note that in nearly all cases of a distinct lesion the symptoms presented fall easily into one of two groups. One of these may be designated as the acute symptom complex and the other as the chronic set of symptoms.

The acute group would include not only inflammation but also such conditions as tubal pregnancy, endometriosis, and tumor with a twisted pedicle, for these conditions have many symptoms in common, such as sudden onset, sharp pain, tenderness on examination, and remissions or recurring attacks. The chronic symptoms would include gradual onset, dull pain or dragging sensation, absence of tenderness, and gradual increase in symptoms; these would apply to a uterine or ovarian tumor, prolapse or other uterine displacement, or relaxed pelvic floor.

In complicated cases there may, of course, be a combination of conditions, with a consequent mixture of symptoms, but uncomplicated lesions usually drop readily into one or the other of these two symptomatic classes.

There are, however, gynecologic patients without any organic lesion. Their disturbances constitute a third class—the functional group. The symptoms may simulate those of either class of lesions or they may be a mixture. The functional group includes endocrine and nutritional disorders, allergic manifestations, postural or occupational strain, and neurologic or psychosomatic disturbances. Appropriate additional information acquired from special examinations or tests will help to establish the diagnosis. In psychosomatic problems the diagnosis must sometimes be made by elimination of an organic lesion or other cause for the complaint. The suffering that these patients have is very real to them, and, although some will be relieved when assured in an intelligent way that there is no serious organic lesion present, others will merely seek further medical help until they finally have someone perform an unnecessary operation. In this latter type, suggestive treatment with vitamins, iron, and mild nerve sedatives will frequently work wonders, much to the relief of the patient and doctor. In complex neurologic and psychiatric problems the patient should be advised to seek the proper consultant promptly.

Pitfalls of diagnosis

Before taking up the details of diagnosis it is well to call attention to some of the pitfalls that the practitioner will encounter. Forewarning may put him on the alert and diminish the number of bitter surprises that come with experience. If gynecologic diseases always followed a typcial course and the patient always picked out from her subjective disturbances the identifying ensemble of symptoms, gynecologic diagnosis would be an easy process in which the tyro could proceed confidently and safely, and the experienced gynecologist would have to look elsewhere for the difficult problems and unexpected findings that give spice and interest and development to life. However, there is no necessity to go elsewhere for difficult problems or stimulating surprise. As every gynecologist can testify, gynecologic diagnosis furnishes plenty and some to spare. It has been said that "the abdomen is the greatest surprise box ever opened," and the pelvic portion of it is not the least disconcerting.

The particular diagnostic difficulties pertaining to each disease will be considered in the chapter dealing with that disease, but it may be helpful to call attention here to certain difficulties having a general bearing. Keeping these in mind constitutes a part of that diagnostic alertness or eternal vigilance that must be exercised in working safely through the maze of diseases and their combinations and associated conditions.

ERRORS ABOUT HISTORY

The information obtained from the patient occupies a large place in the diagnosis in most cases, and in some cases certain items are of decisive importance. The history, however, is largely a subjective matter. The stated "facts" are the patient's interpretation of recalled sensations that often were, even at the time, not clearly defined in content or origin. In addition there are the suggestive and other psychic factors to be considered. Occasionally also there is attempt at deception, with the patient endeavoring to build up a claim for damages for some alleged accident, pretending acquired disease as a cause for divorce, or hoping for abortion from some instrumental examination or treatment.

ERRORS ABOUT PELVIC MASS

A common error is to interpret a mass as something that it is not. The nature of a pelvic mass must be determined *indirectly*. We cannot see it or touch it directly, except through the danger of peritoneal invasion. There are no simple sounds that identify it (except in latter part of pregnancy or aneurysm). Our palpation of it must be through intervening tissues, which may obscure its outlines or give a false impression as to its size and consistency. Attempts to overcome these difficulties have been of some aid, but they have not removed the necessity for trained palpation or for gray-matter activity concerning the possible interpretation of what is felt. After preliminary instruction and practice in technique of examination under the guidance of a qualified teacher, repeated use of this knowledge in examining patients and interpreting pelvic findings is needed in order to acquire the "educated touch." At every opportunity conditions found at operation or autopsy should be used to check the preoperative pelvic appraisal.

The *apparent size* of a mass under vaginoabdominal palpation depends largely on the thickness, consistency, and tension of the intervening tissues, particularly the abdominal wall. The *apparent consistency* may be misleading because of the intervening tissues or because of failure to palpate completely. The *apparent tenderness* of the uterus or other pelvic mass must be interpreted with caution. For example, when pressure on the cervix causes pain, do not jump to the conclusion that the cervix is tender. Consider other conditions that may cause pain when the cervix is moved or pressed on, such as a tender tube or ovary. Again, tenderness may be due also to neuritis in the area. Remember, too, that pain is a subjective symptom and may be a referred psychic phenomenon or possibly a deliberate attempt to deceive.

FACTS AND ASSUMPTIONS

Owing to the hiatuses in our knowledge of deep-seated conditions in a patient even after a careful examination, some assumptions are usually necessary in marking a diagnosis. For example, in palpating a pelvic mass, there are some portions for which the outlines can be clearly felt and other portions for which the outlines cannot be felt. To complete the diagnosis we assume a certain approximate outline in the nonpalpable area, endeavoring to avoid error by careful interpretation of all the findings. The outline of the palpable portion represents a fact, while the outline of the nonpalpable portion represents an assumption. Unless constantly on guard we are likely to overlook the relative dependability of the two in working toward a conclusion. It is so easy to allow the probable to slip into the positive class, to be used later as a positive factor in deciding between diagnostic possibilities that this process not infrequently leads to a wide error in diagnosis. The reason for the error become apparent as one traces back from the operation findings through the ways in which the erroneous diagnosis was reached, but it is better to recognize the pitfall before the fall-in.

ERRORS ABOUT TESTS

When by the history and pelvic examination the diagnosis has been narrowed down to two or three conditions, decisive differential diagnositc information may often be furnished by one of the various special tests. An important point to keep in mind, however, is that in many instances the diagnositc significance of the result of a laboratory test depends on the associated clinical findings. The test simply furnishes one item on information, and for use in clinical diagnosis this test item must be correlated with the items obtained from the history and the examination. Even the test item itself (pathologist's interpretation of what he sees) may need to be evaluated with the clinical findings. Consequently helpful cooperation between the clinician and pathologist is necessary to avoid serious mistakes on each side.

IGNORING UNACCOUNTED FOR SYMPTOMS

Unaccounted for symptoms and examination findings are danger signals one must learn to heed. The symptom or examination sign that will not fit into the otherwise satisfying diagnosis is an irritating nuisance to the careless diagnostician but a stimulating question mark to the careful one. An unaccounted for symptom indicates that there is something still unknown about the case, and as long as its cause remains unknown it throws doubt on the correctness or completeness of the diagnosis. "A word to the wise is sufficient."

Tenderness in right lower abdomen

As an example of these methods in diagnosis, let us discuss the differential diagnosis of conditions causing pain and tenderness in the right lower quadrant. First, we would consider the pelvic lesions and then other conditions that could account for the symptoms and signs.

In *pelvic conditions* one of the normal processes in which the pain may be severe enough to be confused with acute appendicitis is ovulation. The ratio of appendicitis to ovulation in patients admitted to hospitals because of right lower quadrant pain has been found to be about one case of ovulation to thirteen of acute appendicitis. Pain with ovulation occurs halfway between the periods in women having a 28-day cycle and is accompanied by other signs or symptoms of ovulation. In diseases of the tube, ovary, or broad ligament the tenderness is most marked low in the side near Poupart's ligament (the tubo-ovarian region). It does not ordinarily extend to the appendix region, although it may in exceptional cases involve both regions. A mass may be felt on vaginoabdominal palpation between the uterus and the pelvic wall. There is a history of uterine and pelvic inflammation or other pelvic disturbance. Tenderness on transvaginal uterine movement or adnexal pressure is present.

Neuralgia of the superficial nerves of the abdominal wall is evidenced by hypersensitivity when either light pressure is applied or the skin is pinched or the skin surface is scratched. If the involvement is one-sided, there is a sharp line of demarcation at the midline, and by testing with a pinprick it is possible to outline the area supplied by the involved nerve.

In acute *appendicitis* the pain usually starts in the epigastric area, later shifting to the umbilical area and finally to the right lower quadrant. There may be a history of recurring attacks with nausea. The patient does not desire to eat. (If she has a good appetite, she does not have appendicitis.) Acute tenderness to pressure over the appendix is noted. Rebound or sudden release of the depressed abdominal wall causes pain if the parietal peritoneum is inflamed. The pulse is elevated and the leukocyte count is usually over 12,000, with a Schilling shift to the left.

With *diseases of the ascending colon* or cecum the tenderness is not localized but extends over the region of the colon.

With *pyelitis* the point of tenderness is in the costophrenic angel. With *ureteritis* the point of tenderness is between the umbilicus and McBurney's point. With *stone* the pain is excruciating, often accompanied by vomiting, and the patient constantly moves about while in pain, seeking a more comfortable position. Urinary examination should clinch the diagnosis.

All the possibilities have not been considered, but enough material has been included to show the method of differential diagnosis.

SELECTED REFERENCES

Abou-Shabanah, E.H., and Plotz, E.J.: A biochemical study of the cervical and nasal mucus phenomenon, Am. J. Obstet. Gynecol. **74:**559, 1957.

Ashenburg, N.J.: Total patient care, GP **12:**111, 1955.

Barbot, J., Parant, B., and Dubuisson, J.B.: Contact hysteroscopy: another method of endoscopic examination of the uterine cavity, Am. J. Obstet. Gynecol. **136:**721, 1980.

Beacham, D.W., and Beacham, W.D.: Culdocentesis, New Orleans Med. Surg. J. **103:**283, 1951.

Becker, K.L.: Endocrine and metabolic disorders. In Raphael, S.S., et al., editors: The laboratory in clinical medicine, Philadelphia, 1976, W. B. Saunders Co.

Bennett, A.E.: Faulty management of psychiatric syndromes simulating organic disease, J.A.M.A. **130:**1203, 1946.

Bertalanffy, L. von, Masin, M., Masin, F., and Kaplan, L.: Detection of gynecological cancer, use of fluorescence microscopy to show nucleic acids in malignant growth, California Med. **87:**248, 1957.

Clarke, L., and Gilmore, H.L., Jr.; Endocervical curettage; aid in diagnosis of early cervical cancer, Obstet. Gynecol. **7:**634, 1956.

Cohen, M.E., Robins, E., Purtell, J.J., Altmann, M.W., and Reid, D.E.: Excessive surgery in hysteria; study of surgical procedures in 50 women with hysteria and 190 controls, J.A.M.A. **151:**977, 1953.

Coppleson, M., Pixley, E., and Reid, B.: Colposcopy: a scientific and practical approach to the cervix and vagina in health and disease, Springfield, Ill. 1978, Charles C Thomas., Publisher.

Crossen, R.J.: Wide conization of cervix; follow-up of one thousand cases, six hundred from two to fourteen years, Am. J. Obstet. Gynecol. **57:**187, 1949.

Daro, A.F., Gollin, H.A., and Nora, E.G., Jr.: New methods and concepts of the Schiller test, GP **12:**71, 1955.

Decker, A.: Culdoscopy: its diagnostic value in pelvic disease, J.A.M.A. **140:**378, 1949.

Donovan, J.C.: Some psychosomatic aspects of obstetrics and gynecology, Am. J. Obstet. Gynecol. **75:**72, 1957.

Doyle, J.B.: Use of pelviscope in culdotomy; aid to early diagnosis and relief of pelvic disorders, J.A.M.A. **151:**605, 1953.

Erickson, C.C., Everett, B.E., Jr., Graves, L.M., Kaiser, R.F., Malgren, R.A., Rube, I., Schreier, P.C., Cutler, S.J., and Sprunt, D.H.: Population screening for uterine cancer by vaginal cytology, J.A.M.A. **162:**167, 1956.

Ford, E.C.: Human cytogenetics, its present place and future possibilities, Am. J. Hum. Genet. **12:**104, 1960.

Gardiner, S.H.: The role of the gynecologist in psychosomatic illness, Clin. Obstet. Gynecol. **5:**298, 1962.

Hart, A.D.: Psychosomatic diagnosis, J.A.M.A. **136:**147, 1948.

Hayden, G.E.: Progesterone-induced withdrawal bleeding as a simple physiologic test for pregnancy, a confirmatory diagnostic tool, Am. J. Obstet. Gynecol. **69:**931, 1955.

Jordan, M.J., and Bader, G.M.: New cannula for obtaining endometrial material for cytologic study, Obstet. Gynecol. **8:**611, 1956.

Josey, W.E., Thompson, J.D., and Te Linde, R.W.: Ten years' experience with culdoscopy: an analysis of 594 cases, South. Med. J. **50:**713, 1957.

Kroger, W.S.: Psychosomatic aspects of obstetrics and gynecology, Obstet. Gynecol. **3:**504, 1954.

Kroger, W.S., and Freed, S.C.: Psychosomatic gynecology, ed. 3, Los Angeles, 1962, Wilshire Book Co.

Lang, W.R.: Colposcopy—neglected method of cervical evaluation, J.A.M.A. **166:**893, 1958.

Li Volsi, V.A.: Practical clinical cytology, Springfield, Ill. 1980, Charles C Thomas, Publisher.

Lock, F.R., and Donnelly, J.F.: The incidence of psychosomatic disease from a private referred gynecologic practice, Am. J. Obstet. Gynecol. **54:**783, 1947.

MacDonald, R.R.: Scientific basis of obstetrics and gynecology, New York City, 1977, Churchill Livingstone.

Mandy, T.E., Weinberg, P., Rudolph, A., and Mandy, A.J.: Psychosexual conflicts: their implications in functional pelvic disorders, South. Med. J. **48**:533, 1955.

McCormick, C.O.: A young woman seeks premarriage counsel, Obstet. Gynecol. **4**:355, 1954.

Miller, W.R.: Psychogenic factors in pelvic pain, J.A.M.A. **134**:938, 1947.

Moore, K.L., and Barr, M.L.: Smears from the oral mucosa in the detection of chromosomal sex, Lancet **2**:57, 1955.

Muller, P.F.: Group premarital counseling; a follow-up study, Am. J. Obstet. Gynecol. **73**:941, 1957.

Novak, E., Jones, G.S., and Jones, H.W.: Novak's textbook of gynecology, ed. 9, Baltimore, 1975, The Williams & Wilkins Co.

Osborne, R.H., and Yannone, M.D.: Plasma androgens in the normal and androgenic female: A review, Obstet. Gynecol. Surv. **26**:195, 1971.

Papanicolaou, G.N., and Bridges, E.L.: Simple method for protecting fresh smears from drying and deterioration during mailing, J.A.M.A. **164**:1330, 1957.

Papanicolaou, G.N., Traut, H.F., and Marchetti, A.A.: The epithelia of women's reproductive organs, New York, 1948, Commonwealth Fund.

Roland, M.: The fern test; a critical analysis, Obstet. Gynecol. **11**:30, 1958.

Rosenfeld, S.S., Schwartz, A., and Steckel, S.: Shave biopsy of the cervix, Am. J. Obstet. Gynecol. **75**:904, 1958.

Ruddock, J.C.: Peritoneoscopy: a critical clinical review, Surg. Clin. N. Amer. **37**:1249, 1957.

Sabbagha, R.E.: Diagnostic ultrasound applied to obstetrics and gynecology, Hagerstown, Md., 1980, Harper & Row, Publishers Inc.

Sears, N.P.: Relation of ureteral pain to menstruation, Am. J. Obstet. Gynecol. **37**:685, 1939.

Semm, K.: Atlas of gynecologic laparoscopy and hysteroscopy, Philadelphia, 1977, W.B. Saunders Co.

Ullery, J.C., and Shabanah, E.H.: The cervical-mucus smear during pregnancy and the fate of conception, Obstet. Gynecol. **10**:233, 1957.

Word, B.: Pitfalls of uterine curettage, South. Med. J. **47**:38, 1954.

Yen, S.S.C., and Jaffe, R.B.: Reproductive endocrinology, Philadelphia, 1978, W.B. Saunders Co.

Chapter 3

MALFORMATIONS

EMBRYOLOGY

Except for the bladder, the genital and urinary structures develop simultaneously from the urogenital ridge. Two ducts, the mesonephric (wolffian) and the paramesonephric (müllerian), are formed in the urogenital ridge. The gonad anlage is also formed on this ridge. Differentiation into ovary or testis normally occurs. The primary sex cords may persist to become seminiferous tubules or disappear except for vestigial rests in the ovarian medulla. The secondary cortex becomes the permanent ovarian cortex containing primordial follicles. If an attempt at development of both male and female types continues, an ovotestis is formed. At times sex cords more characteristic of testicular architecture persist in the ovary. These potentially male cells may give rise to arrhenoblastomas or masculinizing hilar cell (Leydig) tumors. Undifferentiated embryonal-type cells are the probable origin of dysgerminomas.

The paramesonephric (müllerian) ducts remain open at their cephalic ends, the eventual fimbriated portions of the oviducts. The upper portions form the oviducts. The middle and lower portions fuse in the midline to form the uterus, cervix, and vagina. The fusion may be incomplete in varying degrees and result in various uterine and vaginal anomalies. Partial or complete aplasia of one müllerian duct may lead to anomalies of rare type. The solid cords of the early stage of the müllerian tissue growing caudally may fail to form ducts, resulting in the absence of the vagina.

The vaginal epithelium is an ingrowth from the urogenital sinus. The hymen is formed from the infolding of the urogenital sinus. Usually an opening is left, but a complete membrane may form, causing an imperforate hymen.

The mesonephric (wolffian) duct forms the collecting portion for the male genital system (epdididymis, vas deferens, seminal vesicle, and ejaculatory duct), but it disappears in the female except for the Gartner duct (cysts), paroophoron, epoophoron, and vesicular appendices.

The ureters, renal pelvis, calyces, and collecting tubules are derived from a bud

Table 3-1   GENITAL HOMOLOGUES

Male	Female
Penis	Clitoris
Uretheral surface	Labia minora
Corpora cavernosa penis	Corpora cavernosa clitoridis
Corpus cavernosum urethrae	Vestibular bulbs
Scrotum	Labia majora
Scrotal raphe	Posterior commissure
Lower prostatic urethra	Vestibule
Prostatic utricle	Lower vagina
Prostate gland	Paraurethral ducts
Bulbourethral glands	Bartholin's glands

growing off the mesonephric duct near the urogenital sinus. Often deformities of the urinary tract develop simultaneously with genital deformities. This correlation is expected when the close association of the paramesonephric and mesonephric ducts is considered.

A study of the homologues listed in Table 3-1 is valuable for understanding external genital malformations.

MALFORMATIONS
Imperforate hymen

Unless detected during a thorough examination, an occluding hymen is not likely to attract attention until puberty. A collection of menstrual flow leads progressively to hematocolpos, hemometra, hemosalpinx, and hemoperitoneum after months or years. An abdominal mass may appear. The hymen bulges, as shown in Figs. 3-1 and 3-2. Incision of the hymen is curative, but danger of infection before and after drainage must be combated by antibacterial agents.

Ectopic urethral and ureteral openings

The urethra may open into the vagina. Very rarely this is associated with imperforate hymen and urine collects in the vagina. If a ureter opens into the vagina, dribbling of urine begins at birth and continues until a partial nephrectomy and ureterectomy are performed or until atrophy of the upper pole of the kidney drained by the anomalous ureter occurs.

Absence of vagina

In partial absence of the vagina the lower portion does not form, and the upper portion is a cavity into which the cervix protrudes. With a functioning uterus he-

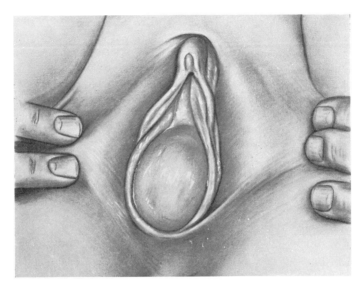

Fig. 3-1. Imperforate hymen. Note the bulging caused by vaginal distention.

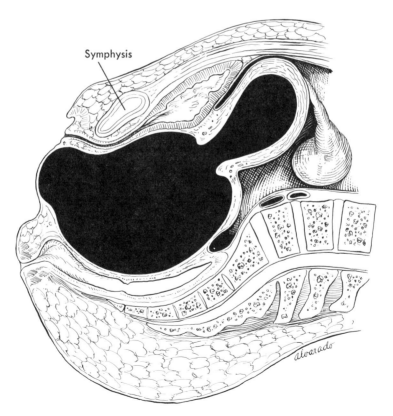

Symphysis

Fig. 3-2. Hematocolpos occurs with imperforate hymen or atresia of the lower vagina. Hemometra and hemosalpinx can also occur as shown in this drawing.

matocolpos can occur without bulging of the hymen. In complete absence of the vagina the uterus is usually absent or represented as a very small bit of fibromuscular tissue. Commonly the *external genitals appear normal*, and the appearance is that of an imperforate hymen. Careful rectal palpation allows one to decide whether there is any midline structure that could be the uterus or a hematocolpos. If no midline structure can be palpated and secondary sexual developments are typically those of a female, the patient usually has functioning ovaries. One must always be observant of other associated anomalies when the vagina is absent. The patient should at least have chromocenter studies done. When other types of anomalies are suspected or when abnormal chromocenters are observed, the karyotype must be known. Urinary anomalies are common in patients without vaginas or with other genital anomalies, and the kidneys and ureters should be properly investigated. Absence of the uterus with presence of normal ovaries is the most common anomaly with complete absence of the vagina, and laparotomy is unnecessary. If there is some doubt concerning the internal genitals, laparoscopy can be performed; however, total visualization of some internal anomalies requires laparotomy. The ovaries should be removed only when there is evidence of Y chromosomal material. Its presence is associated with development of dysgerminomas.

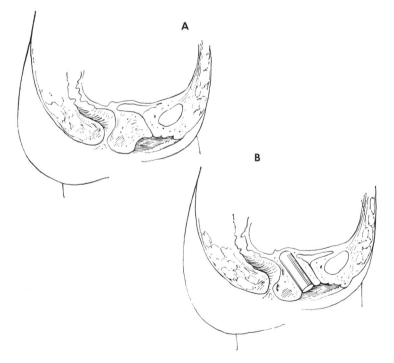

Fig. 3-3. A, Absence of the vagina. **B,** Mold in space for artificial vagina.

A study of the urinary tract by endoscopy and pyelography and a determination of the state of the internal genitals (by laparotomy, if necessary) are in order before construction of an artificial vagina. A vagina may be formed by separation of the bladder and rectum, with or without skin grafting (Fig. 3-3). The operation is best done a few months before marriage, lest adequate size not be maintained.

Septate vagina

Vaginal examination is necessary to palpate or visualize a partial or complete vaginal septum attached to the anterior and posterior walls of the vagina. Dyspareunia may or may not occur, depending on the size of the spaces available for coitus. Tearing of the septum with delivery may occur. The septum can be removed by division in its midportion. The portions attached to the anterior and posterior vaginal walls will gradually retract.

Congenital stricture of the vagina is very rare and may require vaginoplasty.

Uterine anomalies

Improper fusion of the müllerian ducts leads to the various formations shown in Fig. 3-4. If there is a pathway for egress of menstrual flow, obstetric complications are the primary concern. Recurrent abortion calls for hysterography. Removal of the uterine septum to create a cavity of normal shape increases the likelihood that pregnancy may progress to term.

The uterus may be absent, represented by a thickened strand of tissue, or it may be very small. With amenorrhea and a patent cervix, bleeding produced by estrogen therapy will prove the presence of endometrium. A hypoplastic (infantile) uterus may cause infertility. Many uteri smaller than average are not associated with sterility; therefore prognostication by size alone is inaccurate.

Rudimentary uterine horns may be sites for ectopic pregnancies.

Anomalies of the female fetus occur when the mother has received diethylstilbestrol. Original interest centered on clear cell adenocarcinoma, which developed in daughters whose mothers had received diethylstilbestrol during pregnancy. These have been very few in number. More important are the changes that have been identified in the vagina, cervix, uterus, and tubes. Changes in the uterus include a T-shaped cavity, small cavities, and constriction rings involving the endometrial cavity as viewed after hysterosalpingography. The principal concerns are those of pregnancy wastage with increased incidence of ectopic pregnancy, early and late abortions, and premature labor. The cervical and vaginal changes are adenosis of the vagina and endocervical-type tissue presenting as collars or cock's combs on the cervix. These changes tend to regress with time under estrogen influence and seldom require any therapy. Cytologic and colposcopic studies are indicated to find those rare patients who develop carcinoma.

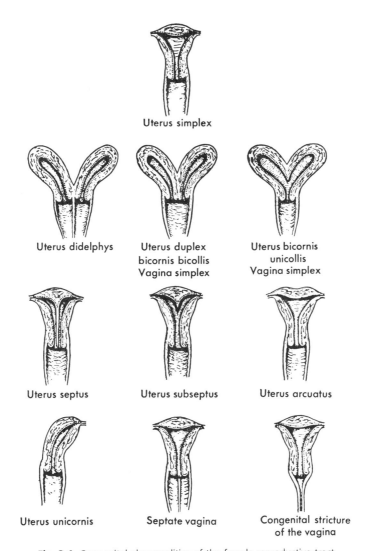

Fig. 3-4. Congenital abnormalities of the female reproductive tract.

Reproduced in part from Jarcho, J.: Am. J. Surg. **71**:106, 1946; from Fenton, A.N., and Singh, B.P.: Am. J. Obstet. Gynecol. **63**:744, 1952.

Ovarian dysplasia

Turner's syndrome includes primary ovarian insufficiency, decreased stature, webbed neck, cubitus valgus, little or no genital hair, and a small vagina. Streak ovaries containing only ovarian stroma are found. Experimental embryology indicates that, if the gonad does not develop, the müllerian ducts differentiate while the wolffian ducts regress. This indicates why the vagina and uterus are found in persons with this syndrome. Chromocenters are usually not found, and the patient is considered to be a genetic male. Usually 45 chromosomes are found, with no Y chromosome present. Estrogen administration will cause breast development and uterine bleeding and should be given to most of these patients.

Intersexuality

Disorders of sexual behavior may be psychic, endocrine, or genetic in origin. Malformations result from genetic, endocrine, and unknown causes.

True hermaphroditism is diagnosed when ovarian and testicular tissues are found unilaterally or bilaterally in the same person. Chromocenter and chromosomal counts more commonly reveal female types or combinations of types. In this exceedingly rare condition a hypospadiac phallus and small vagina are usually developed. The gonads may be in the labial or scrotal folds.

Male pseudohermaphroditism,—testicular feminization,—appears to be a genetic disorder and occurs in siblings; however, many variations occur. A hypospadiac phallus, a small vagina, and scant pubic hair are found. The testes are intraabdominal, inguinal, or labial. Breasts are well developed. These patients do not respond to testosterone, and their primary disturbance is failure of end-organ response to androgens. The 17-KS levels are normal or elevated and fall after gonad removal. Chromatin study reveals male type (see Fig. 3-5).

Female pseudohermaphroditism is most often caused by congenital adrenal hyperplasia (Fig. 3-6). Chromatin study reveals female findings. Excessive androgens produced by the adrenal glands cause enlargement of the clitoris and persistence of the urogenital sinus, so that the appearance of the external genitals is that of a hypospadiac male. The primary disturbance is an enzymatic defect with failure of hydrocortisone production. This enzyme disturbance is most often failure of 21-hydroxylation, which leads to virilism when incomplete, whereas the complete blockage leads also to impaired aldosterone secretion and excess salt loss. Since hydrocortisone is the principal inhibitor of ACTH production, in adrenal hyperplasia the ACTH continues to be produced in larger than normal amounts. When hydrocortisone or one of its immediate family is administered, the ACTH levels fall and adrenal function decreases. The ovary then begins to receive adequate stimulation, since FSH is no longer inhibited by high androgens. The 17-KS levels are usually elevated and decrease after administration of hydrocortisone.

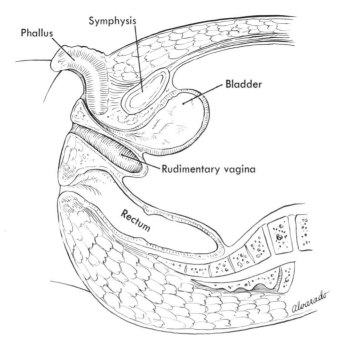

Fig. 3-5. Sagittal section view of a male pseudohermaphrodite.

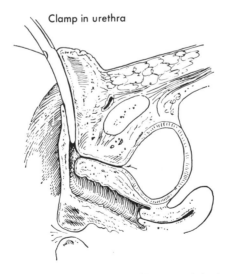

Fig. 3-6. Female pseudohermaphrodite caused by congenital adrenal hyperplasia.

Congenital adrenal hyperplasia, if recognized during infancy or the first few years of life, may be controlled by administration of cortisone or its derivatives. Amputation of the enlarged clitoris and incision of the perineal septum yield a feminine-appearing vulva. If the patient has been reared as a boy and is well adjusted, hysterectomy may be the procedure of choice.

True hermophroditism and male pseudohermaphroditism are best managed by performance of necessary surgery to allow the patients to function as the sex they prefer to be. Reproduction is not possible. The gonads should be excised because of the frequency of dysgerminomas.

TUMORS AND CYSTS ORIGINATING FROM VESTIGIAL STRUCTURES

Parovarian cysts arise in the broad ligament between the ovary and the tube and cause the tube to be stretched over the cyst as noted in Figs. 3-7 and 3-8. A study of their epithelial lining reveals that they may be of mesonephric duct origin or from paramesonephric derivatives. Usually unilocular, with a smoothly lined cavity filled with serous fluid, they are diagnosed clinically as ovarian cysts. Removal should be accomplished to least disturb the tube and ovary.

Pedunculated cysts (hydatids of Morgagni) are most often of paramesonephric origin. Attached to the fimbria of the salpinx, these common small cysts rarely undergo torsion and produce pain.

The mesonephric duct may persist and form *Gartner's duct cysts* in the lateral

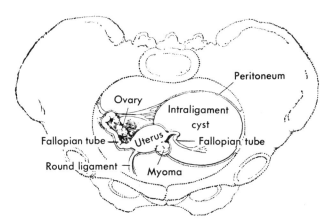

Fig. 3-7. Parovarian cyst (broad ligament cyst) of the left side. Note how it separates the layers of the broad ligament and also displaces the uterus.

From Kelly, H.A.: Operative gynecology, New York, D. Appleton & Co.

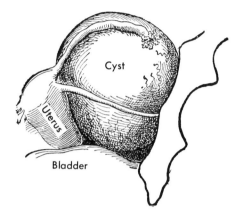

Fig. 3-8. Parovarian cyst forming a large mass and displacing the uterus.

From Ashton, W.A.: Practice of gynecology, Philadelphia, W.B. Saunders Co.

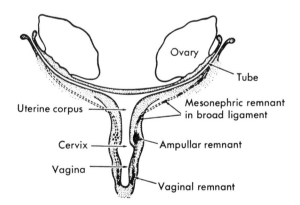

Fig. 3-9. Diagram showing degeneration of the mesonephric duct, which begins during the latter stages of fetal development. This degeneration may be complete; or remnants may be left in the vaginal wall, the cervix, the uterine wall, the broad ligament, or near the ovary.

From Huffman, J.W.: Am. J. Obstet. Gynecol. **56:**23, 1948.

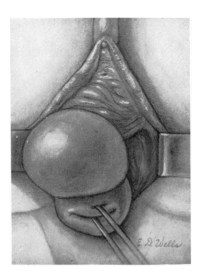

Fig. 3-10. Gross appearance of Gartner's duct cyst, anterior view.

From Kotz, J.: Am. J. Obstet. Gynecol. **30:**854, 1935.

vaginal wall or paracervically (Fig. 3-10). The benign unilocular, serum-filled structures are asymptomatic unless large. Excision is justified at times and is curative.

Novak and associates have indicated that *mesonephromas* and *clear cell adenocarcinomas* are of mesonephric origin.

Neoplasms originating in the broad ligament are very rare. Myoma, fibroadenoma, serous cystadenoma, Brenner tumor, granulosa-theca cell tumor, and adenocarcinoma have been found.

SELECTED REFERENCES

Arey, L.B.: Developmental anatomy, Philadelphia, 1954, W.B. Saunders Co.

Bercu, B.B., and Schulman, J.D.: Genetics of abnormalities of sexual differentiation and of female reproductive failure, Obstet. Gynecol. Surv. **35:**1, 1980.

Brewer, J.I., Jones, H.O., and Culver, H.: True hermaphroditism, J.A.M.A. **148:**431, 1952.

Bryan, A.L., Nigro, J.O., and Counsellor, V.S.: One hundred cases of congenital absence of the vagina, Surg. Gynecol. Obstet. **88:**79, 1949.

Capraro, V.J., and Gallago, M.V.: Vaginal agenesis, Am. J. Obstet. Gynecol. **124:**98, 1976.

DeCosta, E.J.: Endocrinology, disorders of sex. In Brewer, J.I.: Textbook of gynecology, ed. 2, Baltimore, 1958, The Williams & Wilkins Co.

Gardner, G.H., Greene, R.R., and Peckham, B.M.: Normal and cystic structures of the broad ligament, Am. J. Obstet. Gynecol. **55:**917, 1948.

Gardner, G.H., Greene, R.R., and Peckham, B.M.: Tumors of the broad ligament, Am. J. Obstet. Gynecol. **73:**536, 1957.

Grumbach, M.M., van Wyk, J.J., and Wilkins, L.: Chromosomal sex in gonadal dysgenesis (ovarian agenesis): relationship to male pseudohermaphroditism and theories of human sex differentiation, J. Clin. Endocrinol. **15:**1161, 1955.

Jarcho, J.: Malformations of the uterus, Am. J. Surg. **71**:106, 1946.

Jones, H.W., Jr., and Scott, W.W.: Abnormal sexual development: hermaphroditism, genital anomalies and endocrine disorders of gonads and adrenals, Baltimore, 1958, The Williams & Wilkins Co.

Kaufman, R.H., Adam, E., Binder, G.L., et al.: Upper genital tract changes and pregnancy outcome in offspring exposed in utero to diethylstilbestrol, Am. J. Obstet. Gynecol. **137**:299, 1980.

Moore, K.L., and Barr, M.L.: Smear from the oral mucosa in the detection of chromosomal sex, Lancet **2**:57, 1955.

Tomkins, P.: Treatment of imperforate hymen with hematocolpos, J.A.M.A. **113**:913, 1933.

Wharton, L.R.: Congenital absence of the uterus and associated developmental defects, Surg. Gynecol. Obstet. **40**:31, 1925.

Chapter 4

DISEASES OF THE VULVA

The vulva is subject to most of the skin diseases that may occur in other portions of the body. Dependent on endocrine stimulation for development and maintenance and influenced by variations in vaginal, urethral, uterine, and anorectal conditions, the pudendum must be considered with the viewpoints of dermatology, urology, protology, sexual psychology, and gynecology.

VULVITIS

In vulvitis sensory perception is acute. Pruritus, burning, and tenderness are the principal symptoms. All or one or two of these symptoms may be present. Pruritus vulvae may be marked without gross or microscopic tissue changes. Psychosomatic etiology and generalized diseases such as diabetes mellitus, leukemia, infectious hepatitis with jaundice, avitaminosis, or uremia may be involved. Excessive moisture caused by tight, nonabsorbent clothing or obesity and inadequate cleansing increase inflammation in this area.

Candidiasis (moniliasis)

Candidiasis is common and usually causes intense pruritus. Occasionally only cutaneous involvement occurs, and response to nystatin or clotrimazole cream is good. More commonly vaginal involvement is associated. (See discussion of vaginitis, Chapter 5.)

Trichomoniasis

Trichomoniasis is common with a variable degree of pruritus. (See discussion of vaginitis, Chapter 5.)

Pediculosis pubis

Crab lice with eggs can be seen attached to hairs near the roots as brownish particles about the size of hair. The axillae and eyebrows should be checked. Transmission is by coitus or on clothing or toilets. The patient should dust 10% chlorophenothane (DDT) into pubic hairs or apply 1% lindane (Kwell) ointment.

Scabies

Scabies is diagnosed by finding the burrows of *Saroptes scabiei*. The fingers or other typical areas should be searched. One may recover mites under the nails of the patient for microscopic examination. The use of 1% Kwell ointment or 10% benzyl benzoate lotion is effective.

Oxyuriasis

Pruritus begins in the perianal area. Diagnosis can be made by microscopic identification of eggs gathered on clear plastic adhesive (Scotch) tape. All members of the household should be checked and treated if necessary. Piperazine salts (Antepar) for 7 days or pyrvinium pamoate (Povan) in a single dose is usually effective.

Trichophytosis

Commonly tinea cruris (epidermophytosis inguinale) is noted with the vulval lesion of trichophytosis. Scrapings in 10% potassium hydroxide solution may reveal mycelium and a few spores. Culture may be required. When secondary bacterial infection is present, it should be eradicated. Tolnaftate (Tinactin) in 1% solution applied twice daily is often very effective as a fungicide.

Neurodermatitis

The lesions of neurodermatitis are caused by scratching, secondary infection, and reaction to chemicals or radiation used for treatment. Diagnosis depends on excluding other causes and determining the psychosomatic mechanism. Immature attitude, prejudices, and lack of education about sexual functions are common causes. Masturbation, cancerophobia, fear of pregnancy, guilt complex, or marital discord may be found. Psychotherapy, tranquilizers, and antipruritic drugs and bland applications are in order. Creams containing cortisone derivatives may give relief.

Behçet's syndrome of recurrent ulcerative vulvitis, stomatitis, and uveitis can be considered in this category. Oral corticoids give excellent response, but recurrence is likely.

Bacterial infections

Infection of the vulva results in a variety of leisons that differ according to the invading bacteria.

1. Gonorrheal (see discussion of vaginitis, Chapter 5).
2. Staphylococcal—Folliculitis, furuncles, carbuncles, hidradenitis suppurativa.
3. Streptococcal—Erysipelas, cellulitis. Edema may be marked.
4. Tuberculous lesions are very rare and usually are ulcers and/or sinuses. Diagnosis requires smears, culture, biopsy, or guinea pig inoculation.

5. Mixed flora—*Fusobacterium fusiforme* with *Borrelia vincentii*, diphtheroids, *Bacillus coli*, enteric streptococci, anaerobic bacilli, and *Haemophilus vaginalis*, may be pathogenic, with tissue resistance lowered by debility, trauma, or local irritation. Inadequate local cleansing or urinary or fecal incontinence may induce mixed bacterial vulvitis.

Ideal management requires identification of bacteria and the local or systemic administration of a specific antibacterial agent. Drainage of pus, cleansing of the area, avoidance of irritation (chemical or scratching), and relief of debility, if possible, should be accomplished. Keeping the vulva dry with perineal heat or a fan usually aids healing. Oral analgesics and antipruritics may afford comfort to the patient.

Chemical irritations

Tolerance of the vulvar skin is less than that in most areas of the body. Mucous membranes are particularly susceptible to salicyclic acid, phenolic compounds, local anesthetic agents, bichloride of mercury, deodorants, and some patented preparations (self-treatment).

Traumatic lesions

Repeated scratching may cause marked changes (lichenification). Fissures of the fourchette may occur with coitus. Girls may fall while straddling fences or chairs, causing lacerations and particularly hematomas of this vascular area. Seldom do hematomas require ligation of vessels. Cold applications early and heat later are in order.

Viral infections

Viral vulvitis produces vesicular lesions that become shallow ulcers. *Herpesvirus hominis* exists as Types I and II. Type I causes most nongenital herpetic lesions, e.g., herpes labialis, gingivostomatitis, and keratoconjunctivitis. Lesions caused by Type I virus may occur on the vulva of children, particularly concurrent with lesions on the lips and in the mouth.

Type II *Herpesvirus hominis* is recovered almost exclusively from the genital tract of coitally active patients. Although antibodies develop, they do not prevent recurrent lesions. With primary infection from Type II virus the lesions are more numerous, larger, and apt to be found not only on the vulva but also in the vagina and cervix with enlargement and tenderness of the inguinal lymph nodes. Similarly there is likely to be more systematic reaction. With recurrent lesions the areas of involvement are less numerous and smaller, and there is less likely to be any systemic reaction. The incubation period of primary infection is from 2 to 7 days. The lesions usually persist for 7 to 10 days; however, in secondary bacterial or mycotic infection, lesions may persist for 2 to 6 weeks. Most rapid clinical responses are obtained when 0.1% neutral red dye is applied followed by fluorescent light for 20 minutes; however, there is concern that modification of the virus by this treatment may possibly render it oncogenic. Usually when the patient is seen the vesicles have ruptured and superficial ulcers are present with secondary infection. The treatment is then that of the secondary bacterial or mycotic infection with locally applied agents unless the patient has extensive lymphadenitis. Under those circumstances systemic antibacterial agents are in order. When lesions have been contaminated with the indigenous flora of the mouth through oral-genital sex. the extent of secondary infection is much more marked and the patient experiences more pain, edema, and other local reactions.

The varicella-zoster virus *(Herpesvirus varicellae)* may cause painful vesicular lesions on the vulva in older adults; however, this is a rather uncommon occurrence. It is a form of "shingles" with a unilateral grouping of vesicles over one to three dermatomes. It is now recognized as a latent virus activated in adults. This syndrome is not apt to be confused with the infection from Type II *Herpesvirus hominis*.

Allergic reactions

Deodorants, medications, and nylon, rayon, or other sythetics are possible contact antigens. With eczema, vesicles rupture and pruritic lesions become encrusted. One should avoid the allergen. Antihistamine and/or adrenal corticoids may be used locally or orally.

Radiation reactions

Pudendal tissues have low tolerance to x-ray film or other types of external radiation; consequently radiation is now seldom used. Its use should be abandoned. Epilation, telangiectases, decreased vascularity, and decreased cellular replacement occur. The area should be protected, and bland local applications should be used.

WHITE LESIONS AND CHRONIC DYSTROPHIES OF THE VULVA
Evaluation

In the past many of the white lesions of the vulva have been called "leukoplakia." This term has had considerable difference in meaning in various parts of the world, and we contend that the term should be discontinued. First, let us consider how white lesions of the vulva come about. There may be an absence of pigmentation in the cells. There may be thickening of the cornified outer layer of the epidermis. Scarring or subepithelial fibrosis (collagenization) may cause the area to become relatively avascular.

Vitiligo (leukoderma) is a congenital condition in which the pigment is absent in the cells of otherwise normal skin. Scars can result from injury caused by lacerations or incisions, or scarring may develop following prolonged recurrent infection and with ulcerations of the vulva such as occur with granulomatous infections. Hyperkeratosis may develop because of scratching and rubbing, as occurs with neurodermatitis or any lesion associated with pruritis, or it may be a response to dermatoses (seborrheic, fungal, etc.). If it is caused by a condition that can be eradicated, then it may be temporary; however, the condition causing the disease may be unknown or may be chronic, and the hyperkeratosis then becomes a manifestation of a chronic growth problem in the skin and can be called a dystrophy. Subepithelial collagenization is usually a chronic condition and is more frequently associated with a growth problem in the epidermis as well as the dermis. It usually represents a manifestation of a chronic dystrophy.

It thus becomes apparent in evaluating white lesions of the vulva that it is important to recognize whether there is an etiologic situation that can be corrected and particularly whether the condition is chronic. If the condition represents a chronic dystrophy, then the likelihood of malignancy being present or developing is increased. These particular types of white lesions should be investigated by biopsy.

As just mentioned, dystrophies may appear as white areas on the vulva; however, they may also be red areas. To be properly called a dystrophic lesion they must have been present for a considerable time—usually for a year or more. A relatively common dystrophy is lichen sclerosus. This condition is occasionally seen in young girls; however, it is much more prevalent in patients over 40 years of age and becomes more common as they grow older. There may be associated atrophy of the epithelium and dermis. Under these circumstances the term "atrophicus" is added. Keratotic plugging of the follicles may be noted, and areas may become edematous. When patients with these lesions are observed over a long period, it is found that carcinomatous change rarely occurs.

Areas showing thickening of the skin over a long period frequently exhibit hyperkeratosis, and when these areas are moist they are apt to appear whiter. Hyperplasia of the epithelium may be evident with white or red areas and can only be diagnosed by microscopic evaluation. Various areas on the same vulva may present different microscopic appearances. Erythroplasia of Queyrat is a red lesion presenting hyperplasia or even carcinoma in situ on the mucous membrane.

When the hyperplasia exhibits definitely atypical cells and lack of stratification of epithelium, it is termed "dysplasia." When this process is marked, it is properly called carcinoma in situ. At times the hyperplasia is principally limited to the basal cells, and consequently the term "basal cell hyperplasia" is used.

From the foregoing discussions of white lesions and dystrophies, it is evident that to manage patients with vulvar changes the physician must see the patients frequently enough to determine the course of their disease. Particularly, vulvar changes must be investigated as to etiology, and proper therapy when available must be applied. The liberal use of biopsy is emphasized because it is only when the pathologist has analyzed the tissue that a diagnosis of the lesion can be certain. Areas that are chronically too thick or too thin, persistent masses, persistent ulcers, and areas taking deeper nuclear staining are candidates for biopsy. When 1% aqueous toluidine blue is applied and washed away 1 minute later with 1% acetic acid solution, the areas of highest nuclear concentration will stain blue.

Therapy

When malignancy has been ruled out by biopsy, symptomatic therapy is in order. Local application of hydrocortisone or its derivatives usually relieves pruritus and buring. Antihistamines may be applied or taken orally with relief of symptoms. Any associated dermatitis or vaginitis must be relieved if practical. Cold applied to the area will give some relief from intense itching.

Frequent follow-up examination, with repeat biopsy of any area that does not heal readily or exhibits increased nuclear staining, is mandatory because of the increased incidence of carcinoma associated with these lesions.

If conservative therapy does not yield adequate response, vulvectomy may be required, particularly when there have been extensive areas of scarring. If a chronic dystrophy is present, recurrence after vulvectomy is common.

KRAUROSIS

Shrinkage of the vulvar structures and introitus occurs (1) with senile hypoestrogenism leading to atrophy with or without recurrent vulvitis and (2) with some chronic dystrophies.

Enlargement of the introitus surgically after control of vulvitis may be required to cure dyspareunia. In lesser degrees of contracture, local applications of estrogen creams may afford relief.

ULCERATIVE DISEASES

Ulcers may be found as complications of most types of vulvitis. These simple ulcers will heal with definitive therapy of their respective conditions. Certain diseases begin with or usually form an ulcer.

The diagnosis of vulvar ulcerative diseases requires laboratory tests (Table 4-1).

Chancroid

"Soft chancre" has an incubation period of 1 to 10 days and is caused by Ducrey's gram-negative, nonmotile bacillus. The lesion is painful, has a necrotic base, is "punched out," and has red margins. Inguinal lymphadenitis (bubo) is common. Spread is by direct contact, usually sexual.

Diagnosis is suspected by appearance and history and proved by smear and

Table 4-1   DIFFERENTIAL DIAGNOSTIC LABORATORY TESTS USED

1. Darkfield examination (*Treponema pallidum* and fusospirochetes)
2. Serologic tests for syphilis
3. Direct smear, gram stain *(Haemophilus ducreyii)*
4. Culture for *Haemophilus ducreyii*
5. Biopsy for (a) malignancy, (b) condyloma acuminatum, (c) tuberculosis, (d) mycotic infections, (e) tissue type, (f) granuloma inguinale
6. Frei test (lymphogranuloma)
7. Smear-type biopsy for granuloma inguinale (superior)
8. Smears for inclusion bodies (herpes)
9. Rabbit inoculation, eye (herpes)
10. Guinea pig inoculation *(Mycobacterium tuberculosis)*
11. Culture for *Mycobacterium tuberculosis*
12. Tuberculin tests
13. Direct examination of material for fungi *(Actinomyces, Blastomyces, Candida)*
14. Fungus and bacterial cultures

From Thomas, W.L.: Am. J. Obstet. Gynecol. **61**:790, 1951.

culture. Therapy includes cleansing and administration of oral sulfonamides or tetracyclines.

Syphilis

The incubation period for syphilis is 3 to 8 weeks. The chancre, or primary lesion, may be found on the vulva, vagina, or cervix. Usually it is painless, clean, firm, and slightly raised. One may note edema of the surrounding area. Most often it is overlooked and heals spontaneously. A chancre should be searched for in all cases of gonorrhea. Darkfield examination allows identification of the *Treponema pallidum*. Serologic tests, although negative with an early chancre, should be repeated later, since they will become positive in untreated patients.

Condylomata lata are the secondary lesions that consist of moist slightly raised patches. These lesions are likely to occur on the thighs and buttocks. One should look for them also in the pharynx. Diagnosis can be made by darkfield examination or biopsy with stain for spirochetes. Results from serologic tests are usually positive.

Gumma or syphilitic ulcer of the vulva or vagina is rare. Serology and biopsy allow diagnosis.

For therapy to be adequate, it is necessary to maintain a sufficient blood level of the agent over a period of 10 days or more. Benzathine penicillin G can be given as one dose of 2.4 million units. For patients sensitive to penicillin, erythromycin can be given orally in the dosage of 2 grams per day for 10 to 15 days, or a tetracycline can be given in the dosage of 3 grams per day for 10 to 15 days. Repeated serologic tests are essential to diagnose failures or relapse. The isolation technique should be used for primary and secondary lesions. A search for active syphilis in contacts is the best method of finding new cases.

Granuloma inguinale (Donovan bodies)

Granuloma inguinale, a chronic ulceration of the vulva and inguinal regions, is found in tropical and temperate climates. More commonly it occurs in blacks. At times lesions are found in the mouth, cheek, neck, or extremities.

The first, small, papular lesion is followed in a few weeks by ulceration tending to be serpiginous. The surface of the ulcer is seropurulent without secondary infection. Bubo is rare. Pseudobubo (subcutaneous granuloma) is more often found.

Usually there is little or no pain. Soreness, pruritus, or burning may be annoying. Masses may develop in patients with the less common hypertrophic type of case.

Diagnosis is made by smear or biopsy for Donovan bodies. The patient should be examined for other venereal diseases. Biopsy is indicated because carcinoma may develop in the involved tissues.

Therapy may be relatively successful with streptomycin, chlortetracycline (Aureomycin), and chloramphenicol (Chloromycetin). Vulvectomy is needed for large lesions and for cosmetic reasons.

Lymphogranuloma inguinale or lymphopathia venereum

Lymphogranuloma inguinale is a disease caused by an obligate intracellular parasite, a bedsonia, that affects lymph channels and nodes. It is more common in blacks. The primary lesion of the vulva or vagina, single or multiple papules, is likely to be overlooked. The most frequent secondary manifestation is the inguinal bubo (lymphadenitis), which is often chronic and may be attached to or break through the overlying skin. With secondary infection suppuration ensues, and incision and drainage may be indicated. Recurrent ulceration and chronic edema with elephantiasis may occur. As a result of the lymph drainage from the vagina and perineum to the rectum. rectal wall involvement with stricture formation may develop.

Diagnosis is made by the Frei skin test. There is no specific histologic finding.

Therapy includes administration of sulfadiazine and/or streptomycin, chloramphenicol (Chloromycetin), chlortetracycline (Aureomycin), or oxytetracycline (Terramycin). Oral estrogens may soften rectal strictures to avoid colostomy for intestinal obstruction. In acute obstruction colostomy is needed. After the infection has been cleared, vulvectomy may be in order to remove the masses. The increased incidence of carcinoma with this disease demands biopsy as a routine.

Actinomycosis, tularemia, typhoid fever, tuberculosis, and foreign bodies may cause ulcerations of the vulva.

CARCINOMA

Cancer of the vulva may originate in red or white lesions with or without symptoms. Thickened areas, chronic ulcerations, skin or mucosal masses, and areas that stain with toluidine blue (a nuclear stain) should be suspect, and biopsy should be performed. Lymphogranuloma and granuloma inguinale are chronic diseases of the vulva that may have areas of cancer. Intraepithelial carcinoma may present as a mass. Any portion of the vulva may be the primary site. More commonly a squamous cell growth on the labia, clitoria, or vestibule or in the Bartholin gland. If untreated, vulvar carcinoma invades the lymphatics, resulting in spread to the inguinal nodes, then to the femoral, iliac, and aortic nodes, or (via the vagina) to the obturator nodes. At times spreading to the perirectal lymphatics is found. The anastomoses of vulvar lymphatics allow metastases to contralateral lymph nodes.

Multiple intraepithelial growths are cured by vulvectomy. Single small lesions may be adequately excised. Topical fluorouracil has been reported to eradicate small lesions.

Invasive cancer requires total vulvectomy and excision of the inguinal, femoral, obturator, and iliac nodes. Vaginectomy and resection of the anorectal region may be required. An overall 5-year survival of 60% should be attained.

Paget's disease may be found on the vulva. Origin in the apocrine gland is postulated. Wide local excision has been advocated; however, Norman F. Miller and Conrad G. Collins have advised total vulvectomy.

Basal cell carcinoma of the vulva may be treated by local excision.

Metastatic vulvar cancer may occur from choriocarcinoma, cervical or uterine cancer, hypernephroma, and mamary carcinoma. Melanomas of the vulva are uncommon; however, all nevi should be excised.

BENIGN VULVAR CONDITIONS
Stasis hypertrophy

Stasis hypertrophy may be caused by (1) lymphatic blockage of chronic infections or (2) filariasis (prevalent in certain regions). After infection is cleared, vulvectomy is the means of eradication of the remaining masses.

Varicose veins

Varicose veins are rarely troublesome except during pregnancy. If persistent and symptomatic, they may require excision in nonpregnant patients.

Bartholin cysts

Bartholin cysts (Fig. 4-1) are caused by duct obstruction and may or may not be preceded by abscess. Gonococcus is sometimes the cause. They are syptomatic only if large. With abscess formation, incision and drainage are indicated to relieve the

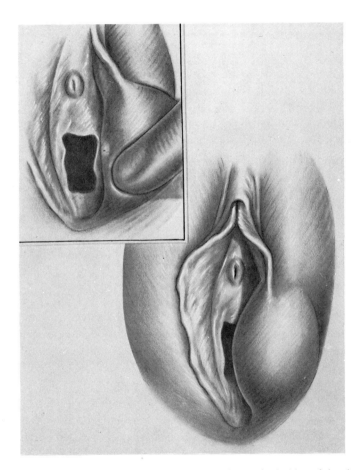

Fig. 4-1. An infected Bartholin cyst. The inset shows the site for incision of the abscess.

severe pain. Cure can be effected by (1) removal of the cyst and gland in the hospital, (2) cystostomy by suture of the cyst wall to the overlying mucosa of the introitus, or (3) a small incision of the cyst and the introduction of a Word bag distended with 1 to 3 ml of water. This gadget is left in place for about 4 weeks until a new ostium is well established by epithelialization. In cases of recurrent infection with persistent induration one should suspect carcinoma.

Condylomata acuminata

Condylomata acuminata (pointed, moist, wartlike growths) are common on the vulvar and anal regions. Although these are called venereal warts, any irritating discharge may be associated. With eradication of the discharge the lesions may not recur. After the associated vulvovaginitis has been cleared, the growths should be removed with podophyllin in tincture of benzoin, by cryotherapy, or electrosurgical excision and fulguration. Molluscum contagiosum appears to be similar to condylomata acuminata except that it occurs on the skin as a raised smooth lesion with a dimple in the center. After the surface is broken they can be cleared in the same manner.

Hematomas

Hematomas of traumatic origin may be large but rarely require ligation of bleeding vessels. After liquefaction, aspiration hastens healing.

Inguinal and labial masses

Femoral hernias turn cephalad over the inguinal ligaments. Inguinal hernias may be present in the labia majora. Inguinal nodes, peritoneal cysts (canal of Nuck), and varicosities may cause confusion. Pudendal hernia very rarely occurs via the obturator foramen.

Urethral caruncle

Urethral caruncle is a small, deep red, very sensitive, papillary growth protruding from the meatus. Essentially it is a vascular tumor associated with chronic urethritis or skenitis. Dysuria and dyspareunia are common. The lesion may bleed on contact. Treatment requires excision.

Prolapse of urethral mucosa

Prolapse of urethral mucosa is a condition distinguished from caruncle by absence of tenderness and pediculation. If the prolapse is marked, excision is required.

Paraurethral cyst

Cysts of Skene's glands may appear at the introitus. Cure is effected by excision.

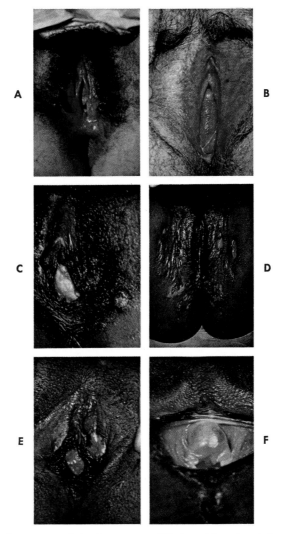

Plate 1. Types of vulvitis: **A,** Psoriasis. **B,** Acute candidiasis and hyperkeratosis with hyperplasia in a diabetic patient. Ulcerative diseases: **C,** Chancre. **D,** Lymphopathia venereum. Carcinoma and cyst of the vulva: **E,** Intraepithelial squamous cell carcinoma. **F,** Skene cyst.

Courtesy Dr. Conrad G. Collins and others, Tulane Medical School Vulvar Clinic, New Orleans, La.

Miscellaneous

Sebaceous cysts, verrucae, nevi, fibromas, lipomas, hemangiomas, neuromas, lymphangiomas, chondromas, myxomas, leiomyomas, myoblastomas, accessory breasts, hidradenomas, areas of endometriosis, and wolffian duct cysts are cured by complete excision, but they require histologic study for accurate diagnosis. Hidradenoma should not be confused with adenocarcinoma by a competent pathologist.

SELECTED REFERENCES

Baker, R.L.: Treatment of condyloma acuminatum, Obstet. Gynecol. **10**:611, 1957.

Buscema, J., Woodruff, J.D., Parmley, T.H., and Genadry, R.: Carcinoma in situ of the vulva, Obstet. Gynecol. **55**:225, 1980.

Collins, C.G., Collins, J.H., Cassidy, R.E., and Burman, R.G.: Malignancies involving the vulva, Dallas Md. J. **43**:675, 1957.

Creadick, R.N.: Severe chronic pruritus vulvae, J. Fla. Med. Assoc. **42**:1007, 1956

Gardner, H.L., and Kaufman, R.H.: Benign diseases of the vulva and vagina, Boston, 1981, G.K. Hall.

Greenblatt, R.B.: Management of chancroid granuloma inguinale, lymphogranuloma venereum in general practice, United States Department of Health, Education, and Welfare, Public Health Service Publication No. 225, 1953.

Huber, C.P., Gardiner, S.H., and Michael, A.: Paget's disease of the vulva, Am. J. Obstet. Gynecol. **62**:778, 1951.

Hunt, E.: Diseases affecting the vulva, ed. 2, St. Louis, 1943, The C.V. Mosby Co.

Jeffcoate, T.N.A. Chronic vulva dystrophies, Am. J. Obstet. Gynecol. **95**:61, 1966.

Jeffcoate, T.N.A.: Pruritus vulvae, Br. Med. J. **2**:1196, 1949.

Miller, N.F., Parrot, M.H., Stryker, J., Riley, G.M., and Curtis, A.C.: Leukoplakia of the vulva, Am. J. Obstet. Gynecol. **54**:543, 1947.

Miller, N.F., Riley, G.M., and Stanley, M.: Leukoplakia of the vulva, Am. J. Obstet. Bynecol. **64**:768, 1952.

Noojin, R.O.: The dematologic management of pruritus, South. Med. J. **49**:149, 1956.

Novak, E., and Stevenson, R.R.: Sweat gland tumors of the vulva, benign (hidradenoma) and malignant (adenocarcinoma), Am. J. Obstet. Gynecol. **50**:641, 1945.

Parks, J., and Martin, S.: Reactions of the vulva to systemic disease, Am. J. Obstet. Gynecol. **55**:117, 1948.

Sarma, V.: Gynaecological and obstetrical aspects of tropical disesases, Mediscope **4**:1, 1961.

Schock, E.P., Jr., and McCuiston, C.H.: Diagnostic and therapeutic errors in certain dermatoses of the vulva, J.A.M.A. **157**:1102, 1955.

Thomas, W.L.: A clinical study of granuloma inguinale with a routine for the diagnosis of lesion of the vulva, Am. J. Obstet. Gynecol. **61**:790, 1951.

Ulfelder, H.: Radical vulvectomy with bilateral inguinal, femoral, and iliac node resection, Am. J. Obstet. Gynecol. **78**:1074, 1959.

Ward, J.: Five cases of basal-cell carcinoma of the vulva, Am. J. Obstet. Gynecol. **63**:697, 1956.

Way, S.: The anatomy of the lymphatic drainage of the vulva and its influence on the radical operation for carcinoma, Ann R. Coll. Surg. Engl. **3**:187, 1948.

Wilder, E.M.: A simple method of treating vulvovaginal (Bartholin) cyst and abscess, South. Med. J. **46**:460, 1955.

Word, B.: New instrument for office treatment of cysts and abscesses of Bartholin's gland, J.A.M.A. **190**:777, 1964.

Chapter 5

DISEASES OF THE VAGINA

VAGINITIS

The passageway from the vulva to the cervix is particularly influenced by the condition of the cervix. In recurrent and resistant vaginitis, cervical disease is usually found. Evaluation of vaginal status must also include evaluation of discharges originating in the uterine cavity. The complete inspection of the vagina and the microscopic examination of vaginal material are essential for an accurate diagnosis. Failure of proper diagnosis and employment of "shotgun" preparations are deplorable.

Trichomoniasis

Trichomoniasis vaginitis occurs in 15% or more of all married women, with symptoms varying as to duration and extent. Typical patients have a greenish yellow profuse discharge with bubbles, a red tender vulva and adjacent portion of thighs, and marked pruritus and buring. The patient is often awakened because of the pruritus. The discharge persists in spite of douching. The vaginal mucosa is red, tender, and rough, with small hemorrhagic spots. The paraurethral glands, urethra, and vulvovaginal glands are not as likely to be acutely involved as with gonorrhea. As in other vaginitides, Döderlein's bacilli decrease in number. Along with the protozoan a large number of leukocytes and bacteria are found.

The extent of involvement varies in a given patient from time to time and varies greatly in individuals. Increase in symptoms may be noted before, during, and after menstruation. Diagnosis is suggested by the typical type of discharge and is established by finding the motile, flagellate, oval-shaped protozoan in a wet, unstained smear. One should place 1 drop of discharge on a slide, dilute it with 2 drops of normal saline solution or water, and examine it immediately with the light of the microscope decreased.

Therapy. Metronidazole (Flagyl) administered orally, 250 mg either twice or three times daily for 10 days, is highly effective in the eradication of this troublesome protozoan. No local therapy is required with this oral medication. The tricho-monacides used for vaginal application are as follows:

1. Phenylmercuric acetate—Nylmerate jelly, Lorophyn jelly
2. Iodine compounds—diiodohydroxyquin (Floraquin) tablets, iodochlorhy-droxyquin (Vioform) tablets
3. Chelating, wetting, detergent agents—Vagisec jelly and liquid

Since metronidazole has become available and is well tolerated by the majority of patients, there is little need for vaginal application of trichomonacides. An accurate diagnosis is essential.

Recurrence. Most often reinfection is from the coital partner. Incomplete therapy and involvement of paraurethral, vulvovaginal, or cervical glands may be causes of recurrent infection. Eradication of chronic infection, treatment of the male with metronidazole, or the use of a condom by the male for 3 months is essential in the management of trichomoniasis. When trichomoniasis is found in a woman, her coital partner should be treated with metronidazole. The identification of the organism in the male is very difficult, and frequently the male patient is asymptomatic.

When trichomoniasis has been diagnosed, it is well to think of the possiblity of other venereal diseases, gonorrhea in particular. When the patient has recurrent trichomoniasis or there is knowledge that either she or her coital partner has other partners for coitus, cultures should be obtained from the cervix and the anal canal for the gonococcus.

Candidiasis (moniliasis)

Candidiasis is common during pregnancy and with untreated diabetes mellitus. Combined estrogen-progestogen oral contraception increases the occurence. The yeastlike organism *Candida (Monilia) albicans* thrives in a "sweet" environment. Wide-spectrum antibiotics may destroy normal bacteria and allow this fungus to increase. In a typical patient the discharge is thick, white, and curdy and is associated with intense pruritus. The vagina and vulva are red and swollen. Small, white patches adhere to the vagina. Mycelia and conidia may be seen on a plain wet smear or after adding 10% sodium hydroxide solution (Fig. 5-1).

Typical smears reveal few leukocytes. Culture can be used to identify the organism. In less typical cases the patients present a thin watery discharge and are found on examination to have a whitish sheen of the vagina and labia minora. Microscopic examinations of wet smears in these cases seldom reveal the conidia or mycelia. The diagnosis is made by finding the organism on culture (Nickerson's medium is excellent), together with the observance of response to the application of fungistatic agents. In atypical cases recurrence may be without apparent cause. In evaluating cultures it is important to remember that positive cultures can be obtained from the normal vagina, the normal skin, or the normal mouth.

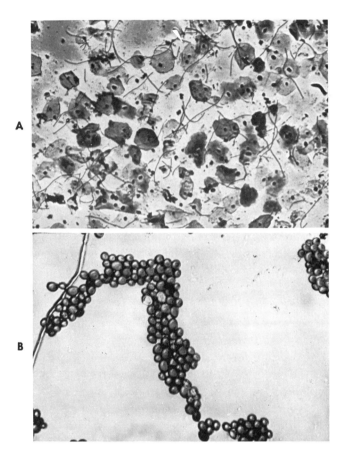

Fig. 5-1. A, Mycelia of *Candida albicans* seen on suspension of vaginal exudate. Silver carbonate stain. (×100.) **B,** *Candida albicans.* Suspension made from colony and stained with methylene blue. (×450).

From Campbell, R.M., and Parrott, M.H.: Am. J. Obstet. Gynecol. **59:**1005, 1950.

Therapy. To stop the growth of *Candida albicans* (*Monilia albicans* is the term some prefer) applications in the vagina are used for 1 week or longer. One of the following effective preparations in tablet, cream, or gel can be used: (1) nystatin, (2) clotrimazole, (3) chlordantoin, (4) candicidin, (5) proprionic acid and salts, (6) gentian violet, or (7) miconazole. A 5% gentian violet solution may be applied by the physician; however, the occasional marked reaction to this preparation has decreased its popularity. Application of 0.5% hydrocortisone cream to the vulva usually gives symptomatic relief. Plain water or acid douches usually give temporary comfort. Investigation to ascertain whether the patient has diabetes mellitus is important in nonpregnant patients. Glucose tolerance tests are needed to diagnose preclinical diabetes. With proper diabetic management candidiasis is usually successfully treated.

Elimination of candida in the intestine by oral nystatin and elimination of infection from the male may be required to prevent recurrence.

Nonspecific vaginitis

When trichomoniasis, moniliasis, and gonorrhea are not diagnosed, some physicians use the term "nonspecific vaginitis." There is considerable variation in the vagina's appearance and in the amount of vaginal discharge. Colposcopic findings may elicit acute and subacute inflammatory changes. Smears reveal an increase in the concentration of bacteria. Many patients with nonspecific vaginitis respond to the application of triple sulfonamide creams. Some patients exhibit a mucopurulent discharge from the cervix that may respond to oral administration of tetracycline; these patients may harbor *Chlamydia*.

A number of patients diagnosed as having nonspecific vaginitis have previously been considered to have *Haemophilus vaginitis*. This organism has recently been renamed *Gardnerella*. Some patients without symptoms have *Gardnerella* organisms in their vaginas. Cultures of this organism are not commonly done; diagnosis has been mainly made when squamous cells have large numbers of adhering bacteria ("Clue cells"). Local applications of sulfonamides and local or systemic administration of tetracyclines have failed to eradicate *Gardnerella* organisms in the majority of patients. Metronidazole has been found to be effective and to relieve symptoms in symptomatic patients.

Senile vaginitis

Postmenopausal atrophy of the vagina renders it less resistant to trauma and infection. Ulcerations of the thin epithelium, if on opposing surfaces, may result in adhesions. Early these are easily broken to separate the walls but, if left undisturbed, become firm and may partially obliterate the vagina.

Trichomoniasis, candidiasis, *Gardnerella* (formerly called *Haemophilus*) vaginitis, and nonspecific bacterial infection may involve the vulnerable senile mucosa. In addition to the specific therapy for these conditions, estrogen stimulation by local and, at times, oral means must be used. It is essential that estrogens be continued until mucosal resistance is adequate and all inflammation is gone.

Gonorrheal vaginitis

Neisseria gonorrhoeae, when placed on the vaginal mucosa, may after a few days cause an acute inflammatory reaction. In the adult the delicate mucous membranes of the urethra, vulvovaginal glands, and endocervix are the sites of most marked reaction. When the profuse yellow discharge exudes over the vulva, burning, pruritus, and tenderness may be pronounced. Dysuria and frequency indicate urethral reaction. If a vulvovaginal abscess develops, pain is severe and tumefaction occurs.

Extension is primarily along and just beneath the mucous membranes. In children and postmenopausal women infection rarely extends beyond the cervix; however, during and following menstruation acute endometritis and salpingitis may occur unless treatment has been adequate. Although extension is characteristically along the mucosa, bacteremia can occur with gonorrhal arthritis and endocarditis, the most likely types of distant focal infections. The bacteria may be carried by the hands or on fomites to the eye and cause a severe conjunctivitis.

Diagnosis. In children any purulent vaginal discharge should routinely be examined by gram-stained smears and culture. Many women tolerate the annoyance or discomfort of lower genital tract gonorrhea and wait until the acute pain of salpingitis compels them to seek the aid of a physician. Women often act as asymptomatic carriers. In surveys of large groups of women 80% of those with positive cultures for the gonococcus are found to be asymptomatic.

Accurate diagnosis requires identification of the diplococci. Smears made by expressing pus from the endocervix or urethra in acute cases reveal many intracellular gram-negative organisms without the variety of secondary invaders that commonly obscure the other organisms in smears of vaginal leukorrhea. During the incubation period (3 to 14 days) and in patients with chronic cervictis and urethritis, smears usually are not diagnostic. In subacute and chronic cases cultures and repeated examinations are needed for diagnosis. Material should be obtained from the endocervix and the anus for culture. Special culture media that contain substances to suppress the growth of irrelevant bacteria, such as Thayer Martin media containing vancomycin, colistin, and nystatin, should be used. This type of medium can be supplied in closed bottles containing carbon dioxide so that this delicate organism can be transported from the examining room to the laboratory. Fluorescent antibody techniques provide rapid and more effective identification in direct smears or in smears from early cultures.

In acute cases one should carefully search for chancre or condylomata lata. This is particularly true because penicillin is often used and may cause these syphilitic lesions to heal rapidly and yet not be sufficient to eradicate the spirochetes. Frequently other venereal diseases are found in the woman with gonorrhea.

The person from whom the disease was contracted should be tactfully sought, and, if found, he should be treated. The coital partner is best treated prophylactically.

Therapy. Penicillin is the treatment of choice if the patient is not sensitized. A high concentration of penicillin is needed over a short period. Procaine penicillin G should be used as a single does of 4.8 million units. For a patient who cannot tolerate penicillin, tetracycline should be administered, utilizing 1.5 grams for the first dose and 0.5 gram every 6 hours for five more doses. If syphilis is present with gonoorhea, additional long-acting penicillin or prolonged treatment with tetracycline must be provided, since cure of syphilis requires adequate blood levels for 10 days or more.

Chronic cervicitis, skenitis, or bartholinitis may require excision or destruction of involved tissues.

The criteria of cure include (1) lack of clinical evidence of disease after five monthly examinations, (2) three or more cervical cultures that are negative, and (3) absence of infection in the male sexual partner.

Gonorrhea in children usually responds to antibiotics. Rarely estrogenic stimulation may be needed to increase vaginal resistance.

Reaction to foreign bodies

In children, foreign bodies in the vagina should be searched for as a cause of vaginitis. Rectal palpation and vaginal inspection through an infant proctoscope or Kelly urethroscope can be used. In adults "forgotten" or "neglected" pessaries, diaphragms, or tampons may be the causes.

Chemical reactions of vagina

Reaction may occur as a result of therapeutic or contraceptive agents applied. Concentrated gentian violet and particles of potassium permanganate tablets are common offenders. Severe hemorrhage caused by such tablets used to attempt abortion has been more commonly seen.

TUMORS

Cysts of the vagina in anterolateral locations are usually Gartner's duct cysts. The cysts found in the outer third of the posterior vaginal wall are usually inclusion cysts. Since these cysts have no ostia, infection rarely occurs and they rarely cause symptoms.

Solid, nontender masses are usually myomas or fibromas. Benign vaginal tumors can be cured by complete excision.

Adenosis has been found in teenagers who were exposed to diethylstilbestrol while a fetus. The ectopic columnar epithelium in the vagina presents as marked cervical ectopia and, in some, as separate areas of the upper vagina best seen with the colposcope. Rarely clear cell adenocarcinoma is associated.

Primary malignant tumors of the vagina are very rare. Squamous cell carcinoma can occur. Secondary cancers are more often found. These metastatic growths may have spread from carcinoma of the cervix, adenocarcinoma of the endometrium, or choriocarcinoma. If therapy is surgical, it should be extensive excision (exenteration). Radiation is more commonly used.

A urethral diverticulum usually appears as a tender cystic mass beneath the urethra. Enlargement causes it to lie between the bladder and vagina. With infection its urethral opening may be closed, so that its contents cannot be expressed. Small diverticula or those with adequate urethral openings may not appear as masses and can be found by urethrography. Recurrent, unexplained urethritis may occur when a small diverticulum is present. Consequently such patients should be investigated. Cure results from complete excision.

FISTULAS

Vesicovaginal fistulas allow constant or intermittent leakage of urine into the vagina. Surgical trauma is now their most common cause. This cause can be eliminated by recognition and repair of bladder injury when it occurs. Formerly, obstetric injuries (operation, prolonged dystocia, and infection) were common cases. Sloughing of carcinoma with or without radiation may cause fistulas. *Urethrovaginal* fistulas are most often caused by surgical injury. *Ureterovaginal* fistulas are usually caused by surgical injury or postoperative ischemia. They have become more common with the increased performance of the Wertheim hysterectomy and lymphatic resections. *Ureterocervical* or *vesicocervical* fistulas may occur from surgical injury or malignancies, and urine escapes from the cervix (Fig. 5-2). Vesicouterine fistulas after cesarean section result in some loss of menstrual blood through the bladder but usually no loss of urine through the cervix.

For diagnosis, cystoscopy and ureterography are essential. Small fistulas of recent origin may heal spontaneously. In the absence of malignancy and severe radiation injury, most can be repaired by adequate mobilization and primary suture. Ureteral fistulas may require reimplantation of the ureter into the bladder. If renal damage is extensive, nephrectomy may be required.

Rectovaginal fistulas allow escape of gas, liquid stool, or feces into the vagina. Surgical and obstetric injuries are the most common causes. Surgical repair is usually successful.

Colovaginal fistulas may develop after pelvic abscess from diverticular infection of the sigmoid colon and appear in the posthysterectomy scar of the vagina. Separation and repair of the colon provides cure.

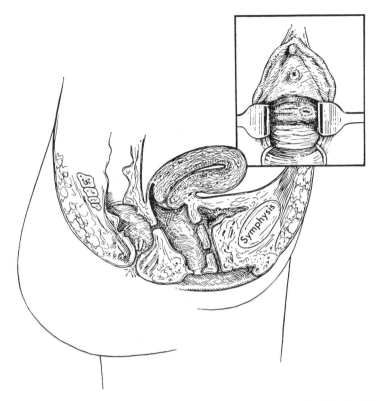

Fig. 5-2. Sagittal section illustrates urethrovaginal vesicovaginal, and rectovaginal fistulas. The inset depicts the vaginal opening of a fistula that proved to be ureterovaginal.

The time to repair genital fistulas of traumatic origin that are too large for spontaneous healing to be expected is governed by the period required for associated tissue inflammation to subside. With proper antibacterial agents and the use of synthetic adrenal corticoids, this period is shortened.

Proper hemostasis and adequate mobilization of tissues to avoid excessive tension of sutures are required. After repair of vesicovaginal fistulas, the bladder must be kept constantly empty with an indwelling catheter to avoid tension on suture lines until healing is adequate.

LACERATION AND RELAXATION OF PELVIC OUTLET

The pubococcygeal portions of the levator ani muscles with their fasciae are the principal supports of the pelvic outlet. The transverse perineal muscles and the fascia of the urogenital diaphragm are located superficial to the levator muscles and add support. The bulbocavernous muscles are superficial to the vestibular bulbs and act as constrictors of the introitus.

These supporting structures normally maintain the introitus and lower vagina in a position sufficiently anterior so that the vaginal axis is as shown in Fig. 1-1. When the upper vagina and cervix are held sufficiently posterior, the resulting effect is that intra-abdominal pressures are not transmitted in the axis of the vagina, i.e., through the vaginal lumen.

Lacerations may infrequently occur with direct accidental trauma or with rape; however, parturition is the common cause. Difficult or improper forceps extractions, precipitate delivery, and failure of adequate repair are the principal factors. Episiotomy should be used to prevent lacerations. Women with excellent obstetric care seldom develop outlet relaxation.

The extent of perineal laceration is classified as first-degree when only the mucosa and superficial connective tissue are involved. With second-degree tears the perineal body muscles are interrupted. Third-degree extent indicates laceration through the anal sphincters.

Trauma that injures the perineal body can also result in tears in the pubococcygeus muscles and urogenital diaphragm lateral to the vagina. Repeated delivery tends to cause lengthening of the vaginal outlet supports because of stretching without obvious tears. Lack of exercise can lead to attenuation and weakness of muscles.

When the introitus is enlarged, there is less support for the vaginal walls, and the patient may notice the sensation of "something falling out." Indeed intra-abdominal pressure is transmitted more directly toward the orifice, and with time protrusion of the anterior or posterior vaginal wall can result. Coitus is likely to be less pleasurable for both participants.

Exercise of the bulbocavernosus and pubococcygeus muscles, performed regularly for several weeks, can result in better support if the unrepaired tears were not too deep. When a considerable portion of the perineal body has been lost, perineorrhaphy is in order; however, it is usually done at the time of a future delivery or in conjunction with other genital surgery.

Complete perineal (third-degree) tear results in fecal incontinence. In modern obstetrics third-degree tears are repaired immediately and usually heal well. Delayed repair is similarly successful.

Vaginal relaxations

As indicated previously, the posterior and lateral portions of the lower vagina are supported by the same structures as the pelvic outlet. It should be particularly noted that the perineal body supports the lowermost 4 or 5 cm of the vagina. Anteriorly the lower vaginal wall is fused with the supports of the lower urethra, which are the urogenital diaphragm, deep transverse perineal muscles, and some fibers from the bulbocavernosus muscles. The upper vagina is fused with the cervix

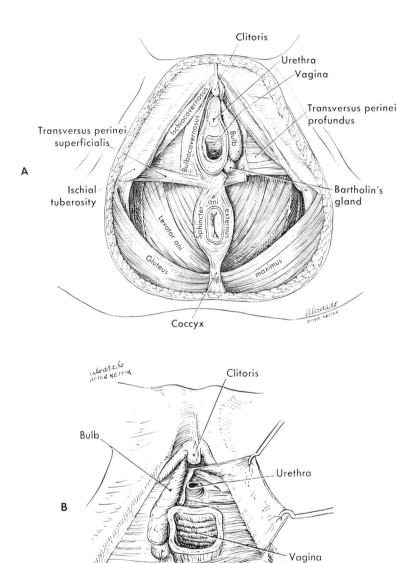

Fig. 5-3. The muscles of the pelvic outlet are shown as viewed from below.

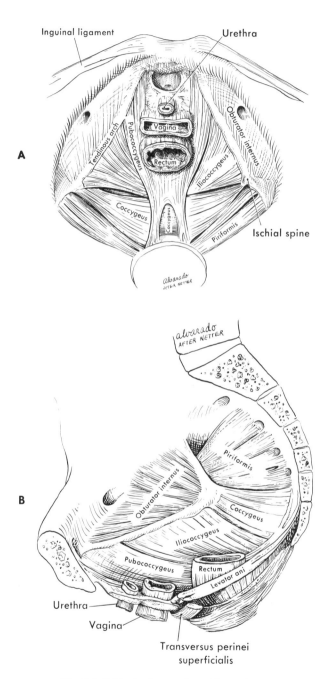

Fig. 5-4. Pelvic diaphragm viewed from above.

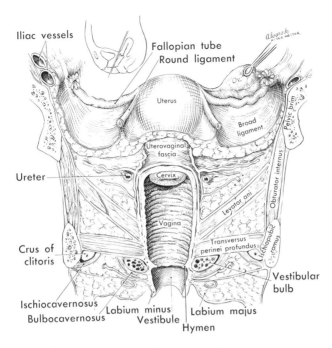

Iliac vessels

Fallopian tube
Round ligament

Uterus

Broad
ligament

Pelvic brim

Uterovaginal
fascia

Cervix

Ureter

Obturator internus

Levator ani

Vagina

Ischiopubic ramus

Crus of
clitoris

Transversus
perinei profundus

Vestibular
bulb

Ischiocavernosus
Bulbocavernosus
Labium minus
Vestibule
Hymen
Labium majus

Fig. 5-5. Ligaments and fascial support of the vagina and cervix.

and is supported anteriorly and laterally by the lower portions of the cardinal ligaments, whereas posteriorly the uterosacral ligaments are of major importance. These ligaments are condensations of endopelvic connective tissue, which also continues downward as part of the vaginal wall. Anteriorly this strong tissue is attached to the pubic bones and has been popularly termed pubocervical fascia.

Cystocele

When the portion of the vaginal wall that is between the cervix and the urethra and the base of the bladder adjacent (but not densely adherent) to it herniate inferiorly, a cystocele is formed. The defect in the anterior vaginal wall is caused by trauma, usually obstetric, or by an inherent weakness that is most likely to be manifest postmenopausally when estrogen is lacking.

With small cystoceles no symptoms result. A large herniation may cause a sensation of pressure in the vagina or present as a mass at or through the introitus. If the bladder herniates far enough, residual urine may lead to cystitis.

Urethrocele

Urethrocele is recognized by finding inferiorly a bulging of the anterior wall adjacent to the urethra. A cystocele is likely to be associated; however, often cystoceles develop with little or no urethrocele formation.

Should the support of the upper urethra be sufficiently involved, the base of the bladder will rotate posteriorly and inferiorly away from the symphysis pubis, so that (1) the urethrovesical junction is the lowest portion of the bladder and (2) the posterior angle formed by the urethra and the trigone of the bladder is lost. Stress incontinence (with coughing, sneezing, laughing, or straining) commonly develops under such conditions. Cystograms made during straining reveal funneling of the upper urethra and more descent of the bladder base than is normal. Cinefluorographic records of the normal bladder and urethra, as well as motion pictures demonstrating stress incontinence, allow the observer to better understand bladder function. Real-time ultrasonography allows the physician to see the urethra's motion.

As indicated in the previous paragraph, stress incontinence of urine occurs with sudden increases in intra-abdominal pressure. Urge incontinence is the involuntary loss of urine after the desire to void has been felt. At times there is a combination of these types of incontinence. Urge incontinence is more likely to occur with cystitis and urethritis, and it indicates the necessity for proper urinalysis and, at times, for visualization of the urethra and bladder by endoscopy. Patients with diseases or injury that affects the nerve supply of the bladder are subject to incontinence. With upper motor neuron lesions the bladder is hypotonic. Coarse bladder trabeculation occurs along with large amounts of residual urine after voiding. With lower motor neuron lesions a hypotonic bladder develops with a large bladder capacity. Some patients have an unstable bladder (detrusor dyssynergia), and a sudden increase in abdominal pressure is apt to trigger bladder contraction in these patients; incontinence may result. This short discussion is given to emphasize that anatomic disturbance discovered at examination, particularly without endoscopy, even with a careful history of incontinence, may not be sufficient to decide on the advisability of surgical suspension of the proximal urethra and bladder.

Rectocele

Herniation of the anterior rectal wall and the posterior vaginal wall may present as an intravaginal mass at the introitus or through the introitus. Weakness of the involved walls results from the same causes as indicated for cystocele.

A sensation of pressure in the vagina, a protruding mass, or difficulty emptying the rectum may occur. If a firm fecal mass is in the anterior rectal hernial pouch, the woman may at times use her fingers to reduce the rectocele and direct the mass toward the anus to allow defecation.

Therapy

Obstetric trauma or attenuation of pelvic fasciae, muscles, and ligaments commonly involves the outlet; the vaginal, vesical, and rectal walls; and the uterus simultaneously, so that relaxation of the outlet, cystocele, rectocele, urethrocele, and uterine prolapse often occur at the same time.

Minor relaxations of the vaginal outlet may be corrected by proper exercises. Stress incontinence can be cured in many cases if the exercises are properly performed and continued. The patient must be instructed by the physician's placing his fingers on the muscles to be exercised and having the patient identify them by contracting the muscles being palpated. A perineometer (Kegel) may be used to determine improvement in the strength of contraction of the vaginal constrictors. When exercises fail to give relief and when the herniations are marked, surgical correction is justified. With minor anatomic changes and no associated disturbance of bladder or anorectal function, surgery is not justified. When stress incontinence is the principal complaint, urethroscopy and cystoscopy along with cystometrograms and urethrometrograms should be done before colporrhaphy or retropubic vesicourethral suspension lest vesical polyps, calculi, infection, or neurologic dysfunction be overlooked.

Anterior colporrhaphy is accomplished (1) by separating the anterior vaginal wall from the bladder and urethra, (2) by placing sutures in the bladder wall to reduce its herniation and in the paraurethral tissue (urogenital diaphragm and voluntary muscle fibers) to reduce the urethrocele (additional sutures being placed to bring additional support under the posterior urethra and neck of the bladder), and (3) by excising the excess (thinned out) vaginal wall before its closure. If vaginal hysterectomy has been done, the uterosacral ligaments and/or the cervical portion of the cardinal ligaments should be sutured to the anterior vaginal wall to add support.

If the region of the internal sphincter of the urethra is adequately elevated, the stress incontinence is usually cured. When a cystocele is repaired without adequate repair of the support of the posterior urethra, stress incontinence may begin even though it was not previously present.

Should the posterior rotation of the bladder not be corrected by colporrhaphy or should there be little cystocele, retropubic urethrovesicopexy may be used to relieve the incontinence of urine. This suspension may be accomplished by suturing the paraurethral tissues and bladder to the periosteum of the pubes (Marshall and associates) or by placing a sling of rectus abdominis fascia beneath the urethra (Aldridge).

Posterior colporrhaphy for rectocele is performed in a manner similar to that used for anterior colporrhaphy, as regards separation and independent repair of the rectum and vagina. Perineorrhaphy is essential to give support to the lowermost part of the posterior vaginal wall and should include approximation of the levator ani muscles in the midline.

Enterocele (posterior vaginal hernia)

Enterocele, a type of hernia, is an extension of the cul-de-sac as a peritoneal sac between the rectum and vagina and may contain omentum, small intestine, or the sigmoid colon. The two types of enterocele are as follows:
1. The rare congenital type in which the sac extends down to the perineal body
2. The acquired type that either presents as a bulge into the upper posterior vagina, usually above a rectocele, or is associated with vaginal prolapse occurring after hysterectomy

The symptoms are a pressure sensation in the vagina or a mass appearing at or through the introitus.

The surgical correction must obliterate the peritoneal sac and utilize the uterosacral ligaments as support. The approach is usually vaginal as other repair is needed. With vaginal prolapse after hysterectomy, colpectomy may be done if coitus is no longer desired. When the vagina is to be preserved and the cardinal and uterosacral ligaments are inadequate, fascial strips from the anterior abdominal wall may be attached to the deepest portion of the vagina as the principal support.

SELECTED REFERENCES

Aldridge, A.H.: Transplantation of fascia for relief of urinary stress incontinence, Am. J. Obstet. Gynecol. 44:398, 1942.

Alter, R.L., Jones, C.P., and Carter, B.: The treatment of mycotic vulvovaginitis with propionate vaginal jelly, Am. J. Obstet. Gynecol. 53:241, 1947.

Burch, J.C.: Urethrovaginal fixation to Cooper's ligament for correction of stress incontinence, cystocele and prolapse, Am. J. Obstet. Gynecol. 81:281, 1961.

Burch, T.A., Rees, C.W., and Reardon, L.: Diagnosis of trichomonas vaginalis vaginitis, Am. J. Obstet. Gynecol. 77:903, 1959.

Counseller, V.S., and Haigler, F.H., Jr.: Management of urinary-vaginal fistula in 253 cases, Am. J. Obstet. Gynecol. 72:367, 1956.

Gardner, H.L.: *Haemophilus vaginalis* vaginitis after twenty-five years, Am. J. Obstet. Gynecol. 137:385, 1980.

Gardner, H.L., and Dukes, C.D.: Haemophilus vaginalis vaginitis, Am. J. Obstet. Gynecol. 69:962, 1955.

Goldstein, L.Z.: Gonorrhea in female contacts, Obstet. Gynecol. 6:193, 1955.

Green, Thomas H.,Jr.: Development of a plan for the diagnosis and treatment of urinary stress incontinence, Am. J. Obstet. Gynecol. 83:632, 1962.

Gunning, J.E., and Ostergard, D.R.: Value of screening procedures for the detection of vaginal adenosis, Obstet. Gynecol. 47:268, 1976.

Herbst, A.L., Kurman, R.J., and Scully, R.E.: Vaginal and cervical abnormalities after exposure to stilbesterol in utero, Obstet. Gynecol. 40:287, 1972.

Hodgkinson, C.P.: Relationships of the female urethra and bladder in urinary stress incontinence, Am. J. Obstet. Gynecol. 65:560, 1953.

Hutch, J.A.: Anatomy and physiology of the bladder, trigone and urethra, New York, 1972, Appleton-Century-Crofts.

Jones, C.P., Thomas, W.L., and Parker, R.T.: Treatment of vaginal trichomoniasis with metronidazole, a new nitroimidazole compound, Am. J. Obstet. Gynecol. 83:498, 1962.

Kean, B.H.: Urethral trichomoniasis in the female, Am. J. Obstet. Gynecol. 70:397, 1955.

Kegel, A.H.: Physiologic therapy for urinary stress incontinence, J.A.M.A. 146:915, 1951.

Kennedy, W.T.: Urinary incontinence relieved by restoration and maintenance of the normal position of the urethra, Am. J. Obstet. Gynecol. **41**:16, 1941.

Latzko, W.: Postoperative vesicovaginal fistulas, Am. J. Surg. **58**:211, 1942.

Lund, C.J., Benjamin, J.A., Tristan, T.A., Fullerton, R.E., Ramsey, G.H., and Watson, J.S.: Cinefluorographic studies of the bladder and urethra in women, Am. J. Obstet. Gynecol. **74**:896, 1957.

Mark, J.E., Jr., and Lester, A.: Transgrow, a medium for transport and growth of Neisseria gonorrhoeae and Neisseria meningititis, HSMA Health Report **86(1)**:30, 1971.

Marks, H.J.: A double-blind comparison of clotrimazole and nystatin vaginal tablets in Candida vaginitis, Postgrad. Med. J. (Suppl. 1) **50**:105, 1974.

Marshall, V.F., Marchetti, A., and Krantz, K.E.: Correction of stress incontinence by simple vesicourethral suspension, Surg. Gynecol. Obstet. **88**:509, 1949.

Mendell, E., and Haberman, S.: The vaginal ecology and its relationship to symptoms in vaginitis, South Med. J. **58**:374, 1965.

Mengert, W.F.: Vesicovaginal fistula: principles of closure, Am. J. Obstet. Gynecol. **84**:1213, 1962.

Mitchell, G.W., Jr.: Cystometry in the evaluation of urinary incontinence, Clin. Obstet. Gynecol. **1**:678, 1958.

Ostergard, D.R.: The effect of drugs on the lower urinary tract, Obstet. Gynecol. Surg. **34**:424, 1979.

Ostergard, D.R., and McCarthy, T.A.: Diagnostic procedures in female urology, Am. J. Obstet. Gynecol. **137**:401, 1980.

Pace, H.R., and Schantz, S.I.: Nystatin (Mycostatin) in the treatment of monilial and nonmonilial vaginitis, J.A.M.A. **162**:268, 1956.

Peters, W.A., and Thornton, W.N.: Selection of the primary operative procedure for stress urinary incontinence, Am. J. Obstet. Gynecol. **137**:8, 1980.

Phaneuf, L.E.: Genital fistulas in women, life of J. Marion Sims and the history of vesicovaginal fistula—management of rectovaginal fistulas and complete tears of the perineum, Am. J. Surg. **64**:3, 1944.

Pickhardt, W.L., and Breen, J.L.: Identification of and therapy for vaginal candidiasis, Am. J. Obstet. Gynecol. **74**:42, 1957.

Robertson, J.R.: Urethroscopy—the neglected gynecologic procedure, Clin. Obstet. Gynecol. **19**:315, 1976.

Seth, A.: Use of trimethoprim to prevent growth of proteus in the cultivation of N. gonorrhoeae, Br. J. Vener. Dis. **46**:201, 1970.

Smith, F.R.: Primary carcinoma of the vagina, Am. J. Obstet. Gynecol. **69**:525, 1955.

Stanton, S.L., and Cardozo, L.D.: Results of colposuspension operation for incontinence and prolapse, Br. J. Obstet. Gynecol. **56**:693, 1979.

Trussell, R.: Trichomonas vaginalis and trichomoniasis, Springfield, Ill., 1947, Charles C Thomas, Publisher.

Ullery, J.C.: Stress incontinence in the female, New York, 1953, Grune & Stratton, Inc.

Wharton, L.R., and TeLinde, R.W.: Urethral diverticulum, Obstet. Gynecol. **7**:503, 1956.

Chapter 6

MALPOSITIONS OF THE UTERUS

ANATOMY

The uterus is situated at about the center of the pelvic cavity with the body of the organ inclined forward and the long axis of the organ directed to a point about the symphysis pubis. The direction varies in different persons and in the same person at different times. The uterus is not fixed in one position but can be moved easily in all directions—upward, downward, forward, or laterally. It is pressed backward in the pelvis when the bladder is distended and somewhat forward when the upper part of the rectum is distended.

It is seen therefore that the uterus possesses normally a considerable range of mobility, and it is only when it is found beyond the normal range that it can be said to be malplaced.

What holds the uterus in normal positions? The uterus is held in normal positions by (1) the pelvic floor, (2) the broad ligaments (the most important portions of which are the cardinal ligaments), (3) the uterosacral ligaments, (4) the round ligaments, and (5) the normal tone and position of the adjacent pelvic structures.

MALPOSITIONS
Retroplacement

Backward placement of the uterus occurs in two forms—retroversion and retroflexion. In *retroversion* the uterine corpus is tilted (turned) backward and the cervix points forward. In *retroflexion* the body of the uterus is bent backward with little or no change in the position of the cervix.

Etiology. Retroplacements may be developmental, physiologic, or pathologic.

1. Congenital (In about 20% of women the uterus fails to migrate to the usual anterior position.)
2. Pregnancy and delivery (During the first few weeks after delivery 40% of the patients may be found to have retroplacements. If sufficient damage to ligaments has occurred or if the position is congenital, this position may persist.)

   3. Uterine fixation may develop because of
      a. Adhesions of peritonitis
      b. Endometriosis
      c. Pelvic cancer
   4. Displacement can occur with
      a. Distended urinary bladder
      b. Uterine myoma
      c. Ovarian tumor

Symptoms. No symptoms occur in most patients with congenital or postpartum retroplacement. Very seldom does this malposition interfere with conception. Rarely incarceration of the enlarging uterus during pregnancy below the sacral promontory may lead to urinary retention and/or abortion.

Dyspareunia on deep penetration may occur with the ovaries in the cul-de-sac. Pressure in the pelvis and backache can be associated with or without uterine fixation. (See discussion on trial of pessary.) Because of the multiple causes of these symptoms, ascribing them to placement of the uterus can be properly done only after thorough investigations over a period of months. The significance of associated uterine and ovarian varicosities must be considered.

Diagnosis. The degrees of retroplacement are shown in Fig. 6-1. The direction of the cervical axis can indicate the possible position of the corpus, but to be certain palpation must be done.

Determination of uterine mobility is essential to indicate the causes and management. If the uterus is fixed, the associated disease is more likely to be the significant disorder. If the uterus can be placed anteriorly by the manipulations shown in Fig. 6-2, and no other cause for the symptoms is found, a pessary should be inserted to hold the uterus anteriorly (Fig. 6-3). If the patient is relieved with

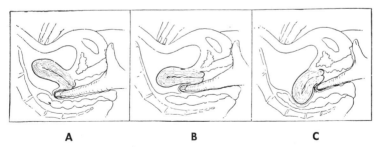

A   **B**   **C**

Fig. 6-1. A, First-degree retroplacement. The corpus uteri is out of reach of the examining fingers, both above and below. **B,** Second-degree retroplacement. Vaginal fingers feel posterior wall of corpus uteri extending directly back. **C,** Third-degree retroplacement. Vaginal fingers impinge on corpus uteri turned down into the posterior cul-de-sac.

From Crossen, R.J.: Diseases of women, St. Louis, C.V. Mosby Co.

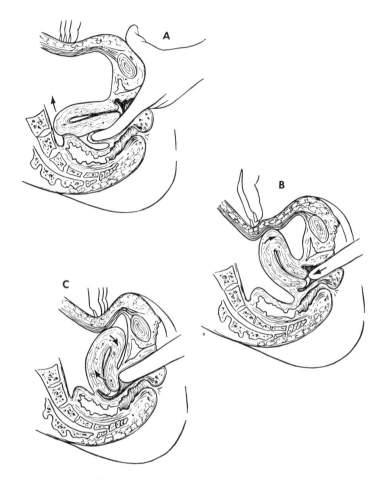

Fig. 6-2. Manual placement of uterus. **A,** Attempting to raise the uterus to determine whether or not it is fixed. This is also the first step in bimanual placement of the uterus. **B,** Bringing the fundus forward and pushing the cervix backward and upward. **C,** Uterus brought forward into position. The diagram also shows the method of taking the backward flexion out of the uterus by bending it firmly over the vaginal fingers.

the pessary in place for 1 month, it is then removed. Should backache or other discomfort return, the pessary is replaced to determine whether relief is again obtained. Observation of this trial with and without the pessary indicates the advisability of its continued use or the rare need for hysteropexy.

Therapy. The pessary may be used in some patients. Should pregnancy occur, the pessary is left in the vagina until the uterus becomes too large to return to the hollow of the sacrum.

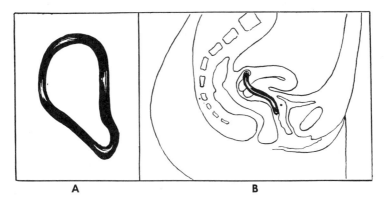

Fig. 6-3. A, Albert Smith pessary. **B,** Pessary in place to hold the posterior vaginal fornix, and with it the attached cervix, well backward and upward in the pelvis.

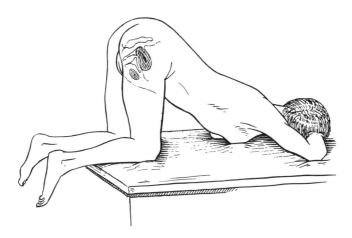

Fig. 6-4. Knee-chest position: thighs perpendicular, chest on bed, knees 1 foot apart.

The knee-chest position (Fig. 6-4) may bring the uterus forward temporarily. Sleeping on the abdomen may aid in the return of the uterus to an anterior position, particularly during the first 6 postpartum weeks. When the uterus appears to be incarcerated the patient should stand on her head with assistance. This maneuver will succeed, particularly for the enlarged, gravid uterus, when other methods have failed.

Hysteropexy is rarely justified as a primary procedure. More often suspension should be done to hold anteriorly a liberated uterus that had been fixed posteriorly by endometriosis or adhesions caused by infections. Plication of the uterosacral ligaments and shortening of the round ligaments by drawing them through the internal inguinal rings and suturing them to the anterior rectus sheath is the most popular method.

Prolapse

Prolapse of the uterus is that condition in which the uterus sinks decidedly below its normal level in the pelvis. It is known also as procidentia uteri and is frequently referred to by the patient as "falling of the womb."

In the usual case of prolapse the uterus is found retroplaced, the pelvic floor is lacerated, and chronic cervicitis is present. The vaginal walls are relaxed and thrown into folds by the uterine position and may project outward at the introitus as an anterior or posterior colpocele. Cystocele and rectocele are usually associated.

Ulcers of the cervix are likely to appear with third-degree prolapse because of irritation of clothing and interference with circulation. Persistent edema and recurrent ulceration with associated infection may lead to fibrosis and thickening of the prolapsed vaginal wall. All of the ligaments of the uterus are stretched until they give practically no support, and the lower pelvis is occupied by the intestines instead of the reproductive organs. Coils of intestine may lie in the cul-de-sac outside the introitus, forming a posterior cul-de-sac hernia.

Prolapse may occur in nulligravidas. Postmenopausal atrophy of pelvic ligaments and other tissues dependent on estrogen stimulation causes an increased rate of uterine descent; therefore conditions of second- and third-degree prolapse are more common in older women. Estrogen administration may reduce the degree of prolapse in some patients.

Etiology. The trauma of parturition and the atrophy of the cardinal and uterosacral ligaments are the main causes for prolapse. The cervix may elongate in older women, so that the upper vagina descends while the body of the uterus remains in almost normal position.

The uterus normally has considerable up and down movement. Respiration causes movement of the uterus, which is noticeable during the speculum examination, especially with the patient in the Sims position.

There may be considerable exaggeration of the usual downward placement without any symptoms, and that could hardly be called pathologic. The condition is not called prolapse unless there is marked downward placement, which is almost always accompanied by backward placement of the uterus. The cervix may elongate, so that the external os presents at the introitus while the corpus is near its normal position.

If the cervix is still well within the vagina, the condition is designated as pro-

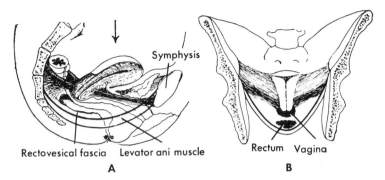

Symphysis

Rectovesical fascia   Levator ani muscle

Rectum   Vagina

A   B

Fig. 6-5. A, Upper and lower diaphragms of the pelvis with the sling action shown anteroposteriorly. In the upper diaphragm the anteroposterior sling is formed by the uterosacral ligaments posteriorly and the uteropubic fascial plane anteriorly. In the lower diaphragm the anteroposterior sling is formed by the levator ani muscles and surrounding fasciae, with supplementary muscles in front and behind. Also indicated in the diagram is the deflecting action of the corpus uteri, which receives the intra-abdominal pressure upon its posterior surface and distributes it toward the margins of the supporting diaphragm. **B,** Upper and lower diaphragms of the pelvis with the sling action shown transversely. In the upper diaphragm the transverse sling is formed by the broad ligaments, particularly by the strong supporting structures forming the lower portion of the broad ligaments. In the lower diaphragm the transverse sling is formed by the levator ani muscles and surrounding fasciae.

From Crossen, H.S., and Crossen, R.J.: Operative gynecology, St. Louis, The C.V. Mosby Co.

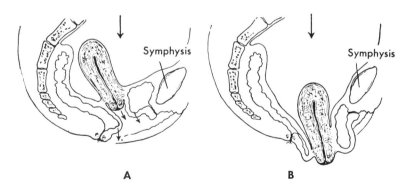

Symphysis   Symphysis

A   B

Fig. 6-6. A, Disarrangement of the deflecting mechanism by retroplacement of the corpus uteri, accompanied by relaxation of the pelvic floor. In the presence of such conditions the development of prolapse is ordinarily only a question of time, for there is no adequate resistance to intra-abdominal pressure. **B,** Prolapse of uterus and bladder. The intra-abdominal pressure tends to push the structures farther and farther out of the pelvis.

From Crossen, H.S., and Crossen, R.J.: Operative gynecology, St. Louis, The C.V. Mosby Co.

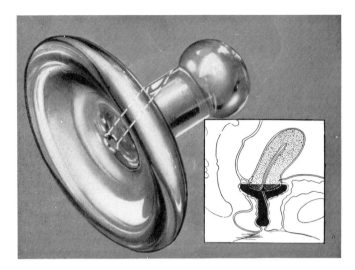

Fig. 6-7. Blair modification of the Gellhorn pessary.

Courtesy A.S. Aloe Co.

lapse of the *first degree*. If the cervix protrudes from the vaginal orifice, it is classed as *second-degree*. If the uterus lies outside the pelvis, it is called *third-degree* or complete prolapse.

Symptoms. Since descent is gradual, symptoms are usually of gradual onset. Many patients become accustomed to a protruding mass and seek advice only because of fear of a tumor. A sensation of something falling out and mild aching pain may be present. Often the accompanying cystocele and/or rectocele produce the most annoying symptoms.

Therapy. Palliative measures include the clearing of local inflammation by cleansing douches, and the administration of local or systemic estrogens, and the use of pessaries to hold the uterus within the pelvis. If enough of the pelvic floor is present to support a pessary, one of the Gellhorn, "doughnut," or "bee cell" type may be introduced (Fig. 6-7). Pessaries of these types obstruct the outlet, whereas pessaries used for maintaining the uterus in an anterior position do so by placing the posterior fornix and cervix backward and upward.

Curative measures require surgery. Usually definitive therapy can be done in a postmenopausal patient or in one who has completed her childbearing. Vaginal hysterectomy, partial obliteration of the cul-de-sac, colporrhaphy, and perineorrhaphy are in order. With complete procidentia, colporrhaphy may require decreasing the size of the vagina. After proper approximation the uterosacral and cardinal ligaments are used to support the vaginal cuff and posterior fornix. The Manchester operation (cervical amputation with plication of the cervical portion of the cardinal ligaments) and the Le Fort operation (colpocleisis) are seldom used in most areas of the United States. If childbearing is to continue, an operation is best deferred until the desired number of children have been born.

Inversion

Inversion of the uterus is more commonly of the acute type that occurs as a complication of the third stage of labor, and the organ can usually be manually replaced. Chronic inversion may occur because a submucous myoma pulls the fundus through the cervix. Vaginal hysterectomy is usually required for chronic inversion.

SELECTED REFERENCES

Bell, J.E., Jr., Wilson, G.F., and Wilson, L.O.: Puerperal inversion of the uterus, Am. J. Obstet. Gynecol. **66**:767, 1953.

Conger, G.T., and Keetel, W.C.: The Manchester-Fothergill operation, its place in gynecology, Am. J. Obstet. Gynecol. **76**:634, 1958.

Gilliam, D.T.: Round ligament ventrosuspension of the uterus, Am. J. Obstet. **41**:299, 1900.

Javert, C.T.: Combined procedure for anteroversion of retroverted uteri, Am. J. Obstet. Gynecol. **52**:865, 1946.

Kennedy, J.W., and Campbell, A.D.: Vaginal hysterectomy, Philadelphia, 1944, F.A.Davis Co.

Mattingly, R.F.: Te Linde's operative gynecology, Philadelphia, 1977, J.B. Lippincott, Co.

Stearns, H.C.: Surgical treatment of prolapsus uteri, West J. Surg. **63**:420, 1955.

Taylor, E.S., McCallin, P.F., and Snow, R.H.: Results of vaginal hysterectomy; immediately and two and one-half to seven years after operation, Am. J. Obstet. Gynecol. **68**:428, 1954.

Chapter 7

PELVIC INFECTIONS

Pelvic bacterial inflammatory diseases are considered by physicians according to the clinical situations in which they develop. In the coitally active woman without evidence of pregnancy, recent surgery, neoplasm, or genital trauma, salpingitis is the most likely disease. In early pregnancy with uterine bleeding after intrauterine manipulation or with rupture of the amnion, the evidences of inflammation are apt to be manifested as endometritis, parametritis, and salpingitis. Infections after hysterectomy, culdotomy, curettage, or partial cervicectomy vary from cellulitis to abscess. Cervical neoplasms and tumors that obstruct or dilate the cervix may cause endometritis, pyometra, or cellulitis. The bacteria causing the disease processes can be predicted with good probability in these various clinical situations. Gram-stained smears and carefully obtained and grown cultures of specimens from the cervix, endometrial cavity, cul-de-sac, abscesses, or inflamed tissue often improve the accuracy of bacteriologic diagnosis. Antibacterial therapy should be started after proper clinical diagnosis and may be changed if the clinical course and cultures more clearly indicate the bacteria involved.

INFECTIOUS AGENTS

Infectious agents producing lesions of the vulva and vagina were discussed in Chapters 4 and 5. This chapter will examine infections causing disease of the uterus, salpinges, ovaries, and pelvic peritoneum.

Neisseria gonorrhoeae, Group A β-hemolytic streptococci, *Mycobacterium tuberculosis*, and *Chlamydia trachomatis* are not normal inhabitants of the vagina and the cervix and should be considered pathogenic when found on smear or culture. The indigenous bacteria that on occasion become important pathogens are the Bacteroidaceae, anaerobic streptococci, *Escherichia coli*, group B hemolytic streptococci, group D hemolytic streptococci, and the *Proteus* group. *Staphylococcus epidermidis*, *Staphylococcus aureus*, nonhemolytic streptococcus, *Pseudomonas*, *Klebsiella*, *Fusobacterium* species, *Clostridium* species, *Mycoplasma hominis*, and *Ureaplasma urealyticum* may at times be pathogenic. *Gardnerella* and diptheroids are rarely pathogenic. The lactobacillus is not pathogenic and is very important during a woman's reproductive years for maintenance of the acidity of the vaginal secretions, which is antagonistic to pathogenic bacteria. It should be noted that the indigenous genital bacteria are essentially those that are indigenous in the rectum, anus, and perianal areas; however, the density of the bacterial population in the vagina is considerably less than that in the intestines, particularly for the anaerobic bacteria. Although little is known about the quantitative bacteriology of the vagina and cervix, it would appear logical that higher concentrations of the more pathogenic indignous bacteria would cause more disease. Fecal contamination, infrequent bathing, soiled clothing, frequent coitus, oral-genital contact, trichomoniasis, and vaginal foreign bodies appear to increase numbers of potentially pathogenic bacteria.

Many factors have been shown to influence the microecosystem of the vagina. The importance of the lactobacillus has already been suggested. Its growth depends on the glycogen, which becomes available through the estrogenic stimulation of the vagina and cervix. Lactobacilli are less frequently found or are absent in children and postclimacteric women. Bacterial antagonism in the indigenous flora involves the competition for nutrients, the production of bacteriocidins, and the production of substances unfavorable to other bacteria. Studies show that estrogens tend to increase the abundance of bacteria in the vagina. This in part may be caused by the increased vascularity with enhancement of nutrition as well as increased production of mucin that may enhance bacterial growth. Conversely since progestogens oppose the effects of estrogens there is some decrease in bacteria and in the rate of infections under the influence of progesterone. Concentrations of bacteria are lower in postmenopausal women. This could possibly be explained by the decrease in estrogenic effects. It has been documented that the indigenous flora changes with vaginal surgery. It has also been demonstrated that antibiotics have effects on the indigenous flora, which may or may not be of aid in the prevention of disease caused by indigenous bacteria.

ANTIBACTERIAL DEFENSES

The vaginal mucous membrane is an excellent mechanical barrier. Similarly the functional closure of the cervix and the viscosity of the endocervical mucus, particularly under progestogen influence, ordinarily offer protection for the endometrium. During menstruation this protective barrier for the cervix is diminished and, indeed, the bleeding endometrium becomes more vulnerable to the possibility of inflammatory reaction. Vascularity of the vagina and cervix allows for excellent phagocytic activity. Similarly the capability for inflammatory response when organisms become invasive allows for better attempts at localization of infection. The delivery of antitoxins and beneficial antibodies to the area is usually good as well.

Conversely the mechanical barrier does not exist once the bacteria are established within the endometrial cavity since surface spread may occur through the salpinges into the peritoneal cavity. IUDs offer surfaces for colonization and increase endometrial infection. Other host variations that are involved in pelvic infection will be discussed under the various clinical types of inflammatory processes.

INFECTIONS
Salpingitis

Acute salpingitis is most often caused by *Neisseria gonorrhoeae* or *Chlamydia trachomatis*. The indigenous vaginal pathogenic bacteria can cause salpingitis without the gonococcus or chlamydia. Indigenous bacteria are commonly found along with the primary organisms when suppuration in the tube and peritoneal cavity is noted.

The subjective manifestations are lower abdominal and back pain, fever, and sometimes chills; at times there are nausea and/or vomiting, pain with voiding, and an increased vaginal discharge. Objective findings are acute tenderness on both sides of the lower abdomen, marked tenderness on motion of the uterus and adnexa, elevated temperature, tachycardia, and increased cloudy cervical exudate. The patient may or may not have had recent evidence of gonorrheal or chlamydial vaginitis and urethritis and may or may not know of an infected consort. (In some groups studied 80% of women and 20% of men with positive cultures were asymptomatic.)

When urethritis and vaginitis occur the onset is apt to be 3 to 10 days after coitus with an infected individual. The onset of salpingitis caused by gonorrhea is more common during or immediately after menstruation. The history of a previous episode of salpingitis may be elicited.

As shown in Fig. 7-1, gonococcal and chlamydial inflammation proceeds along the mucous membranes. Once the inflammation reaches the salpinx, first the lining and later the entire tubal wall become involved in the inflammatory process. A purulent exudate escapes from the end of the tube if it is open. The bacteria spread to the adjacent peritoneum to produce the inflammatory reaction that causes pelvic pain.

Diagnosis. The clinical diagnosis is made with reasonable certainty when the majority of the subjective and objective manifestations previously discussed are found. In a minority of patients purulent material can be expressed from the urethra or from the cervix, and gram-stained smears will allow identification of the bean-shaped, gram-negative, intracellular diplococci. For the majority of patients smears will not be diagnostic, and cultures should always be taken from the endocervix. Anal cultures are needed if anal coitus has occurred. If the manifestations of peritonitis are more severe and evidence of disease exists outside the pelvis, aspi-

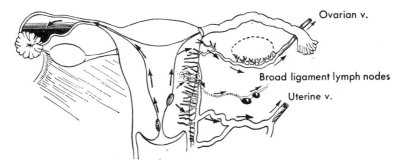

Fig. 7-1. Routes of spread of pelvic infection. On the left is shown the spread of gonococcal inflammation along the mucous membranes, endocervix, endometrium, and endosalpinx. On the right is shown the spread of streptococcic, staphylococcic, and other bacterial inflammation via the uterine and ovarian veins and via the lymphatics.

ration of the cul-de-sac is desirable with proper culture for the gonococcus, chlamydia, and the bacteria that are indigenous to the vagina.

Diagnostic efforts should include not only continuing observation of the febrile response and pulse and abdominal changes, along with the subjective manifestations, but also pelvic palpation every 1 or 2 days to try to determine as early as possible evidences of abscess formation. Failure of response to antibiotics should increase the search for an abscess. If pus is obtained by aspiration or incision, proper smears and cultures should be made, as these may be of particular assistance in decisions concerning the use of various available antibacterial agents. Blood cultures are advised for patients with chills and high fever.

The identification of *Chlamydia* requires culture with tissue culture cells that have been treated to render them more susceptible to this type of inoculation. The organism produces characteristic intracytoplasmic inclusions in the cells. For the serologic diagnosis of genital chlamydial infections microimmunofluorescent tests are used. At present laboratory means for diagnosing chlamydial infections are becoming available. Clinicians suspect the diagnosis when gonococci cannot be cultured in patients with salpingitis or cervicitis and in patients who do not respond to penicillin.

When one contrasts the manifestations of gonococcal and chlamydial infections, it is evident that both can exist asymptomatically and can be found on cervical or urethral cultures. Gonorrheal salpingitis appears to manifest itself more commonly immediately after menstruation, whereas chlamydial infections have their onset at other times as well. Pain and fever with chlamydial involvement are apt to be milder and may take longer to develop.

Therapy. In addition to analgesics, rest, and attention to fluid, electrolyte, and nutritional needs, various plans of antibacterial therapy are available. For the patient seen within 24 to 36 hours of the onset of acute pelvic pain, 4.8 million units of penicillin G should be administered intramuscularly. For those sensitive to penicillin, 4 grams of spectinomycin should be given intramuscularly as a single injection. For the patient who has evidenced infection over a longer period, particularly with more severe manifestations of peritonitis, hospitalization is required with intravenous administration of medications. The first dose of aqueous penicillin G (80,000 units per kilogram of body weight) should be given over 1 hour. Then a similar dose should be given gradually every 6 hours. If the patient has shown a previous allergic reaction to penicillin, tetracycline should be administered intravenously. Currently 200 mg of minocycline is being used initially followed by 100 mg every 12 hours. Tetracyclines are the agents of choice for treatment of chlamydial infections and should be used when chlamydia is identified on culture or suspected because of the absence of the gonococcus. In the severely ill patient it appears justified to add intramuscular administration of gentamycin. This is done because of the frequent association of *E. coli* and other enteric organisms. When *Bacteroides* is suspected or diagnosed the choice is among metronidazole, clindamycin, carbenicillin, and chloramphenicol.

When abscesses form that are accessible in the cul-de-sac, they should be

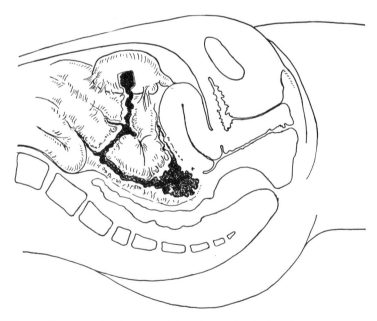

Fig. 7-2. Diffuse pelvic suppuration from pyosalpinx. The pus has broken through the tube wall, spread among the intestinal coils, and gravitated to the cul-de-sac. A window cut in the distended tube shows the connection of the suppurating tract with the tubal cavity.

drained by posterior culdotomy. In some instances extraperitoneal drainage can be accomplished by inguinal incision. If the abscesses cannot be entered by these two approaches, it is necessary on occasion to perform a laparotomy for the excision of tubo-ovarian abscesses, thus avoiding the high mortality of rupture causing peritonitis. If rupture has occurred, it is even more important that the laparotomy be performed with excision of the abscesses as completely as possible, lavage of the abdomen, placement of drains, and intensive antibacterial therapy.

Septic pelvic thrombophlebitis may occur with salpingitis and peritonitis. (See postabortal infection.)

Sequelae. After the patient recovers from the acute phase of salpingitis and/or abscess formation, she may have sufficient tubal damage to cause infertility. With repeated salpingitis and occlusion of the fimbriated end of the tube, hydrosalpinx may occur. Adhesions of the bowel and omentum within the pelvis, of the adnexa, and of the uterus may reduce mobility of the pelvic organs. Chronic lower abdominal pain, back pain, and menstrual irregularity may develop. The patient who has

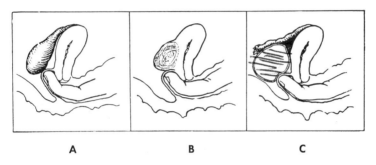

A   B   C

Fig. 7-3. Differential diagnosis of pelvic inflammation with rounded mass rather high in cul-de-sac. **A,** Tubal mass. **B,** Small myoma on posterior wall of uterus. **C,** Small ovarian cyst.

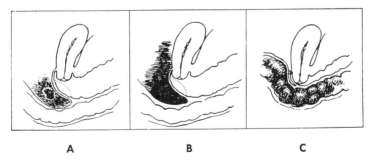

A   B   C

Fig. 7-4. Differential diagnosis of pelvic inflammation with mass low behind cervix. **A,** Inflammatory mass filling cul-de-sac. **B,** Blood from ruptured tubal pregnancy filling cul-de-sac. **C,** Fecal mass distending rectum back of cervix.

had an attack of acute salpingitis is more likely to have recurrent attacks. She should be taught and motivated to avoid recurrent infection. When the pain is chronic and mild, full effort at conservative therapy should be used. Frequent warm douches may give comfort. The decision as to the surgical therapy for the residues of pelvic infection are best based on the degree of disability of the patient who has been observed over a considerable time.

Masses that persist after pelvic infection may be chronic tubo-ovarian abscess containing sterile fluid, pyosalpinx, ovarian abscess, pelvic abscess, or adherent omentum or intestine. Hydrosalpinx may develop over several months. These masses that result from inflammation are likely to be confused with neoplasms and when persistent for several months require excision even if asymptomatic. Figs. 7-3 and 7-4 illustrate how confusion can result.

It should be emphasized that, in patients with recurrent or acute pelvic infections, uterine-bleeding disturbances occur either because of infection of the endometrium or because of ovarian changes.

Pelvic abscess

Pelvic abscess not only may follow purulent salpingitis but also may develop following rupture in suppurative appendicitis, ruptured gastric ulcer, ruptured colonic diverticula, ectopic pregnancy with hematocele, or intra-abdominal operation. A prolonged febrile course after pelvic surgery leads one to suspect pelvic abscess. An intra-abdominal foreign body left at the same time of operation may be a contributing factor. As indicated in the management of these abscesses following salpingitis, drainage is desirable. If drainage cannot be accomplished, laparotomy may be required to remove the abscess partially or completely to effect cure.

When infection of a cystic ovarian structure occurs, the term "ovarian abscess" is used. These abscesses may follow pelvic infection or may occur in endometrial cysts that penetrate through the bowel wall. An ovarian abscess should be suspected when repeated drainage fails to cure the abscess. This type requires excision for cure.

Postoperative infections

All surgeons performing minor or major operations of the pelvis are responsible for the preventive, diagnostic, and therapeutic functions required to lower the mortality and morbidity of bacterial disease. When possible vaginitis and acute cervical infection should be effectively treated before endometrial biopsy, IUD insertion, tubal insufflation, dilatation and curettage, hysterectomy, or elective culdotomy for adnexal surgery. When possible wounds of the cervix (conization or extensive biopsy) should be allowed to heal before hysterectomy. Complete evacuation of the products of gestation is imperative when the uterine cavity has been invaded. Personnel with group A β-hemolytic streptococci should not be in the operating room. Adequate sterilization and the avoidance of contamination are always required.

Surgical techniques to ensure minimal accumulation of blood and minimal devitalized tissue is essential, particularly when indigenous vaginal bacteria are contaminants. Mechanical cleansing of the vulva, vagina, and skin decreases extent of contamination. Local application of antibacterial chemicals affects surface bacteria. Contamination by endocervical secretions, feces (anal and perianal), and infected urine may occur during surgery. The bacteria within tissue are not killed or removed by cleansing or local applications.

When vaginitis and cervicitis are present or when the patient's defense is decreased, antibiotics given in high dosage to provide good tissue levels before surgical spread of bacteria may decrease the severity of postoperative infection. Use of selected antibacterials is in order when intra-abdominal operations involve abscesses, areas of cellulitis, or fecal contamination. The routine use of antibacterial agents postoperatively will not prevent all infections. There is no safe combination of drugs to cover all pathogens.

Bacterial contamination and small accumulations of blood result in a high incidence of cellulitis and cuff abscesses after vaginal hysterectomy. The occasional development of pelvic abscesses, peritonitis, and thrombophlebitis, particularly caused by anaerobic bacteria, has been a continuing postoperative threat. Recent studies have revealed that the extent of morbidity has decreased with preoperative, intraoperative, and postoperative use of antibacterials. Open cuff procedures or use of drains may be indicated.

Gynecologic surgeons must search daily for evidence of postoperative infection. Identification and drainage or removal of abscesses are essential. Pus should be studied by gram-stained smears and careful culturing. Blood cultures should be obtained for patients with chills or other evidence of bacteremia. Use of antibacterial agents requires knowledge of bacteriology and pharmacology of agents available, coordinated with the pathophysiologic changes of the patient.

Postabortal and postpartum infections

After abortion or delivery there is usually a mild degree of self-limiting endometritis of no clinical significance. Following instrumentation and severe uterine contamination a pathogenic endometritis may develop. The common offending organisms are streptococci, staphylococci, *Escherichia coli*, *Bacteroides fragilis*, and other gram-negative enteric pathogens and occasionally *Clostridium welchii*. The vascular uterus of pregnancy with a physiologic wound at the placental site offers little resistance, so that the usual spread of infection is rapid through the uterine wall and lymphatics, into the parametrial tissues to cause cellulitis, into the vascular spaces of the uterus to cause bacteremia, and into adjacent uterine and ovarian veins to cause suppurative thrombophlebitis. Pelvic peritonitis via the salpinges or a perforated uterus may occur.

The patient is apt to develop chills and high fever. Pain may be severe with peritonitis but usually is not as severe as with gonorrheal salpingitis, since the extent of early peritoneal reaction is not as marked with postpartal and postabortal infection. The serosanguinopurulent material from the cervix may or may not be foul. In addition to tenderness, when cellulitis is marked, the parametria may become ligneous.

When gram-negative bacteria are involved, septic shock may occur because of liberation of endotoxins. Hypotension with restlessness and fast pulse may rapidly be followed by pallor, vomiting, diarrhea, and a clammy skin with weak pulse. Oliguria may progress to anuria. A semicomatose state may precede death.

Endotoxic shock can be best understood as a disturbance of the microcirculation. Precapillary and postcapillary spasm occur; however, the venospasm is more marked so that there is a pooling of blood in the capillary bed. This may also occur in the splanchnic veins. The failure of venous return leads to decreased cardiac output and decrease in the arterial pressure. If the amount of endotoxin initially liberated is not too great, the principal response will be hypotension and tachycardia. If the amount of endotoxin is greater, the condition rapidly proceeds to greater impairment of the microcirculation. Intravascular coagulation occurs to cause microthrombi. Although formation of intravascular clots seldom depletes fibrinogen to the level that clinical bleeding problems occur, the microthrombi, along with decreased circulation, appear to be important regarding injury to the adrenals, kidneys, liver, and other vital organs. A generalized Shwartzman reaction may occur. Study of the changes in coagulation and of the appearance of split fibrin and fibrinogen products can be correlated with the severity of involvement.

When septic thrombophlebitis develops, septic embolization, particularly to the lungs, is expected. With numerous small emboli, marked tachycardia and dyspnea develop. Roentgenograms of the chest are apt to reveal small scattered areas of increased densities and an enlarged heart. Isotopic lung scans reveal decreased perfusion. Electrocardiograms may indicate right ventricular strain. Small metastatic abscesses may form in the lungs, brain, or kidneys if the disease is not arrested.

Early employment of effective antibacterial agents and early evacuation of placental tissue from the uterus will interrupt the progression of the pathologic processes and manifestations just described.

Management. Cervical smears and cultures and blood cultures should be taken to identify the pathogens; however, in acutely ill patients, agents effective against commonly encountered organisms must be started without delay. After identification of bacteria, if such can be done, the antibacterial agents may be changed.

The drugs of choice are penicillin G or ampicillin and an aminoglycoside. If the patient is unable to receive penicillins, cephalosporins or cefoxitin are substituted. When bacteroides are identified or suspected because of the clinical course, penicillin should be changed to carbenicillin and the possibility of the administration of metronidazole, chloramphenicol, or clindamycin should be entertained. (See the section on antibacterial drugs for urinary and pelvic infections.)

Chest examinations, lung scans, and x-ray films are needed to determine pulmonary complication, in particular evidence of septic emboli to the lungs.

If the patient has had an unskilled induced abortion, tetanus toxoid or antitoxin and polyvalent gas gangrene antitoxin should be given prophylactically.

If placental tissue remains in the uterus, it should be removed as soon as practical. With early pregnancy, gentle dilation and finger evacuation may be done, or curettage and sponge forceps removal may be required. Oxytocin (Syntocinon) administered by infusion may allow expulsion of the placenta and/or fetus in more advanced pregnancy. With septic shock caused by endotoxins or with tetanus the advisability of hysterectomy must be entertained and may be lifesaving. When septic emboli are leaving the pelvis, vena cava and ovarian vein ligation may be required.

Patients may require transfusions when anemia is marked or blood loss rapid. If the peritonitis causes ileus, parenteral fluids with nothing to be taken orally are in order. Gastric suction may be needed.

In severely ill patients, particularly those with hypotension not caused by acute blood loss, care necessitates constant monitoring of respiration, blood pressure, pulse rate, and urinary output. Central venous pressure determination via a catheter left in the superior vena cava allows more accurate determination of blood available to the heart or its failure as a pump. Blood volume determination with venous pressures allows a better decision as to the intravenous fluid administration. Evaluation of electrolytes and carbon dioxide–combining power aids in choosing electrolyte solutions for corrections of acidosis, etc. if needed. For severe acidosis, sodium bicarbonate given intravenously is required.

If septic shock is present, hydrocortisone administered intravenously and/or intramuscularly in large dosages of 2 to 4 grams per 24 hours has been associated with improved heart action, increased renal output, and more effect of vasopressors when used. The dosage of antibacterials must be increased with severe infections.

Oxygen should be used for patients with shock. Rapid digitalization may be in order with persistent venous pressure over 15 cm of water. Some authorities have advocated isoproterenol with constant ECG monitoring for patients with acute heart failure.

Vasopressors may be required despite the knowledge that peripheral vasoconstriction is one of the principal pathologic changes found with septic shock. Metaraminol bitartrate (Aramine), phenylephrine hydrochloride (Neo-Synephrine), and angiotensin II are usually effective and may be required for several days. Patients appear to particularly do well with vasopressors when they are administered in the warm stage of septic shock.

Once tissue perfusion has markedly decreased and the patient has become cool and pallid, the use of vasodilating drugs is in order, and their use can result in dramatic improvement in some moribund patients. Before and along with the use of chlorpromazine given intravenously to block α-receptors and cause vasodilation, dextran solution, normal saline solution, and blood must be used to expand the plasma volume so that the patient can tolerate the peripheral vasodilation. The value of hypothermia to decrease metabolic rates in vital organs is questioned. With marked impairment of renal function dialysis may be required. In a few instances, although the damage is so extensive as to cause cortical necrosis of the kidney, the patient may recover with recurrent renal dialysis.

When the acute phase of this disorder has subsided, the patient may be left with considerable debility associated with pelvic cellulitis. The administration of adrenal corticoids and oral proteolytic enzymes in combination with the effective antibacterial agents is advocated to hasten the resolution of the tissue reaction. Perisalpingitis may have occurred and have resulted in some distortion of the salpinx, but it is not so marked as that which occurs with purulent salpingitis.

Toxic shock syndrome

During menstruation women using tampons (particularly the more absorbent tampons) and leaving them in place for longer times have occasionally suffered from a multisystem toxic response called toxic shock syndrome (TSS). Fever over 102° F, malaise, vomiting and diarrhea, erythema, and subsequent exfoliative dermatitis are the principal manifestations.

Cultures from the vagina usually reveal *Staphylococcus aureus*. The exotoxin produced is called an "exfoliatin" because of its ability to cause skin exfoliation in mice. The multisystem involvement suggests a generalized vasculitis. A similar syndrome has been caused in men and children by a penicillin-resistant *Staphylococcus aureus*.

About 9% of women reported to have had TSS have died. The reported incidence of 3 per 100,000 menstruating women may be low. Recurrence rate has been about 30%.

If a woman using a tampon experiences fever, vomiting and diarrhea, and a rash, she should discontinue tampon use and consult a physician. Cultures from the vagina and cervix for *Staphylococcus aureus* and administration of a β-lactamase-resistant antistaphylococcal antibiotic are in order.

Infections associated with pelvic malignancies are discussed in Chapter 9. In some cases the infection associated with submucous myomas that act as large foreign bodies in the uterine cavity will subside only after total hysterectomy.

Tuberculosis of reproductive system

Tuberculosis of the pelvic organs is usually secondary to lesions elsewhere in the body. The primary site may be the lung, the intestine, the urinary tract, or the retroperitoneal glands. Peritoneal tuberculosis may involve pelvic structures. Although tuberculosis may be introduced through the vagina, the route of spread is most often the hematogenous one. In the majority of instances no active lesion can be demonstrated in any of the primary locations at the time of diagnosis.

The severity of infection varies greatly. In mild cases there are no gross abnormalities found on pelvic examination and there are no symptoms. Some of these cases are diagnosed when sterility investigations are performed. Biopsy of the endometrium reveals tuberculosis. At times the diagnosis is obtained on curettage when the patient is thought to have functional uterine bleeding. In some instances a very severe infection results, in which there may be localized peritonitis with many dense tough adhesions binding together the abdominal and pelvic viscera.

The endosalpinx is the most commonly involved tissue. Next in frequency are the endometrium and ovary. Chronic ulcerations or sinuses of the cervix, vagina, or vulva are lesions of very rare type. When symptoms occur, they are generally chronic; however, at times acute exacerbations are noted, and the disorder may be confused with other inflammations of the pelvis. Rarely is the diagnosis made before surgery. Failure of inflammatory processes to respond to the usual treatment should bring to mind the consideration of the likelihood of tuberculosis. Accurate diagnosis requires identification of the *Mycobacterium tuberculosis*, which is accomplished by smears, cultures, and guinea pig inoculation. Histologic diagnosis is sufficient to indicate management.

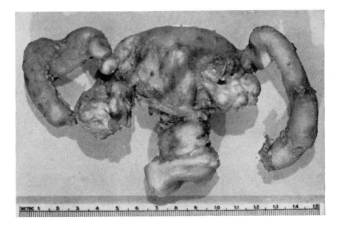

Fig. 7-5. Pelvic tuberculosis. Note the tubercles on the tubes.

From Willson, J.R., Beecham, C.T., Forman, I., and Carrington, E.R.: Obstetrics and gynecology, St. Louis, The C.V. Mosby Co.

Therapy. Treatment of pelvic tuberculosis, if the diagnosis is made preoperatively, is essentially the same as the treatment of tuberculosis elsewhere. When genital tuberculosis is limited to the endometrium or tube, regimen of isoniazid and ethambutol administered orally is used over many months. If more advanced tuberculosis is found at surgery, intramuscular use of streptomycin is required and is continued along with isoniazid and ethambutol over many months. The incidence of normal pregnancy after medical treatment remains exceedingly low. The likelihood of recurrent abortion is great. The best chance of cure is the surgical excision of the involved genital structures, particularly in combination with the use of the drugs previously mentioned; however, many medically treated patients have been followed for years without evidence of reactivation of pelvic lesions. With persistent peritoneal tuberculosis, salpingectomy has been associated with arrest of the disease process.

Actinomycosis

Actinomycosis, a chronic disorder, may involve the pelvic organs. It is extremely rare, and the causative organism is thought to gain access by way of the bowel. Sinus formation may occur, and, should the tract open into an accessible area, the possibility of the diagnosis being made by microscopic examination of the ray fungus is more likely.

Therapy. When the diagnosis is made after surgical removal of the masses found in the pelvis, the intramuscular use of long-acting penicillin preparations such as benzathine penicillin G, 1,200,000 units weekly for 6 to 8 weeks, is advocated if the excision has not been complete. Aqueous penicillin, 2,000,000 units daily, should be used for severe infections.

ANTIBACTERIAL DRUGS USED FOR URINARY AND PELVIC INFECTIONS
Sulfonamides

Sulfonamides are bacteriostatic chemical substances that act as competitive antimetabolites to impair folic acid synthesis. They are the drugs of choice against *Haemophilus ducreyi* causing chancroid and *Bedsonia* causing lymphogranuloma and are commonly used to treat cystitis, for which they are usually effective when *Escherichia coli*, *Klebsiella-Aerobacter*, *Proteus mirabilis*, or enterococci are involved. Resistance commonly develops during prolonged suppressive therapy, and sulfonamides should not be continued. Since resistant strains are encountered on initial or continuing use, culture and sensitivity tests are ideal for all urinary infections and essential with failure of response and recurrent infection.

Pyelonephritis, gonorrhea, and uterine and adnexal infections are not treated with sulfonamides since more effective and less toxic antibacterial substances are available. Vaginal applications are effective for nonspecific vaginitis.

Adverse reactions. Headache, lassitude, and dizziness are common. Skin reactions varying from macular to urticarial are less common. Nausea and vomiting may occur. Hemopoiesis is depressed, particular with high drug levels, and hemolytic anemia occurs with glucose-6-phosphate dehydrogenase deficiency.

Since sulfonamides are conjugated in the liver and excreted by the kidneys, they are avoided in patients with significant impairments of these organs.

Adverse reaction to one sulfonamide usually indicates adverse reaction to others; therefore they are best avoided in patients with a reliable history of previous adverse reaction.

Use with some drugs should be avoided. Penicillins and cephalosporins may not be as effective when sulphonamides are added. The sulphonamides are bacteriostatic agents that function as competitive antimetabolites that decrease metabolic activity. Penicillin and cephalosporins are most effective against bacteria that are actively synthesizing cell wall; consequently their effectiveness is diminished by the sulfonamides. Tolbutamide, methotrexate, and coumarin are drugs that may have actions enhanced.

Complete blood cell counts should be performed with higher doses and prolonged use.

Preparations. Sulfisoxazole and sulfamethizole are short acting and soluble in acid urine, so that crystalluria is rare. When adverse reactions occur, their rapid elimination is desirable. Longer acting sulfonamides allow doses every 12 hours, unlike the 4- to 6-hour doses of the short-acting drugs; however, when adverse reactions occur, they last longer.

Trimethoprim

Trimethoprim is a synthetic pyrimidine that blocks the production of tetrahydrofolic acid from dihydrofolic acid to interfere with biosynthesis of nucleic acids and proteins. It is available for oral administration every 12 hours. When used alone, it requires doses that cause more frequent rash, pruritus, and exfoliative dermatitis than sulfonamides. It has essentially the same antibacterial effectiveness and adverse reactions as sulfonamides.

When combined with sulfamethoxazole, which also gives effective plasma concentrations for 12 hours, bacteriostatic effectiveness is increased over that of each component and bacterial resistance develops more slowly. The combination blocks two steps in the biosynthesis of nucleic acids and proteins (p-aminobenzoic acid to folic acid and dihydrofolic acid to tetrahydrofolic acid).

Nitrofurans

Nitrofurans, synthetic antimicrobial hydantoins, are bactericidal for *Escherichia coli* and enterococci when high concentrations in urine are obtained. Some strains of *Klebsiella-Aerobacter*, *Proteus*, and *Pseudomonas* are resistant. Nitrofurantoins are commonly used orally to treat cystitis and mild pyelonephritis. Development of resistance during therapy is uncommon, and prolonged use to prevent recurrence of disease is practical. Nitrofurazone is topically applied to the urethra, bladder, and vagina to decrease many indigenous bacteria, thus decreasing odor and avoiding or decreasing inflammation.

Adverse reactions. Nausea and vomiting may be produced. Headache, dizziness, and drowsiness are less common. Hypersensitivity reactions of the skin vary from erythema to urticaria. Rarely, nonfatal anaphylactic reactions involving respiration have occurred. Polyneuropathy is possible with impaired renal function, severe anemia, diabetes, electrolyte imbalance, and nutritional deficiency. Anemia occurs with glucose-6-phosphate dehydrogenase deficiency.

Tests for anemia should be done with prolonged or repeated use. Urine cultures and sensitivity tests are indicated as for sulfonamides. Concurrent use with other urinary antiseptics is illogical. Nitrofurans should not be used for pelvic infections.

Nalidixic acid

Nalidixic acid is used orally to treat urinary tract infections caused by certain gram-negative bacteria. It is effective against *Escherichia coli* and most species of *Proteus* and less effective against other coliform bacteria such as *Enterobacter*, *Klebsiella*, and *Streptococcus faecalis*. *Pseudomonas* and gram-positive bacteria are resistant.

Bacterially resistant organisms emerge in 2% to 14% of patients. The emergence of resistance and the relatively narrow spectrum of effectiveness limit this agent's use.

Adverse reactions involving the CNS range from drowsiness to toxic psychosis. Visual disturbances include overbrightness of lights, change in color perception, and double vision. Other ill effects include nausea, diarrhea, rash, pruritus, urticaria, bullae, and arthralgia.

Penicillins

Penicillins, a group of natural and semisynthetic agents, are bactericidal for many pathogens because they interfere with synthesis and function of bacterial cell walls. To effectively use the various penicillins, the physician must know the individual characteristics.

The effect common to all penicillins is their potential antigenicity. *All* penicillin preparations except certain semisynthetic ones (cloxacillin, dicloracillin, methicillin, nafcillin, oxacillin) are rendered ineffective by penicillinase produced by some staphylococci. Penicillins applied topically frequently cause hypersensitization, and preparations are not marketed for this use in the United States.

Most penicillins are rapidly excreted in the urine, unaltered or as metabolites. Factors to be considered for various penicillins are sensitivity of microorganisms, stability in gastric acid, rates of absorption and excretion, protein binding, blood levels obtained, and effective blood levels needed.

Adverse reactions. Allergic reactions are common (1% to 5% of patients), and the only certain means of avoiding such reactions is to not use penicillins. Penicillins should not be used when a previous reaction has occurred. The patient should always be asked about previous reaction. Sensitivity tests are not sufficiently safe or accurate.

There are two types of reactions: (1) an immediate, profound, anaphylactic shock with acute circulatory failure, syncope, and possible laryngeal edema and (2) a delayed illness with rash, urticaria, fever, and perhaps diarrhea. There are no entirely safe methods of testing for sensitivity. Reactions have occurred with no knowledge of previous contact. Epinephrine should be immediately available. Oxygen, resuscitation, and perhaps tracheotomy may be other life-saving necessities. Adrenal corticosteroids may prevent acute relapse and are the principal therapeutic agents for delayed reactions.

Serious superinfections with resistant organisms (such as *Pseudomonas*, *Proteus*, and *Candida*) may occur with long-term use of any of the penicillins.

Interstitial nephritis is a rare allergic reaction common to penicillins. (Methicillin may cause a direct toxic nephropathy.)

PENICILLIN G SALTS

The penicillin G salts are the drugs of choice for diseases caused by the following:

1. Group A β-hemolytic streptococcus
2. *Neisseria gonorrhoeae*
3. *Streptococcus pyogenes*, *faecalis*, *viridans*, and *anaerobius*
4. *Clostridium perfringens* and *tetani*
5. *Treponema pallidum*
6. *Actinomyces*
7. *Staphylococcus aureus* (the 20% that produce no penicillinase)

In high intravenous dosages about 80% of *Escherichia coli* organisms are sensitive and some *Proteus mirabilis*.

Bacteria not covered are gram-negative bacilli (except those above): *Bacteroides*, *Pseudomonas*, *Enterobacter*, *Klebsiella*, *Citrobacter*, *Escherichia coli*, and indole-negative and indole-positive *Proteus* species. Gram-positive cocci not covered are *Staphylococcus aureus* organisms that produce penicillinase and some enterococci.

Oral penicillin G is absorbed erratically and destroyed by gastric acid and should not be used for genital disease. Intramuscular injection of procaine penicillin G, available in aqueous suspension of 600,000 units per ml, can be given (up to 2.4 million units in a single site or larger amounts in multiple sites) to produce high levels that plateau after about 4 hours and fall slowly for the next 20 hours. Cervical, urethral, and early salpingeal gonorrheal inflammation usually require only one dose of 4.8 million units. It is ideally preceded by 1 gram of probenecid orally to inhibit renal transport of penicillin.

Intramuscular use of 2.4 million units of benzathine penicillin G as a single dose provides low levels over long periods of time (10 days). A single dose is adequate for primary, secondary, or latent syphilis. Three doses at weekly intervals are used for tertiary syphilis and neurosyphilis.

Intravenous administration of potassium salts of penicillin G are used for sever pelvic infections in doses of 80,000 units per kilogram given every 6 hours. Peritonitis and tubo-ovarian abscesses from salpingitis; severe endometritis, parametritis, and peritonitis associated with inflammations of pregnancy; and severe postoperative cellulitis or abscess along with septicemia from the above conditions are principal indications. Necrotizing fasciitis or synergistic gangrene of wounds requires high concentrations and adequate excision of devitalized tissue.

When large amounts of pencillin G salts for intravenous use are given, 1.7 mEq of potassium per each million units is involved, so electrolyte determinations should be evaluated. The dosage may need to be reduced for patients with renal impairment.

AMPICILLIN

Ampicillin, a semisynthetic penicillin, has the same general antibacterial spectrum as pencillin G. It is more effective against the gram-negative bacilli, *Escherichia coli,* and *Proteus mirabilis*. Some enterococci resistant to penicillin G respond. Ampicillin is not the drug of choice over penicillin G for most responding diseases.

Ampicillin is water solubel, acid stable, and readily absorbed by the gastrointestinal tract. Adequate blood levels of 2.5 to 3.0 µg per milliliter are obtained 2 hours after a 500 mg capsule has been taken. Higher levels are attained over shorter periods of time after an intramuscular injection. Intravenous administration yields highest levels and should be used for severe diseases.

Adverse reactions are the same as those with penicillin G except that it is given intravenously as a sodium salt with no fear of hyperkalemia, rashes result more often, diarrhea is more common, and intramuscular injections are more painful.

Amoxicillin is an analogue of ampicillin that has twice the oral absorption of ampicillin.

CARBENICILLIN

Carbenicillin, a semisynthetic penicillin, is used intravenously. It has an antibacterial spectrum similar to that of ampicillin but with additional effectiveness against *Pseudomonas*, indole-positive *Proteus*, and the majority of bacteroides. It is used for severely ill patients.

Adverse reactions are the same as those with ampicillin. Less skin reactions occur, though, and anemia, leukopenia, and thrombocytopenia are more common.

NAFCILLIN AND OXACILLIN

Nafcillin and oxacillin, two semisynthetic penicillins, are used rarely in gynecologic patients for wound infections caused by penicillinase-producing staphylococci.

Cephalosporins

Cephalosporins, semisynthetic antibacterial agents, are chemically related to penicillins and, like them, contain a β-lactam ring. They are bactericidal and interfere with synthesis of the bacterial cell wall.

Cephalosporins are effective against most gram-positive cocci and against many gram-negative bacteria. They are not the drugs of choice over penicillin G aginast gram-positive cocci except where penicillinase is involved. They are not the first choice therapy of gonorrhea. Cephalosporins are commonly effective against *Escherichia coli*, *Proteus mirabilis*, and *Klebsiella*.

Resistance is found with *Pseudomonas*, most indole-positive *Proteus* species, and motile *Enterobacter* species. Enterococci are resistant except to the high concentrations obtainable in urine. *Bacteroides* are resistant.

Adverse reactions. Most patients allergic to penicillins can be safely treated with cephalosporins. Rarely cross-allergenicity has occurred. Minor rashes are uncommon. Severe allergic reactions are rare. All patients should be questioned as to previous reactions. Diarrhea may occur with oral administration. Neutropenia, thrombocytopenia, and hemolytic anemia have been reported. A positive result of the direct Coombs test may occur. Rises in serum glutamic-oxaloacetic transaminase (SGOT) and alkaline phosphatase have been noted. Rises in blood urea nitrogen (BUN) and creatinine have occurred. False-positive results of tests for glucose in urine may occur with Benedict's or Fehling's solutions or with Clinitest tablets but not with Tes-Tape. To avoid overdosage the daily total should be decreased for patients with renal impairment.

CEPHALOTHIN SODIUM

Cephalothin sodium, a form of cephalosporin, is used intravenously every 4 to 6 hours in daily dosage of 4 to 12 grams for moderate to severe infections.

CEFAZOLIN SODIUM

Cefazolin sodium, a form of cephalosporin, has replaced cephaloridine because it is less nephrotoxic and can be given intramuscularly for moderately severe disease. The dosage must be reduced with renal impairment. Cephazolin sodium may be given intravenously.

CEPHALEXIN AND CEPHRADINE

Cephalexin and cephradine are the preferred forms of cephalosporin for oral administration. Urinary and mild pelvic infections may respond to 250 to 500 mg given four times daily. When more than 4 grams per 24 hours is required, parenteral administration is advised.

CEFAMANDOLE NAFATE

Cefamandole nafate is a cephalosporin for intravenous and intramuscular use. It offers an advantage over cephalothin sodium because of its effectiveness against some anaerobes. Most strins of *Bacteroides* are resistant.

CEPHAPIRIN SODIUM

This cephalosporin for parenteral use is comparable to cephalothin sodium.

CEPHAMYCIN

Cefoxitin sodium is a broad-spectrum semisynthetic cepha antibiotic derived from cephamycin C. It is bacteriocidal by inhibition of cell wall synthesis.

Cefoxitin is effective against most gram-positive cocci, both aerobic and anaerobic, and against gram-negative bacilli, both aerobic and anaerobic. It is not inhibited by penicillinases and cephalosporinases. The agent offers the effectiveness of the cephalosporins and is also effective against common anaerobic pathogens. Unlike some cephalosporins, cefoxitin is not administered orally.

Cefoxitin is inactive against most strains of *Pseudomonas aeruginosa* and enterococci and many strains of *Enterobacter cloacae*.

Studies indicate cefoxitin is an effective single antibacterial agent for prevention of serious postoperative infections and is effective for in-hospital treatment of salpingitis. It is not the agent of choice for known *Bacteroides* infection.

Adverse reactions. Previous hypersensitivity reactions to cephalosporins contraindicate the use of cefoxitin. Caution is indicated with penicillin-sensitive patients. Rash, pruritus, eosinophilia, and fever may occur, and anaphylactoid reactions are possible. Renal insufficiency requires reduced doses. False-positive reaction for glucose in urine and false increases in creatinine in serum or urine occur. Elevations in SGOT, serum glutamic-pyruvic transaminase (SGPT), LDH, and alkaline phosphatase have been noted. A positive direct Coombs test may develop. Local reactions include thrombophlebitis, pain, and induration after intramuscular injection. Nausea, vomiting, and diarrhea may occur.

Tetracyclines

Tetracyclines, broad-spectrum antibacterial agents, are bacteriostatic by interference with protein synthesis within the organisms. Semisynthetic chemical modifications affect duration of action and some adverse reactions.

Tetracyclines are drugs of choice in the treatment of infections caused by the following:

1. *Haemophilus ducreyi*
2. *Calymmatobacterium granulomatis*
3. *Bedsonia*
4. *Chlamydia trachomatis*

They may be effective against *Clostridium perfringens, Bacteroides,* and indole-producing strains of *Proteus.* Many strains of *Escherichia coli* respond. They may be used when penicillin cannot be given to patients with gonococcal or spirochetal infections. Some strains of streptococci and staphylococci respond; however, a high percentage are resistant, and tetracyclines should be used only after culture and sensitivity testing for gram-positive cocci. With the exception of chancroid, granuloma inguinale, chlamydial infections, and lymphogranuloma, tetracyclines are not drugs of first choice in gynecologic infection. Since they are usually adequately absorbed by the gastrointestinal tract, are distributed well throughout tissues, and are of relatively low toxicity at a recommended dosage, they are used for urinary and mild pelvic infections. The presence of or emergence of resistant strains indicates that short-term use is preferred.

Adverse reactions. All tetracyclines are of low toxicity at recommended doses. The alimentary tract is the site of the most common reactions, varying from anorexia or nausea to flatulence or diarrhea. Glossitis, enterocolitis, and proctitis can develop with higher doses and prolonged use. Staphylococcal enterocolitis is a rare and serious problem.

Hypersensitivity reactions of the skin are uncommon. Candidiasis of the vulva and perianal area is common.

The antianabolic action of these drugs causes a negative nitrogen and riboflavin balance. Azotemia, hyperkalemia, hyperphosphatemia, and acidosis can develop in patients with poor renal function. Tetracyclines are best avoided for patients with poor renal function and should not be given with diuretics. Oral aluminum and magnesium antacids prevent oral absorption.

Severe hepatotoxicity is a threat with prolonged use and high dosage, especially during pregnancy. Tetracyclines are avoided during early pregnancy because of teratogenic effects on bones and teeth and in late pregnancy because of staining of deciduous teeth.

Rarely neutropenia and hemolytic anemia are caused. The effects of coumarin are potentiated. The synthesis of vitamin K in the intestinal tract is decreased.

Tetracyclines impair the effectiveness of penicillins and cephalosporins.

MINOCYCLINE

Minocycline, a semisynthetic derivative of tetracycline, has a serum half-life of 11 to 17 hours and is administered every 12 hours. It appears to be more completely metabolized than other tetracyclines. At present it has the best record among the tetracyclines against *Bacteroides fragilis*. Intravenous administration is possible.

DEOXYCYCLINE

With a serum half-life of 19 to 20 hours, deoxycyline, a derivative of tetracycline, can be given daily. It appears to be about equal to minocycline in effectiveness and toxicity and may be better if renal function is impaired.

DEMECLOCYCLINE

Demeclocycline is a tetracycline usually given every 12 hours only by mouth.

CHLORTETRACYCLINE, TETRACYCLINE, AND OXYTETRACYCLINE

Chlortetracycline, tetracycline, and oxytetracycline are derivatives available for intravenous and oral use and should be given four times daily.

Metronidazole

Metronidazole is a synthetic bacteriocidal antibacterial agent. Once inside an anaerobic cell the metronidazole molecule is reduced, and the cytotoxic products formed will kill the cell. Although the drug's mode of action is not completely understood, its bacteriocidal activity depends on an environment of reduced oxygen concentration and occurs in both dividing and nondividing cells. The action is specific for obligate anaerobes. Facultative anaerobes, microaeophilic streptococci, most strains of *Actinomyces, Arachnia,* and *Propionibacterium,* and aerobic bacteria are resistant. It has in vitro and clinical activity against the following organisms:

1. Anaerobic gram-negative bacilli: *Bacteroides* species, including the *B. fragilis* group (*B. fragilis, B. distasonis, B. ovatus, B. thetaiotaomicron, B. vulgaris, Fusobacterium* species)

2. Anaerobic gram-positive bacilli: *Clostridium* species and susceptible strains of *Eubacterium*

3. Anaerobic gram-positive cocci: *Peptococcus* species and *Peptostreptococcus* species

Metronidazole is the drug of choice for *Trichomonas vaginalis* and is effective against *Entamoeba histolytica* at all sites in the body.

Metronidazole is a small hydrophilic molecule that is unchanged at physiologic pH, has a low degree of plasma-protein binding (less than 20%), and can diffuse into most tissues. It is absorbed orally, vaginally, and rectally. Recently metronidazole hydrochloride for intravenous administration has become available.

The major pathway of elimination is via the urine (60% to 80%). Fecal excretion accounts for 6% to 15%. With renal and hepatic impairment lower doses should be administered cautiously.

Metronidazole is the drug of choice in most anaerobic infections and may be lifesaving in severe infections. Experience in Europe has led to the use of metronidazole with agents effective against aerobic organisms, for example, (1) infections associated with pregnancy complications or surgical procedures—gentamycin and metronidazole, (2) infections associated with sexually transmitted agents—penicillin G and metronidazole (for *N. gonorrhoeae*), or for nongonorrheal (probable *Chlamydia*)—tetracycline and metronidazole.

Adverse reactions. Convulsive seizures and peripheral neuropathy (numbness or paresthesias) are the most serious reactions and occur with higher doses and prolonged use. Nausea, vomiting, diarrhea, and unpleasant metallic taste occur more often when alcoholic beverages are used. Reversible leukopenia has been noted. Pruritus, erythematous rash, and urticaria have occurred. Fever and darkened urine may result. Candidiasis of the mouth or vagina has been noted. Phlebitis at the injection site may be due to failure to properly neutralize the highly acidic reconstituted solution (pH 0.5 to 2.0).

Accurate care is required for the preparation and administration of intravenous metronidazole.

Chloramphenicol

Chloramphenicol, a highly effective antibacterial drug (formerly natural, now synthetic) is bacteriostatic by interference with protein synthesis within organisms. It is effective against many gram-negative and gram-positive cocci and bacilli. It offers good coverage against bacteroides. It readily enters tissues. Conjugation occurs in the liver. It clears through the kidneys readily and can be used with renal impairment. Serious blood dyscrasias limit its use in gynecology to life-threatening disease caused by bacteroides or unknown or nonresponding mixed infections.

Adverse reactions. Aplastic anemia occurs after courses of therapy with an incidence variously calculated to be 1 in 10,000 to 100,000. Studies of white blood cells are best performed every 48 hours. Anemia of a reversible type may occur with decrease in reticulocyte counts.

Skin and gastrointestinal reactions occur.

Dosage should be decreased with severe liver impairment.

Toxoids and other actively immunizing agents may not be effective when given during chloramphenicol therapy. Less vitamin K production in the intestine is likely. Biotransformation of tolbutamide, diphenylhydantoin, dicumarol, and other drugs metabolized by the microsomal enzymes of the liver may be inhibited. For maximum effectiveness intravenous administration is used.

Clindamycin

Clindamycin is a semiscynthetic antibiotic produced from lincomycin. It is bacteriostatic by preventing peptide bonding in ribosomes. It is an effective agent against *Bacteroides fragilis* and many gram-positive pathogens. It is not effective against *Streptococcus faecalis*.

The principal use of clindamycin in gynecology has been to treat or prevent bacteroides infections. Since pseudomembranous colitis has been reported to occur in up to 10% of patients, use should be limited to severely ill patients. Early proctoscopic diagnosis of pseudomembranous colitis usually due to *Clostridium difficile* allows therapy with vancomycin to treat this severe complication.

Aminoglycosides

Aminoglycosides are bactericidal antibiotics that induce misreading of the genetic code at the ribosomal level. They are effective against aerobic gram-negative bacilli and many strains of *Staphylococcus aureus*. They are not effective against bacteroides and most cocci. Parenteral administration is required as they are not absorbed by the gastrointestinal tract. Streptomycin has been replaced by gentamicin and kanamycin because they are more effective.

Adverse reactions. Damage to the eighth cranial nerve is the most common serious complication. Vestibular damage is the more common change with gentamicin, whereas kanamycin is more likely to cause deafness. Previous damage contraindicates use of these agents. With dizziness, vertigo, and tinnitus, reduction of dosage or discontinuance is in order.

Since aminoglycosides are eliminated by the kidney, creatinine blood levels should be determined before and during therapy and the dosage reduced accordingly. Rapidly acting diuretics should be avoided.

Aminoglycosides may produce neuromuscular blockage and enhance action of neuromuscular blocking agents or general anesthetics used during surgery. Parenteral magnesium in sizable doses and muscle relaxants should not be given. Gentamicin should not be mixed with carbenicillin in solutions, and it precipitates with heparin.

GENTAMICIN

Gentamicin is the first choice for *Pseudomonas aeruginosa*, an organism often hospital acquired, particularly in patients with indwelling urethral catheters.

KANAMYCIN

The drug kanamycin has the same effectiveness as gentamicin except that *Pseudomonas* is resistant to it. It is not absorbed after oral administration but is used to reduce bacteria in the colon before surgical entry into the large intestine.

Spectinomycin

Spectinomycin is an aminocyclitol antibiotic used only as a substitute for the single-dose treatment of gonorrheal urethritis and cervitis. Adverse effects after a single dose occur infrequently as pain at the site of injection, nausea, fever, or urticaria.

SELECTED REFERENCES

AMA drug evaluations, ed. 2, Acton, Mass., 1973, Publishing Sciences Group, Inc.

Bailey, G.L., and Straub, R.L.: Gram-negative septic shock: the new approach, South. Med. J. **59:**1327, 1966.

Charles, D.: Infections in obstetrics and gynecology, Clin. Obstet. Gynecol. **19:**45, 1976.

Collins, C.G., MacCallum, E.A., Nelson, E.W., Weinstein, B.B., and Collins, J.H.: Suppurative pelvic thrombophlebitis; a study of 70 patients treated by ligation of the inferior vena cava and ovarian vessels. I. Incidence, pathology, and etiology, Surgery **30:**311, 1951.

Collins, C.G., Nix, F.G., and Cerba, H.T.: Ruptured tubo-ovarian abscess, Am. J. Obstet. Gynecol. **72:**820, 1956.

Douglas, G.W.: Postoperative infections, Clin. Obstet. Gynecol. **5:**501, 1962.

Gall, S.A., Kohan, A.P., Ayers, O.M., et al.: Intravenous metronidazole or clindamycin with tobramycin for therapy of pelvic infections, Obstet. Gynecol. **57:**51, 1981.

Gupta, P.K., Lee, E.F., Erozan U.S., et al.: Cytologic investigations of *Chlamydia* infection, Actacytol. **23:**315, 1979.

Haines, M.: Tuberculous salpingitis as seen by the pathologist and the surgeon, Am. J. Obstet. Gynecol. **75:**472, 1958.

Halbrecht, I.: The relative value of culture and endometrial biopsy in the diagnosis of genital tuberculosis, Am. J. Obstet. Gynecol. **75:**899, 1958.

Johannisson, G., Lowhagen, G., and Lycke, E.: Genital *Chlamydia trachomatis* infection in women, Obstet. Gynecol. **56:**671, 1980.

Kardos, G.G.: Insoproterenol in the treatment of shock due to bacteremia with gram-negative pathogens, New Engl. J. Med. **274:**868, 1966.

Kitzmiller, J.L.: Septic shock: an eclectic view, Obstet. Gynecol. Surv. **26:**105, 1971.

Knaus, H.H.: Surgical treatment of genital and peritoneal tuberculosis in the female, Am. J. Obstet. Gynecol. **83:**73, 1962.

Lash, A.F.: The indications for surgical treatment in pelvic inflammatory disease, Surg. Clin. N. Am. **30:**299, 1950.

Maclean, L.D.: Pathogenesis and treatment of bacteremic shock, Surg. Gynecol. Obstet. **115:**307, 1962.

Moller, V.R., Westrom, L., Ahrons, S., et al.: *Chlamydia trachomatis* infection of the fallopian tubes: histological findings in two patients, Br. J. Vener. Dis. **55:**422, 1979.

Monif, G.R.G.: Infectious diseases in obstetrics and gynecology, ed. 1, New York, 1974, Harper & Row Publishers, Inc.

Paalman, R.J., Dockerty, M.B., and Mussey, R.D.: Acinomycosis of the ovaries and fallopian tubes, Am. J. Obstet. Gynecol. **58**:419, 1949.

Per-anders, M.: An overview of infectious agents of salpingitis, their biology, and recent advances in methods of detection, Am. J. Obstet. Gynecol. **138**:933, 1980.

Rees, E.: The treatment of pelvic inflammatory disease, Am. J. Obstet. Gynecol. **138**:1042, 1980.

Shands, K.N., Schmid, G.P., Dan, B.B., et al.: Toxic shock syndrome in menstruating women: association with tampon use and *Staphylococcus aureus* and clinical features in 52 cases, N. Engl. J. Med. **303**:1436, 1980.

Sutherland, A.M.: Tuberculosis of the endometrium, Obstet. Gynecol. **11**:527, 1958.

Tedesco, F.J., Gibbs, R.S., and Gallagher, M.: Clindamycin-associated colitis, Ann. Intern. Med. **81**:429, 1974.

Thompson, S.E., Hager, W.D., Wong., K.H., et. al.: The microbiology and therapy of acute pelvic inflammatory disease in hospitalized patients, Am. J.Obstet. Gynecol. **136**:179, 1980.

Yonekura, M.L., and di Zerega, G.S.: Antibiotic-associated colitis, Obstet. Gynecol. Surv. **35**:743, 1980.

Chapter 8

BENIGN LESIONS OF THE UTERUS

LESIONS OF CERVIX (Fig. 8-1)
Congenital ectopia

In congenital ectopia the endocervix (columnar epithelium) extends onto the portio vaginalis of the cervix, so that a red area surrounds the external cervical os. This mild degree of endocervical ectopia is considered normal during premenarchal development. Under estrogen influence and through metaplasia the columnar epithelium is replaced with squamous epithelium in an area that is called the transformation zone. The principal symptom before coitus is an increased amount of mucus. In children this mucus may cause the mother some alarm and may result in vulvitis if *Candida* or pathogenic bacteria grow therein. After coitus is frequent, cervicitis may occur. The increased amount of mucus may favor development of vaginitis. When the amount of mucus is excessive or when chronic cervicitis develops, destruction of the abnormally located endocervix is indicated.

Eversion

Eversion of the cervix is a "rolling-out" of the endocervix, which occurs with lacerations. When the condition is symptomatic, treatment by cryotherapy or electrocauterization may be performed. Should a deep laceration be found several weeks postpartum with no infection of the vulnerable endocervix, trachelorrhaphy may reestablish the cervical canal and reduce the eversion.

Eversion of the endocervix and hypertrophy of ectopia occur with the stimulation of oral contraceptives similar to the eversion and hypertrophy that occur during pregnancy. These changes will regress when the administration of oral estrogens and progestogens is stopped; therefore the decision concerning cryotherapy or cauterization may be better made after discontinuing the oral contraception.

Cervicitis

Acute cervicitis is most often bacterial. Trichomonads, *Candida*, or herpetic virus may be the cause. Specific diagnosis of endocervicitis due to gonococcus or *Chlamydia* requires proper culture (see Chapter 7).

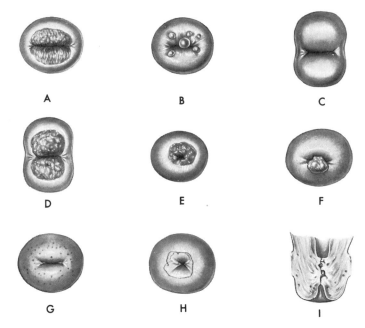

Fig. 8-1. Lesions of the cervix. **A,** Eversion. **B,** Nabothian cysts. **C,** Healed bilateral laceration. **D,** Bilateral laceration with eversion and chronic cervicitis. **E,** Congenital ectopia. **F,** Mucous polyp. **G,** Strawberry cervix of trichomoniasis. **H** and **I,** Cervical stenosis.

After Kleegman, S.J.: Am. J. Surg. **48:**294, 1940.

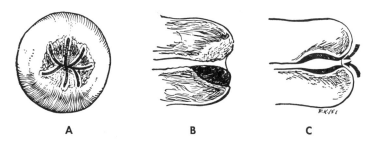

Fig. 8-2. Linear cauterization of the cervix. **A,** The cautery incisions and also the type of lesion suitable for this treatment. **B,** The deepening of the cautery incisions on the inside to secure inversion from the scar contraction. **C,** The correction of the eversion by contraction of the scars.

From Crossen R.J.: Diseases of women, St. Louis, The C.V. Mosby Co.

Chronic cervicitis is very common. The endocervix exposed on the vaginal portion of the cervix, whether as an eversion caused by laceration or as an ectopia, is vulnerable to recurrent infection. Within the cervical canal, foreign-body (stem pessary) reaction and trauma of instrumentation or abortion may invite infection. Repeated gonorrheal inflammation leads to structural changes.

Vaginal discharge is the principal symptom, varying from purulent yellow to clear mucoid. Pain or pressure in the lower abdomen or back may indicate lymphangitis. The cervix may bleed slightly on contact.

Chronic cervicitis undergoes exacerbations and remissions. There is a constant interplay between the squamous and columnar epithelium. The squamous epithelium tends to cover and occlude endocervical glands, so that retention (nabothian)

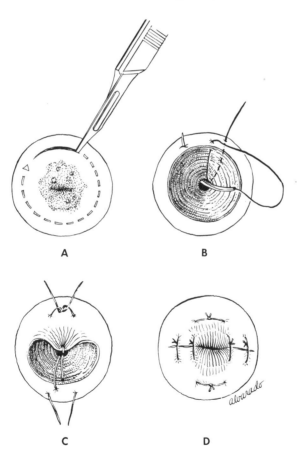

A   B

C   D

Fig. 8-3. Conization of the cervix, when done as illustrated, removes all grossly abnormal tissue for microscopic examination with an ample margin of normal tissue. Sturmdorf sutures are placed for control of bleeding and for repair of the cervix.

cysts filled with mucus form. When retention cysts are numerous, the cervix is enlarged. Squamous cells may be found replacing the cylindric cells of endocervical glands. This process is termed epidermization, squamous metaplasia, or squamous prosoplasia. The last term has been advocated by Fluhmann to indicate that bipotent subcolumnar cells, which become squamous as they grow toward the lumen, are derived from columnar cells.

After cleansing douches are used and acute inflammation, if present, is cleared, chronic cervicitis is treated by (1) electrocauterization in the office (Fig. 8-2), (2) cryoconization, (3) surgical conization (Fig. 8-3), or (4) total hysterectomy, depending on the extent of disease and the desire for childbearing.

Most carcinomas of the cervix occur after chronic cervicitis has been present for years. Eradication of the recurrently inflamed tissue is a means of preventing cancer. Every chronically diseased cervix should be suspected of being carcinomatous, and smears for cytologic study should be obtained before destruction or removal of the involved tissue. If colposcopic or gross findings suggest carcinoma, biopsy is mandatory.

Dysplasia of the cervix is a premalignant lesion. If the atypical hyperplasia has not reached the stage of carcinoma in situ, destruction or excision of the changed tissue should be curative. When areas of dysplasia have been adequately destroyed, the possibility of recurrence of dysplasia necessitates frequent reexaminations.

Cryoconization affords the advantages of little or no pain and of healing with minimal scar. Freezing of the tissue in the desired area is accomplished by heat transfer using liquid nitrogen, freon, carbon dioxide, or nitrous oxide in specially designed probes and is delivered with special equipment.

Endocervical (mucous) polyps

Endocervical polyps may form with chronic inflammatory changes. Mucoid vaginal discharge and bleeding are the usual symptoms. Most mucous polyps can be twisted off in the office. When the base of the polyp is high in the cervical canal, cervical dilation and curettage under anesthesia are required for complete removal. All polyps should be submitted to tissue study, although malignant changes are seldom found.

Cervical stenosis

Cervical stenosis may be developmental (congenital) in origin. Most often, scarring following cauterization, conization, amputation, trachelorrhaphy, or radium application is the cause. Retention cysts, myomas, or polyps may partially obstruct the cervical canal. Postmenopausal atrophy tends toward stenosis and at times complete occlusion. With the latter, pyometra may result. Cancer is the usual cause of obstruction when there is pus in the uterus in postmenopausal women.

Many women with cervical stenosis, which is a normal finding in old women, have no symptoms. Dysmenorrhea, irregular bleeding, leukorrhea, and sterility may result.In the absence of neoplasia, repeated dilations in the office may correct the stricture. Rarely conization is in order, or with accompanying disease hysterectomy may be indicated. Pyometra requires dilation under anesthesia and maintenance of adequate drainage. Bacteriologic study by smear or culture may allow more effective employment of antibiotic therapy.

Hypertrophy

Hypertrophy resulting in marked elongation of the intravaginal portion of the cervix occasionally occurs without infection. If protrusion to or outside the introitus is annoying, amputation should be done if hysterectomy is contraindicated.

LESIONS OF CERVICAL STUMP

The cervical stump remaining after partial hysterectomy may have or may develop the benign diseases discussed in this chapter. It should be excised transvaginally to effect cure.

LESIONS OF UTERUS
Uterine myomas

Except for pregnancy, myomas are the most common cause of uterine enlargement. Since they are of muscle cell origin, they are preferably not called by the term "fibroids." Supporting connective tissue is a secondary component as a rule. However, if such tissue is markedly present, the growth is justifiably termed "fibromyoma." If the myoma contains endometrial glands, it is properly designated "adenomyoma" (see Chapter 11). Uterine myomas have their highest incidence in blacks. They have been diagnosed most frequently in patients between ages 30 and 45. Pregnancy may cause myomas to increase in size but does not favor their genesis, as they are relatively more common in the nulliparous uterus. New tumors do not originate after the menopause, and existing ones usually regress but do not disappear. Rapid postmenopausal increase in size should suggest the possibility of leiomyosarcoma; however, some benign tumors gradually enlarge.

Myomas may be single, but they are usually multiple. Their size varies from microscopic to gigantic. Characteristically they are pseudoencapsulated spherical nodules subject to enucleation; on the cut surface they have a whorled appearance. Microscopically bundles of unstriped muscle cells can be seen in many directions. The shape of the cells varies from round or polyhedral to spindle, depending upon whether the bundles are cut transversely or longitudinally. The nuclei are of the rod type with somewhat rounded extremities.

Secondary changes. The gross and microscopic features of the typical myoma may be strikingly altered by *degenerative processes*, including *hyaline, cystic, fatty, calcareous, infectious, necrotic, necrobiotic (carneous), sarcomatous,* and

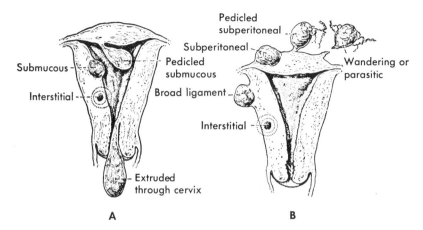

Fig. 8-4. A, Development of different types of submucous myomas. **B,** Development of different types of subperitoneal myomas.

From Crossen, R.J.: Diseases of women, St. Louis, The C.V. Mosby Co.

atrophic. Lymphangiectatic and agniomatous or telangiectatic changes may be observed.

Location. Fig. 8-4 depicts various uterine myomas that are classified as *intramural,* within the myometrium; *submucous,* beneath the endometrium; and *subserous,* beneath the peritoneum. The last two are often pedunculated. Myomas may be *corporal, fundal, cervical, intraligamentary,* or *parasitic.* The parasitic type constitutes one of the curiosities of pathology and is called a *wandering myoma.*

Symptoms and signs. The symptoms and signs depend very largely on the location and size of the uterine myoma. In many patients the status is such that there are no subjective complaints. Submucous growths are the most troublesome as causes of abnormal bleeding and persistent endometrial infection. When the growth disturbs the endometrium, *bleeding* occurs.

The increased bleeding may be caused by (1) increase in the surface area of the endometrium, (2) associated endometrial hyperplasia, (3) ulceration of the endometrium, or (4) venous dilatation and congestion of the endometrium. It is usually first manifested as hypermenorrhea. Later the duration and amount of hemorrhage may cause anemia. A cervical myoma may result in a blood vaginal discharge, and in some instances it causes dyspareunia. When *pressure* is involved, the tumor is encroaching on the bladder, rectum, ovaries, nerves, or some other structure.

Infection, necrobiosis, and *necrosis* cause pain, fever, acceleration of erythrocyte sedimentation rate, and leukocytosis as a rule. *Torsion* is painful and if very marked is likely to produce shock. *Dystocia* results from myomatous obstruction of the birth canal. Other possible childbearing complications of myomas include sterility, abortion, uterine malposition, fetal malpresentation and malposition, uterine inertia, postpartum hemorrhage, and uterine subinvolution. A pregnant myomatous uterus infrequently becomes incarcerated in the pelvis. During pregnancy with increased vascularity, bleeding into and around myomas may occur with resulting pain (carneous degeneration).

Diagnosis. On palpation the uterus is usually enlarged, nodular, and firm. Softening suggests the possibility of pregnancy, necessitating further observation or pregnancy tests. Inflammatory or neoplastic adnexal masses adherent to the uterus may be mistaken for myomas. Omental and intestinal adhesions often obscure the diagnosis. Uterine enlargement may be caused by adenomyosis or subinvolution. Although not enlarged, the uterus may harbor a troublesome submucous myoma that can be diagnosed by curettement or hysterography.

In cases of infertility, especially relative or secondary, the possibility of myoma should be considered.

When myomas are diagnosed, the possibility of associated diseases must still be entertained since myomas are common. Too often the nodular masses in the uterus are thought to be the cause of bleeding when abortion, cancer, or adenomyosis is the unrecognized cause.

Therapy. Small tumors causing no trouble require no therapy. These are ordinarily found at the time of routine examination. In disclosing their presence to the patient one should inform her as to their innocuousness and emphasize that she should be examined at least every 6 months.

There is one class of small myomas that we consider an excpetion to the rule of "no symptoms, no treatment," namely, cervical myomas. Their removal through the vagina is usually comparatively simple. An asymptomatic myomatous uterus of the size of a 12 weeks' gestation requires surgical treatment because of the probability of the development of complications.

In young patients dysfunctional bleeding in association with myomas may be treated with combined estrogens and progestogens, but one should not procrastinate in searching for submucous myomas if the response is not satisfactory.

If the symptoms indicate need for an opeation, the gynecologist must duly consider the age of the patient; her gravidity and parity; her desire for progeny; the location, size, condition, and number of the myomas; and her general condition, including complicating factors. Uterine curettage may stop the bleeding and permit the exclusion of endometrial cancer in some patients. If, however there is marked distortion of the uterine cavity, curettement cannot be expected to be adequate. Cytosmears are mentioned again for emphasis.

Myomectomy, single or multiple, is done in suitable cases when the patient requires definitive treatment and the uterus should be conserved. Certain cases of infertility should be so treated when one is sure that all other possible causes of barrenness have been eliminated. Asymptomatic tumors encountered during oper-

ations involving the pelvic cavity may usually be similarly treated. As a rule my-
omectomies are contraindicated at cesarean section because of the vascularity of the
uterus. Tumors that might interfere with childbearing are best removed when the
patient is not pregnant. During gestation, if a myoma undergoes red degeneration
that does not subside with analgesics, bed rest, and antibiotics administered to
prevent or control associated infection, myomectomy is indicated. Marked torsion
of a tumor requires emergency surgery, and the gynecologist clamps the blood
vessels to prevent the release of thrombi into the circulation upon its manipulation.

A really symptomatic myomatous uterus is usually best removed. Before *hysterectomy* the patient and her husband are entitled to an elucidative discussion of
the purpose and function of the uterus, with care being taken to explain the role of
menstruation. At that time one should discuss ovarian physiology, emphasizing that
the ovaries are glands of internal secretion, which are active after removal of the
uterus, and that consequently they will be left in situ unless the findings absolutely
necessitate their extirpation. A few words regarding the production of "female hormone" by the adrenal glands are appreciated by patients schedules for hysterectomy and bilateral salpingo-oophorectomy. In each case the decision must be made
regarding the type of operation that should be done, but one must not do an incomplete operation by removing the corpus uteri and leaving the cervix. Fortunately
such developments as modern anesthesiology, improvements in surgical technique
and materials, and the availability of antimicrobials have made the total hysterectomy less hazardous than the supracervical variety. In the presence of urethrocys-
tocele, rectocele, enterocele, and/or actual or traction-demonstrable uterine de-
scensus of myomatous uteri not larger than the size of a 12 weeks' gestation, vaginal
hysterectomy is the procedure of choice, provided there is no complicating degree
of pelvic inflammatory disease or endometriosis. Malignancies, ovarian tumors, in-
traligamentous growth, and sizable tumors beneath the bladder are usually considered to be contraindications to the vaginal approach.

Radiation therapy of myomas is reserved for those rare patients for whom there
is an absolute contraindication to surgery but who require intervention because of
bleeding that does not respond to conservative measures. As time has elapsed, this
group has decreased to practically nil. Dr. R.J. Crossen has pointed out the fact
that radium therapy has been erroneously criticized by some investigators because
of the supposed tendency for radiation to cause endometrial carcinoma in later life.
It is generally agreed that the beneficial result of radiation is primarily because of
its castration effect upon the ovaries. This fact causes the gynecologist to perofrm
surgery with conservation of the ovaries unless there is definite indication for their
extirpation or unless the patient is a poor surgical risk. Uterine carcinoma evidently
develops as frequently in myomatous as in nonmyomatous uteri, but the presence
of myomas in the uterus does not seem to predispose the woman to a greater than
average incidence of adenocarcinoma.

Uterine polyps

Uterine polyps include pedicled submucous myomatous and adenomyomatous growths, but the most common are the endometrial polyps, which have a structure like that of the endometrium and are called adenomatous polyps. They are to be compared with the mucous polyps, which constitute the majority arising from the cervix uteri. They may cause a mucous discharge. Novak and Novak have discussed both polyps composed of immature endometrium and polyps composed of functional endometrium, pointing out the difficulties in distinguishing them from the microscopic patterns of adenocarcinoma. Malignant degeneration of a benign polyp is a rare occurrence, but there may be coexisting malignancy. The term "multiple polyposis" is used by them in preference to "polypoid hyperplasia of the endometrium" in cases of endometrial hyperplasia with a uterine cavity full of polypoid masses. Polyps may be single or multiple and small or large enough to fill the uterine cavity. The pedicle may be short or sufficiently long to allow protrusion of the polyp through the cervical canal into the vagina and very rarely through the introitus.

Clinical symptoms are usually not produced by the small polyps, but the large ones or those with long pedicles often undergo degeneration and ulceration with resultant bleeding. Postcoital "spotting" or active bleeding may result from a polyp exposed to the trauma of coitus. In some cases patients have intermenstrual bleeding, particularly premenstrual "spotting." *Adenomyomatous* polyps are obviously a type of endometriosis. *Placental* polyps may form after incomplete abortion and be easily removed by forceps or curet. The placental polyps that are found days or months after parturition of a term pregnancy may be caused by placenta accreta and a hysterectomy may be required.

Therapy. If a polyp is single, its removal is usually simple. The routine procedure performed is cervical dilation and uterine curettement. A Randall stone forceps or a sponge forceps should be used to search for polyps that may be missed by the curet. Obviously the curettage should be thorough, since there may be an associated malignancy within the uterine cavity.

In the case of a symptomatic myomatous uterus with bleeding caused by an infected polyp projecting through the cervical os, it is good judgment to remove the polyp and to treat the infection before to extirpating the uterus; otherwise peritonitis or a wound infection may occur.

Angiomas and cysts

Lymphangioma is a rare uterine lesion, and hemangioma is even more rare. Pedowitz and co-workers have reviewed the literature on vascular uterine tumors, including these and hemangiopericytoma.

Cysts of Gartner's duct and similar topics have already been discussed (see Chapter 3).

SELECTED REFERENCES

Carter, B., Jones, C.P., Ross, R.A., and Thomas, W.L.: A bacteriologic and clinical study of pyometra, Am. J. Obstet. Gynecol. **62:**793, 1951.

Crossen, R.J.: Wide conization of the cervix, Am. J. Obstet. Gynecol. **57:**187, 1949.

Faulkner, R.L.: Blood vessels of myomatous uterus, Am. J. Obstet. Gynecol. **47:**185, 1944.

Fluhmann, C.F.: The histiogenesis of acquired erosions of the cervix uteri, Am. J. Obstet. Gynecol. **82:**790, 1961.

Haskins, A.L., and Sehgal, N.: The mechanism of uterine bleeding in the presence of fibromyomas, Am. Surg. **26:**21, 1960.

Hofmeister, F.J., and Gortley, R.L.: Benign lesions of cervix, Obstet. Gynecol. **5:**504, 1955.

Holden, F.C.: Treatment of cervicitis, particularly by cautery and operation, Am. J. Obstet. Gynecol. **16:**624, 1928.

Kistner, R.W., and Hertig, A.T.: Papillomas of the uterine cervix, Obstet. Gynecol. **6:**147, 1955.

Miller, N.F., and Ludovici, P.P.: Origin and development of uterine fibroids, Am. J. Obstet. Gynecol. **70:**720, 1955.

Miller, N.F., Ludovici, P.P., and Dontas, E.: Problem of the uterine fibroid, Am. J. Obstet. Gynecol. **66:**734, 1953.

Novak, E., and Novak, E.R.: Gynecologic and obstetric pathology, Philadelphia, 1958, W.B. Saunders Co.

Parks, J., and Barter, R.H.: The myomatous uterus complicated by pregnancy, Am. J. Obstet. Gynecol. **63:**260, 1952.

Pedowitz, P., Felmus, L.B., and Grayzel, D.M.: Vascular tumors of the uterus, Am. J. Obstet. Gynecol. **69:**1291, 1955.

Roblee, M.A.: Cervicitis clinic—twenty-five years in review, Am. J. Obstet. Gynecol. **71:**660, 1956.

Romney, S.L., Gray, M.J., Little, A.B., et al.: Gynecology and obstetrics—the health care of women, Hightstown, N.J., 1981, McGraw-Hill Book Co.

Scott, R.B.: The elusive endometrial polyp, Obstet. Gynecol. **1:**212, 1953.

Te Linde, R.W.: Operative gynecology, ed. 3, Philadelphia, 1962, J.B. Lippincott Co.

Chapter 9

CANCER OF THE UTERUS

The three types of malignant neoplasms that may originate in the uterus are carcinoma of the cervix, adenocarcinoma of the endometrium, and sarcoma. Choriocarcinoma is of trophoblastic origin and is discussed Chapter 13.

CARCINOMA OF CERVIX

Cervical carcinoma is second to carcinoma of the breast as the most common cancer of women. It is the most common genital cancer. Formerly it was reported to occur eight times as often as endometrial cancer. More recently it appears to be occurring approximately four times as often as endometrial cancer, and in some groups of patients cervical cancer has been found to be less common than endometrial cancer. It is estimated that 2% of women past 40 years of age will develop carcinoma of the cervix. The majority of these cancers are squamous cell in type (95%). The other 5% occur as adenocarcinoma of the endocervix.

Cervical intraepithelial neoplasia (CIN)

Before menarche the vaginal portion of the cervix is covered in varying degrees with columnar epithelium that is continuous with the endocervix. With increased estrogen production metaplasia occurs, so that the columnar epithelium is converted into squamous epithelium. Metaplasia occurs in varying degrees in patients and is normal process. After coitus begins and there is some degree of cervicitis, changes in cellular morphology, epithelial pattern, and subepithelial vascular arrangement may be found in the transformation zone. (The transformation zone is the area of squamous epithelium that was formerly columnar.) With more years of intercourse, more cervicitis, and more pregnancies, dysplasia becomes more likely. CIN is nonexistent in celibate women. When dysplasia does occur the practicality of eradication by adequate treatment must be considered. Dysplasia may disappear without treatment, may not become more severe, or may develop into carcinoma in situ. When dysplasia becomes more marked, microscopic examination reveals a loss of stratification of the cervical epithelium and the term "carcinoma in situ" is

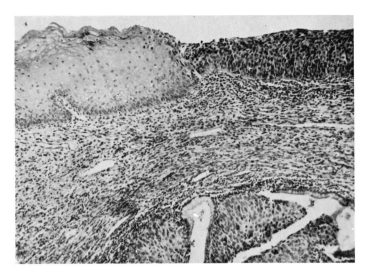

Fig. 9-1. Note the abrupt change between the normal epithelium of the cervix uteri on the left and the malignant change on the right.

Courtesy Dr. John H. Dent and Dr. J.H. Dent, Department of Pathology, Tulane University School of Medicine, New Orleans, La.

used. The mean age of patients with carcinoma in situ at the time of diagnosis is about 35 years. Dysplasia or carcinoma in situ may originate in a single site or in multiple sites within the transformation zone. The upper limits of the transformation zone, i.e., the squamocolumnar junction, are visible in the majority of patients; however, in some it is within the cervical canal and cannot be seen even with a colposcope. If the dysplastic changes extend into the cervical glands and crypts, they are not visible with the colposcope. On tissue section study there may be some confusion as to the possibility of invasion through the basement membrane and hence some difficulty in making an accurate diagnosis.

CIN can occur on the "pretty" cervix. It cannot be diagnosed by ordinary examination. Cytologic study of material obtained by scraping the transformation zone is the most practical method of identifying suspected CIN. Inclusion of mucoid material from the area of the cervix will allow better identification of shed cells. A moist cotton-tipped application can be used when the transformation zone is within the canal. In properly screened groups the most common abnormal smears should indicate dysplasia or carcinoma in situ. (The Papanicolaou smear should not be considered primarily as a means of diagnosing invasive carcinoma of the cervix but should be considered as a means of preventing injury caused by cancer by finding the precursors of the invasive lesions.) Fortunately the time required for the development of dysplasia into invasive cancer is commonly several years, and time exists for repeated cytologic study and diagnosis. The proper therapy for cervical intraepithelial neoplasia should prevent most invasive squamous cell carcinoma.

When large numbers of smears are evaluated statistically it is found that from 10% to 15% of smear reports are falsely negative. Some studies indicate that with colposcopy alone even a higher percentage of CIN may be missed. These statistics indicate that the technique of obtaining cytosmears is of great importance. It also indicates the limitations of colposcopy. When the entire transitional zone is not available for scraping, the likelihood of false-negative reports increases. Distortion of the transitional zone is particularly apt to occur after conization of the cervix, cryoconization, cauterization, and laser therapy. In older patients, particularly menopausal ones, the upper portion of the transitional zone is frequently not accessible. Since neoplastic change develops in deeper crypts and endophytic spread may occur, all invasive cancers cannot be identified in the preinvasive stage. With good screening techniques it is estimated that 5% or more of invasive squamous cell cancers of the cervix occur in patients who have had regular examinations. These lesions are usually Stage IB occult.

Cytology is used to detect change. Biopsy is required to evaluate the type of lesion. Colposcopy allows the evaluation of the borders of the lesion and selection of small sites for biopsy. If the entire squamocolumnar junction and consequently all of the transformation zone can be visualized, then biopsy of abnormal areas will allow accurate diagnosis. When the upper limit of the transformation zone cannot be seen, it is necessary that the endocervical area be curetted and this tissue properly diagnosed.

CIN is treated by removal or destruction of the abnormal areas. Excision with biopsy instruments as an outpatient procedure has been shown to be frequently inadequate in eradicating CIN. When dysplastic change occurs in the transitional zone, it appears justified to destroy the entire zone by freezing, cryosurgery, heat, cautery, electrocoagulation, or surgical conization. Adequate tissue must be removed. Delineation of the lesion's borders particularly by colposcopy is essential. Follow-up by cytology and colposcopy for evidence of primary recurrence or development of new lesions is essential for adequate therapy.

Without the use of colposcopy, diagnostic conization is required. Unfortunately hemorrhage and infection may occur after conization. The risks of anesthesia are involved. For selected patients with CIN, particularly for patients with carcinoma in situ when surgical sterilization is desired or when other diseases of the uterus such as prolapse or leiomyomas coexist, hysterectomy may be justified as a means of eradicating the disease in a preinvasive stage.

Invasive carcinoma of the cervix

The mean age of patients with invasive squamous cell carcinoma is about 47 years. This would lead us to think that in some cases cancer has preexisted for approximately 10 years as carcinoma in situ. The gross lesions that appear may be a type having a small granular area and later developing as a cauliflower-like growth that has been descibed as an exophytic form of cancer. In other patients the growth is principally invasive and endophytic, and the tumor appears as an area of induration and ulceration. The cervix may enlarge.

After invasive cancer has existed for months to years, the patient may develop a water discharge and notice spotting, particularly on contact with the cervix as during coitus.It should be emphasized that when these symptoms occur the cancer is somewhat advanced. As the cancer invades through the tissue spaces into the bases of the broad ligament and along the upper vagina, tenderness and pain may develop. The growth may extend upward into the body of the uterus. The spread fore and aft is somewhat limited by fascial planes that offer temporary protection to the bladder and rectum.

Vein permeation may occur with early degrees of invasion. Blood vessel invasion indicates a bad prognosis. The differentiation of venous spaces from lymphatic spaces may necessitate elastic tissue stains. Invasion of lymphatics tends to occur relatively early, and metastasis to the external iliac nodes, obturator nodes, and internal iliac and common iliac nodes may occur progressively. Tumor may be found in nodes when there is no other tumor histologically identifiable outside the cervix. This status leads to the idea of lymphatic embolism. Lymph nodes may enlarge to cause venous obstruction and edema of the thigh and leg. By direct extension and/or lymphatic extension the ureter is often encircled by the growth. Ureteral obstruction occurs with the development of hydroureter, hydronephrosis, and pyelonephritis. Extension to the lateral pelvic wall with resulting induration and fixation may be associated with an increased amount of pelvic and back pain. When the bladder wall is invaded, the first cystoscopic sign is edema. Ulceration and hematuria may be noted later. Similar effects can occur in the rectum. With necrosis of carcinomatous tissue, fistulas develop.

Sizable carcinomas of the cervix are usually associated with some degree of cellulitis. There may be an associated endometritis and salpingitis. At times the induration of infection and of the fibrosis that follows infection cannot be distinguished on palpation from carcinomatous extension. The growth may block the cervix and be a cause for pyometra. (This is more likely to occur with adenocarcinoma of the endocervix.) Bony metastases occur most frequently in the bodies of the vertebrae and may lead to pathologic fractures.

Distant metastases have been reported in 25% to 45% of autopsy cases. Order of frequency has been listed as liver, bone, lung, bowel, brain, and skin.

As previously indicated, the patient may experience pain and vaginal bleeding. With erosion of sizable cervical or vaginal vessels, this bleeding may be very marked. The more extensive degrees of cancer cause pain from irritation of pelvic nerves or those leaving the cord in instances of spinal metastasis. The majority of

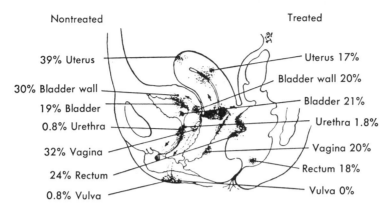

Fig. 9-2. Incidence of organ involvement in 154 nontreated and 202 treated cases of cervical carcinoma. From Henriksen, E.: Radiology **54:**812, 1950.

patients dying from carcinoma of the cervix die as a result of uremia caused by ureteral obstruction and impairment of renal function. Intestinal obstruction may occur because of metastasis.

The course of carcinoma of the cervix is variable. It is correlated somewhat with the histologic grading (Broder) but is more likely to be related to the staging of the disease, which will be discussed later. Some small primary lesions exhibit lymph gland metastasis early, whereas other very large local lesions have no associated lymphatic involvement. Illustrating the extreme variation of this frequently lethal disease, reports from California showed that 13% of the patients whose conditions were diagnosed histologically as carcinoma of the cervix and who were not treated lived 5 years.

Adenocarcinoma of cervix

Endocervical carcinoma may present as a lesion through the cervical os; however, more frequently it is not seen as such. When it is recognized, the extent of its invasion is likely to be greater than that of squamous cell carcinoma even in patients having frequent routine examinations. The tendency of lymphatic spread of this histologic type is similar to that of squamous cell carcinoma. About one half of endocervical adenocarcinomas originate in the endometrium. Since about 50% of adenocarcinomas of the cervix are not suspected by cytology and the lesions usually cannot be seen with colposcopy, bloody and mucopurulent endocervical mucus should be investigated by endocervical curettage.

Etiology

Although the primary cause of cervical malignancy is not known, certain factors seem to be associated with an increased incidence of cancer. Women with chronic cervicitis, more years of coitus, more coital partners, herpes type 2 antibodies, and more pregnancies have more cervical malignancies. Conversely, cervical cancer is almost nonexistent in celibate women and occurs less with adequate treatment of cervicitis. Jewish women have fewer cervical malignancies than non-Jewish women. Indigent women have a high incidence.

Diagnosis

It is desirable that neoplasia of the cervix be diagnosed in an intraepithelial phase. Under these circumstances, though, the patient is asymptomatic, and un-magnified observation of the cervix often reveals no gross lesions suggestive of neo-plasm. It is apparent that cytologic study is required. After coitus begins annual cytologic studies should be made. More frequent examinations are necessary with cervical disease. If there are gross exophytic or ulcerative lesions suggestive of can-cer, biopsy should be performed. When outpatient destruction of benign lesions is planned by cryoconization or cautery, cytologic studies should always be performed and other steps to rule out invasive cancer and to adequately identify the extent of the CIN should be employed before destruction of the lesions When cervical smears are reported to contain atypical cells suggestive of inflammation, cervicitis and vaginitis should be treated and the smears repeated. Persistent atypical cells on smears require colposcopy. When the cytologic findings are consistent with CIN Grade I, II, or III, colposcopically directed biopsy is indicated for any areas sugges-tive or indicative of CIN. When invasive squamous cell carcinoma is suggested by smear examination and no gross lesion is seen, colposcopy and biopsy are required. The limitations of colposcopy and the need for conization and, at times, endocer-vical curettage have been indicated in the discussion of CIN. If minimal invasion is identified on punch biopsy, conization is required to further delineate the extent of invasion before selection of the method of therapy.

When a trained colposcopist is not available, lesions exhibiting atypical cells that persist after treatment for inflammation require biopsy. Biopsy is required with smears consistent with CIN or invasive cancer; it should be directed by iodine staining. When iodine is applied to the cervix, the normal epithelium takes on a mahogany color because of the glycogen contained therein, whereas neoplastic ep-ithelium and some benignly diseased tissues, along with the endocervix, do not take the stain. The endocervix should be curetted for biopsy. When carcinoma in situ is diagnosed without colposcopy, cervical conization for diagnostic purposes is imperative to avoid missing areas of invasion. If microinvasion is found during out-patient biopsy, conization becomes imperative to determine the extent of invasion before selecting the method of therapy. To be certain that there are no areas of invasive cancer, one must remove a cone of tissue from the cervix to eliminate all likely sites of neoplasm. Numerous sections can then be made of this tissue to determine the areas of involvement and the depth of invasion. In patients past menopause, cervical stenosis is more likely and the transitional zone may be within the endocervical canal. Under these circumstances cytologic diagnosis is more in-accurate, and curettage of the endocervix and cervical conizations become neces-sary for the proper diagnosis of cervical neoplasms.

During recent years physicians have become more knowledgeable on the natu-ral course of cervical neoplasms, including recognition of the long preinvasive phase. With the increase in the number of competent colposcopists, more patients are being treated for CIN and minimal invasion, so that the death rate from cervical cancer is diminishing in certain populations.

Clinical staging of cancer of cervix

The international classification of the stages of cancer of the cervix is as follows:

Stage 0
This includes carcinoma in situ, intraepithelial carcinoma.

Stage I
The carcinoma is strictly confined to the cervix (extension to the corpus should be disregarded).

Stage IA
This includes microinvasive carcinoma (early stromal invasion).

Stage IB
This includes all other cases of Stage I; occult cancer should be marked "occ."

Stage II
The carcinoma extends beyond the cervix, but has not extended to the pelvic wall. The carcinoma involves the vagina, but not as far as the lower third.

Stage IIA
There is no obvious parametrial involvement.

Stage IIB
There is obvious parametrial involvement.

Stage III
The carcinoma has extended to the pelvic wall. On rectal examination, there is no cancer-free space between the tumor and the pelvic wall. The tumor involves the lower third of the vagina. All cases with hydronephrosis or nonfunctioning kidney are included.

Stage IIIA
There is no extension to the pelvic wall.

Stage IIIB
There is extension to the pelvic wall and/or hydronephrosis or nonfunctioning kidney.

Stage IV

The carcinoma has extended beyond the true pelvis or has clinically involved the mucosa of the bladder or rectum. A bullous edema as such does not permit a case to be allotted to Stage IV.

Stage IVA

The growth has spread to adjacent organs.

Stage IVB

The growth has spread to distant organs.

There is considerable difficulty in accurately determining the extent of cancer by palpation. As just indicated, the induration of active infection and of the fibrosis that follows infection may be confused with the infiltration of carcinomatous tissue. Associated endometriosis, ovarian tumors, or uterine tumors may cause further confusion. Tumor-bearing lymph nodes of the pelvis usually are not felt and can be found only in surgical specimens properly examined histologically. The following classification gives the postoperative designation of nodal involvement as correlated with the clinical staging of cancer:

Stage I

Nodal involvement 15%

Stage II

Nodal involvement 25%

Stages III and IV

Nodal involvement 30% (determined by exenteration); nodal involvement after radiation 42% (determined by exenteration)

Therapy

If the therapy is to be curative, all malignant tissue must be removed or destroyed. When this cannot be accomplished, the treatment is palliative. When, on conization, microinvasive Stage IA lesions are found and not only the depth of invasion is not in excess of 3 mm, but also there are no confluent tongues and no obvious lymphatic or vascular invasion, abdominal or vaginal hysterectomy is justified therapy; care is necessary to remove sufficient vaginal mucous membranes to include all areas noted as abnormal on colposcopy or as not taking the iodine stain. Cervical lesions that do not meet these rigid criteria should be classified as Stage IB and treated by irradiation or hysterectomy with parametrial excision and gland dissection. When the carcinoma starts to involve the parametrium, it is particularly important to determine the condition of the ureters by ureterography. Whether the therapy is surgical or radiologic, the correction of anemias and the clearing of infection are necessary to give optimum response and to prevent complications. The majority of invasive carcinomas of the cervix are now treated by irradiation. In some centers surgery is employed for selected patients as primary therapy and for use in cases of failure or certain complications after irradiation.

Radiation therapy. Radioactive substances may be placed within the endometrial cavity, within the endocervical canal, or in the vagina adjacent to the cervix or vaginal lesions. Radium 226 is most commonly used for these applications. Cesium 137, iridium 192, and tantalium 182, as well as cobalt 60, can also be used for this purpose. Radiation can be applied from a distance through the skin and tissues of the abdomen to the desired area or by use of cones through the vagina. Radiation machines include the linear accelerator and the betatron. Teletherapy units make use of the radioactive material cobalt 60 or cesium 137, which is housed in a protective barrier; emission of gamma radiation is through a collimator that allows direction of the radiation to a certain area.

The unit of quantity of radiation is the roentgen. It is defined as that quantity of x or gamma radiation that will produce ionization 2.09×10^9 electrons per cubic centimeter of air at normal temperature and pressure. The rad is a unit of absorbed dose. It is a measure of energy imparted to matter by ionizing radiation per unit mass of an irradiated material. It is equivalent to 100 ergs per gram. Radiation causes ionization and excitation with resulting chemical changes within cells involving many substances from water to complex proteins. The histologic evidences of chemical changes are vacuolization, cellular swelling, chromatin changes, disruption of cell membranes, necrosis, endarteritis, and increase in lymphocytes and plasma cells. Later there are formation of fibrous tissue and obliteration of lymph and blood vessels. The tissues are apt to become whiter with loss of vascularity and pigment. Areas of telangiectasis may form.

For radiation therapy to be feasible the effect on neoplastic tissue must be greater than that on normal tissue. If the differential radiosensitivity is such that the neoplasms or the lymphatics are more sensitive, benefits are more easily obtained. Because of the accessibility of cervical and endometrial neoplasia for direct application of radioactive materials, a larger dose can be applied to the tumor area, since the normal tissue is for the most part at a greater distance from the source of radiation. The radiation dose is inversely proportional to the square of the distance from the source. Increasing the distance from 1 to 2 cm reduces the dose to one fourth. When the radium tubes are held in a line by a rubber or plastic container and placed in the cervical canal and endometrial cavity, the term "tandem" is used. When ovoid applicators are placed in the vaginal fornices about the cervix, the term "colpostat" is used (Fig. 9-3). The size of the uterus, cervix, and vagina, as well as the size of the growth, will govern the spatial arrangements of the sources of radiation. It is desired to screen out all but gamma rays and to properly calibrate the amount of radiation that is being emitted from a container. The radium salt or other material is placed in a filtering metal tube and is calibrated for its rate of

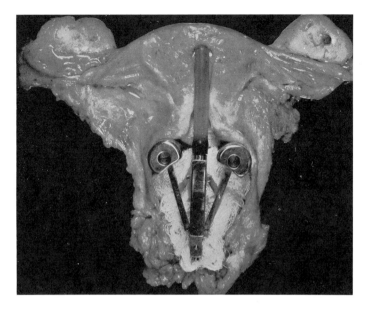

Fig. 9-3. Cross-sectional view of a uterus with colpostat in place showing vaginal packing.

From Ter-Pogossian, M., Sherman, A.I., and Arneson, A.N.: Am. J. Obstet. Gynecol. **64**:937, 1952.

emission. By knowing this calibration and plotting isodose curves by the use of phantoms for various amounts and spatial arrangements of radiation sources, one can predict that amounts of radiation that will reach various points.

As can be seen from the foregoing discussion, it is necessary that radiation applications be performed by a physician with considerable knowledge of radiation physics, since there will be variation from one case to another. It is also necessary that this clinician be well schooled in gynecologic pathology to avoid the problems that occur with necrosis of accompanying myomas of the uterus or ovarian neoplasms. Similarly he must be appraised of the likelihood of adhesions of the bowel about the uterus or cul-de-sac.

For radium applications the cervix is dilated and a tandem holding the source of radiation is placed within the uterus. After the colpostats have been placed in the vagina, the vagina is packed with gauze in an effort to keep the vulnerable bladder and rectum as far as possible away from the radiation source. It is important that the bladder be kept empty with an indwelling catheter and that the rectum and colon be previously emptied and remain so during the application. As indicated

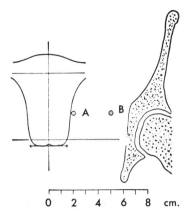

Point "A" receives 200 R per 1 mg. of radium each 24 hrs.

Tubes containing 5 mg. deliver 1,000 R at "A" in 24 hrs.

Using from 8 to 15 tubes, 960 to 1,800 mg. hrs. per day
   are employed.

For 4,400 mg. hrs., point "B" receives approximately
   1,000 R or about 0.2 to 0.4 of the dose at "A".

Fig. 9-4. Cancer of the cervix—radium treatment. Diagrammatic representation of dose falling at specified points for different intensities of irradiation (Manchester system).

From Arneson, A.N.: In Meigs, J.V., and Sturgis, S.H., editors: Progress in gynecology, vol. 2, New York, Grune & Stratton, Inc.

in Fig. 9-4, point A is located 2 cm from the midline of the cervical canal and 2 cm superior to the lateral vaginal fornix. Point B is 5 cm from the midline along the same lateral axis. The amount of radiation reaching points A and B can be calculated by knowing the amount of radium in the applicators and the position of the applicators. The size and location of the cancerous tissue, the variations in the length of the cervical canal, and the size of the vagina must be taken into account in placing the radium. The use of points A and B is of limited value in the calculation of the dose delivered to the neoplastic tissue.

The total amount of radiation to be applied to the pelvis varies with the stage of disease. The applications are planned in order that the sites of known cancer receive the most rads. In Stage IIIB and Stage IVA the maximum amounts of 6000 to 7000 rads are delivered to the pelvis.

Two separate applications appear to accomplish the best result. Either radiation may be inserted for about 48 hours, removed for 24 to 48 hours, and reapplied, so that the hospitalization of 6 to 7 days results, or radiation may be applied for 72 hours and the patient discharged from the hospital to return for a second application 14 days later. This method of two separate applications tends to avoid infection, severe systemic reaction, and undesirable local reaction. When treatment is delayed 2 weeks there may be gross improvement in the size of the lesion, so that the second application is more appropriate.

In addition to the radiation applied directly to the tumor, radiation is applied through the skin in an effort to deliver to the areas of the lymph nodes of the pelvis sufficient radiation to kill tumor tissue or to cause obliteration of lymphatics and trap cancer cells. External irradiation and/or transvaginal irraditation may be used before direct application to the cervix when infection is present or the cervical growth is large. This method avoids mechanical disruption of natural barriers to infection and allows shrinkage of the lesions for better placement of colpostats. Linear accelerators are becoming the most commonly used methods of external radiation. They have the advantage of producing greater depth dosage because of higher energy beams. Linear accelerators are machines producing radiation. A cobalt 60 source has a half-life of 5.3 years. When cobalt 60 is used for teletherapy, the time of application has to be lengthened as cobalt 60 becomes older so that the same number of rads are delivered. Betatrons have a greater strength of penetration than do linear accelerators; however, they are more expensive. Since these excellent sources of external radiation deliver more penetrating rays, the injury to the skin is less of a problem. Even though large doses can be delivered without appreciable skin injury, the danger of injury to the intestinal tract with the likelihood of ulceration or perforation is still present; this danger mainly limits the doses of the more powerful sources of radiation.

In planning radiation therapy for carcinoma of the cervix and for endometrial carcinoma involving the cervix, the amount of radiation to the lymph nodes of the lateral pelvic wall must be estimated as accurately as possible. These computations involve radiation from the internal sources as well as from the external radiation.

Among the advantages of radiation therapy in the treatment of carcinoma are applicability to practically all patients and a very low mortality and low morbidity. The demands on hospital facilities and personnel are usually less than they are when patients undergo surgical procedures.

When the small intestine is adherent in the pelvis and larger amounts of radiation are employed, injuries are expected with symptoms of incomplete intestinal obstruction (crampy pain, distention, diarrhea, and anorexia). Early surgical procedures to correct bowel malfunction and prevent perforation may be required.

Certain disadvantages are encountered in radiation therapy. During the application of external and internal radiation, nausea and vomiting occur. These usually can be controlled with antiemetic medications. Febrile reactions may be annoying and may be caused by radiation per se. Those reactions that occur because of exacerbations of the existing infection can usually be controlled with antibacterial agents; however, occasionally they require cessation of radiation therapy applied directly to the cervix. Rectal irritation, with accompanying diarrhea and tenesmus, is relatively common. If the tolerance of the rectum is exceeded, proctitis may be very marked and ulceration or perforation may occur. As anticipated with ulceration, melena is frequently noted. The bladder is more tolerant to radiation; however, frequency of urination and dysuria are common. The necessity of an indwelling catheter increases the likelihood of cystitis. When carcinomatous tissue has infiltrated the rectum or the bladder and it is destroyed by radiation, fistulas are likely to result. By using instruments (scintillation counter probes) that register directly the amount of radiation going into the bladder and into the rectum during the application, as well as by checking the position of the applicators by x-ray film, one can usually avoid injury of the bladder and rectum. When radiation for destruction of cancer is used, the endocrine function of the ovary is eliminated, thus precipitating menopausal symptoms. As a disadvantage of radiation therapy, the failure to identify nodal metastasis must be acknowledged. Femoral phlebothrombosis may rarely cause massive pulmonary emboli. New cancers may arise in the same areas years later.

Surgical therapy. Although surigcal therapy is the accepted procedure for certain cases of carcinoma in situ and for properly selected microinvasive cancer (Stage IA), opinions differ on the advisability of surgery for the other stages of cancer. When the cancer is limited to the cervix or the adjacent vagina and parametrium, total excision is possible. This can be done by the vaginal approach according to the technique of Schauta, which allows for adequate removal of the uterus and parametrial tissue after mobilization of the ureters but not for excision of the lymph nodes of the pelvis. By the abdominal approach the uterus and parametrium can be removed, along with the adjacent vagina, and the lymph nodes of the pelvis can be dissected from the pelvic arteries and veins. When the tumor has invaded the bladder, cystectomy can be done and the ureters transplanted to a pouch made from the ileum. Similarly, when the rectum has been invaded, the rectum can be excised and a colostomy performed. With the improvements in anesthesiology, the availability of larger quantities of blood, the employment of antibacterial agents, and the knowledge of fluid and electrolyte balance, more extensive operations can be performed with a lower operative mortality. Indeed, exenteration procedures are now being performed with an overall mortality of 10% or less. The operative mortality with procedures of the Schauta and Wertheim types should be no more than 1%.

Among the advantages of surgical excision of cancer in the cervix is the fact that a removed tumor cannot fail to respond. Surgical excision allows for a more accurate diagnosis, which, in turn, permits a more accurate prognosis. Not only can the extent of parametrial infiltration and of nodal involvement be more accurately determined, but also the extent of associated pathology such as intestinal adhesions or other tumors of the uterus and/or ovaries can be ascertained. Surgical therapy for younger women may allow the salvage of ovarian tissues, since it is rare that cervical cancer metastasizes to the ovaries. With exenteration, surgery permits diversion of the urinary stream to improve renal function by proper drainage. Another advantage of surgical excision is that it allows removal of tumor tissue that has not been effectively treated by radiation and, in some instances, allows the removal of tissue that is infected and necrotic as the result of radiation.

First among the principal disadvantages of surgical therapy is the requirement of highly skilled operators. The operative mortality is higher than that of radiation, and the need of expert postoperative care and a prolonged hospital stay is considerably higher. Transfusions are frequently required, and the threat of operative and postoperative hemorrhage must be considered. Hematomas and collections of lymph in the pelvis occur unless proper safeguards are provided. Thrombophlebitis is a threat. In the more extensive procedures ileus is common. Atony of the bladder is to be expected with the extensive dissection that is required to remove the local tumor. This requires prolonged catheter drainage of the bladder. If the tumor area cannot be removed and incisions are made through cancer, it is likely that the rate of spread of the tumor will be increased.

The biggest problem with the Schauta and Wertheim operations and gland dissections is the occurrence of urinary fistulas of the ureteral and vesicovaginal types in 1% to 10% of patients. Should the patient recover from the operative procedure, stress incontinence is fairly common. As anticipated, adequate operation means shortening of the vagina. Of course, with exenteration procedures there is absence of the vagina and coitus is not possible. There are also the inconveniences of the care of the ileal pouch and/or the colostomy.

Selection of method of therapy

Although the exact extent of nodal involvement cannot be determined without a surgical specimen, efforts are made to determine what the response to treatment would be. Efforts in this area include the histologic gradings of the tumor and determination of cytologic, morphologic, and cytochemical changes in cells with radiation. When adnexal tumors, intestinal adhesions, or sizable myomas are associated, the surgical approach appears advisable to avoid the complications of radiation necrosis. The more arden advocates of surgery would apply the surgical approach to all patients. Certain others, such as Meigs and Parsons, suggested that surgical therapy be attempted when the likelihood of cure (as in Stage I and Stage II lesions) can be predicted with relative accuracy. Some have advocated that excision of the uterus and parametrium be limited to those early invasive lesions that are not more than 1 cm in diameter since the likelihood of nodal involvement in even less in these patients. Some state that excision should be reserved for radiation failures. Here the problem is to decide when surgical therapy should be used. When the diagnosis of radiation failure is certain, the optimum time for operation is usually past.

Follow-up examinations

All patients treated for any type of carcinoma of the cervix should have examinations frequently for the first year and thereafter should be examined every 6 months. It is imperative that the early examinations be done to determine the effectiveness of therapy.

After radiation therapy it is particularly important that frequent examinations be done to separate any adhesions that may occur in the vagina and to guide the patient in proper vaginal hygiene. Cytologic studies and biopsies may be used in following these patients. If any lesion appears, patients should undergo biopsy. It is necessary that the urinary tract be evaluated, not only by urinalysis but also by pyeloureterography. Ureteral obstruction may be the first indication of recurrence of disease. Similarly metastatic vertebral bone lesions may be observed on x-ray films. After prolonged periods necrosis may occur following radiaton. This must therefore be distinguished from recurrent cancer with necrosis. If the patient survives 5 years, it is likely that her disease has been arrested. As with other types of cancer, it is important that other areas in the body be searched for malignancies, particularly the vulva and the rectum.

Prognosis

The overall prognosis following radiation therapy for carcinoma of the cervix is indicated in Table 9-1.

With primary surgical therapy in the 5-year survival rate is 82% in Stage I lesions and 62% in Stage II lesions. Among patients having Stage I lesions with positive nodes there is a 40% to 50% survival rate; having Stage II lesions with nodes, a 10% to 20% survival rate; and having ureterovaginal and vesicovaginal

Table 9-1 PROGNOSIS WITH RADIATION THERAPY FOR CARCINOMA OF CERVIX

Stage	Five-year survival rate (%)
I	70-80
II	40-50
III	20-30
IV	Less than 10

fistulas, 10%. As previously stated, exenteration procedures have an overall mortality of approximately 10%. The survival rate for patients submitting to exenteration procedures has been reported as high as 30%. When no lymph node involvement is found at the time of exenteration, the 5-year survival rate is the range of 60%.

Cancer of cervix during pregnancy

The diagnosis of carcinoma in situ during pregnancy is usually made after findng abnormal cells in cytologic smears. Colposcopic examinations should be performed to select areas of biopsy and delineate the extent of lesions. Although biopsies cause no increase in abortion, conization has the risk of increasing bleeding and possibly inciting abortion. If the lesion is found to be in situ, the pregnancy is allowed to continue with the idea that therapy will be performed at the time of or after delivery. It should be noted that a few bona fide cases of carcinoma in situ during pregnancy have been stated to disappear after delivery; however, the cytologic changes in the cervix during pregnancy can easily be confused with carcinoma in situ by inadequately trained pathologists. If invasive cancer is found during the earlier portion of pregnancy, no attempt is made to salvage the pregnancy; the cancer is treated as if the patient were not pregnant, with the exception of the fact that evacuation of the uterus may be necessary if radiation is to be performed. It has been advised by some that, because of an increased likelihood of spread of neoplasia associated with termination of pregnancy, surgical therapy is better than radiation for cervical cancer found during early pregnancy. Some clinical studies have failed to show that invasive cancer is spread by vaginal delivery. When diagnosis is not made until late in pregnancy, the pregnancy is allowed to continue and postpartum therapy is instituted.

Management of patient with expected terminal carcinoma of cervix

Since many of the patients with cancer of the cervix will die of their disease, it is important to consider these patients. One of the principal problems is pain relief. In the earlier stages of the disease mild analgesics may be used. Later, opiates will be required. The advisability of interrupting the nerve supply to this area by alcohol injections in the subarachnoid spaces or by the performance of cordotomy must be entertained; however, these methods are seldom used. The psychotherapy of the fatherly or motherly physician will do much to allay the mental anguish that these patients are otherwise likely to have.

ADENOCARCINOMA OF ENDOMETRIUM

Carcinoma occurring in the endometrium ranks second among the most common forms of cancer of the reproductive organs. With increasing longevity more women have attained ages at which this disease occurs most often. The incidence as related to that of cervical cancer is therefore increasing.

Etiology

Although this form of cancer does occur in younger women, it is uncommon in patients under 40 years of age. Two thirds of the cases have been found in patients between 50 and 70 years of age. It has been noted that many patients developing this disorder are obese and hypertensive and that some have diabetes mellitus.

The facts that patients who develop endometrial neoplasia menstruate longer (menopause at 51 or 52 years as contrasted with 49 years for the average woman) and that patients with estrogen-producing tumors of the ovary have a higher rate of occurrence of this disease suggest that prolonged periods of estrogen stimulation predispose to endometrial neoplasia. Atypical forms of endometrial hyperplasia have been noted when extrinsic estrogens have been administered over a prolonged period. The finding of atypical hyperplasia and what appears to be an increase in occurrence of endometrial adenocarcinoma in patients having dysfunctional bleeding at or near the menopause and in patients with Stein-Leventhal syndrome suggests that endocrines play a part in the development of this disorder.

In patients receiving long-term estrogen therapy when oral progestogens have been administered for 10 days in the form of medroxyprogesterone acetate or norethindrone acetate, the incidence of both atypical endometrial hyperplasia and adenocarcinoma has been reduced. Some studies have shown that montly use of progestogens for 10 days will eradicate endometrial hyperplasia and avoid development of the precancerous or cancerous lesions.

Recognition of the fact that the majority of patients are not found to have endometrial cancer until 1 or more years past the menopause and the fact that many patients have been given extrinsic estrogens for prolonged periods without the development of neoplasia serves to indicate that estrogen stimulation is only one of the factors involved.

Natural history

As indicated in our discussion of etiology, adenocarcinoma of the endometrium is usually diagnosed postmenopausally and seemingly develops in older patients more frequently than does carcinoma of the cervix. The association of endometrial hyperplasia with neoplasia noted at the time of diagnosis, as well as studies revealing the preexistence of hyperplastic states, suggests that endometrial hyperplasia can be a forerunner of adenocarcinoma. The growth may appear simultaneously throughout the entire endometrium, or it may appear as a circumscribed area of overgrowth. The tendency is for polypoid projections to occur. Bleeding is likely to occur at a reltively early stages as contrasted with cervical cancer. The material produced by the growth may contain considerable mucin, and it can be noted that the cervical discharge is mucosanguineous. If some degree of cervical stenosis exists before the development of the growth, it is likely that more complete cervical occlusion may occur with resulting pyometra.

The rate of growth is variable. It has been recently reported that in a particular series 50% of patients having early adenocarcinoma of the endometrium diagnosed histologically have survived 5 years without treatment. On other occasions early myometrial invasion occurs. The extension may occur into the lymphatics of the uterine isthmus when myometrial invasion occurs in this area. Similarly the peritubal lymphatics may be involved. Fortunately lymphatic involvement usually does not occur until symptoms have been present for some time. With the formation of a mass within the uterine cavity or with invasion of the myometrium, the uterus can enlarge. At times the mass may cause cervical dilation to take place.

Studies of blood obtained from the vena cava indicate that rather frequently tumor cells from the endometrium enter the bloodstream during the manipulations of examination; however, in the majority of patients so studied there are not any evidences of distant bloodstream metastasis. This suggests that, although tumor cells do escape into the bloodstream, in some manner host resistance avoids their implantation. If the tumor invades the lymphatics of the cervix, it is assumed that the vaginal lymphatics would soon become involved. This route of spread, along with a direct implantation during surgery in the vaginal wall, would indicate the reasons for postoperative vaginal metastasis being found. With extension through the walls of the uterus, peritoneal spread can occur. Similarly the tumor cells may escape via the salpinges and be implanted on the ovary or within the peritoneal cavity. The order of frequency of more distant metastases involves first the liver and then lung, skin, and bone. Patients dying as a result of endometrial cancer are likely to have intestinal obstruction and invasion of the colon or bladder. In some, ureteral obstruction similar to that found with cancer of the cervix has been seen. Pain may become marked, and the patient may die in a state of emaciation.

Diagnosis

The most important sign of endometrial cancer is abnormal uterine bleeding. Before the menopause it is likely to be manifest as intermenstrual bleeding; however, occasionally only hypermenorrhea has been noted. Any patient with postmenopausal bleeding should be suspected of having this condition, particularly when no abnormality of the cervix is encountered. This is emphasized despite the fact that postmenopausal bleeding may be associated with vulval or vaginal disorders, as well as benign conditions such as cervical or endometrial polyps, or may follow the administration of estrogenic substances. The patient with pyometra and, more particularly, a mucosanguineous discharge should be especially suspected of having endometrial cancer. The uterus may be enlarged. Characteristically the cervical canal is patent to a sound or an endometrial biopsy instrument.

The cytologic study of material obtained from the cervix or vagina may allow identification of malignant cells in from 50% to 74% of patients with endometrial cancer, but a negative result is of no practical value. The use of fluorescent stains on cytologic material will increase the accuracy of diagnosis of endometrial cancer, but, if one desires to markedly improve results in endometrial cytodiagnosis, it is essential that material be obtained from the endometrial cavity by washings or brushing. It is our opionion that, when the uterine cavity is to be invaded in the unanesthesized patient, sampling of tissue is preferred over cytologic study. Biopsy before the patient's admittance to the hospital may expedite proper therapy. To obtain the maximum degree of diagnostic accuracy it is essential that curettage be done. In an effort to determine the extent of the growth it is particularly important that specimens be obtained (1) from the cervix, (2) from the endocervix, (3) from the lowest portion of the uterus, and (4) from the upper part of the uterine cavity. By separate examinations of the tissues obtained from these areas it may be possible to determine the extent of cancer. This knowledge can then be used to determine the type of therapy. In recent years technical advances in obtaining good frozen sections by using the cryostat have allowed more accurate and rapid histologic diagnosis.

The histologic grading of the tissue obtained can be roughly correlated with the rate of invasion, as indicated by the extent and type of the gross lesion. Broder's classification is as follows:

Grade I
The glands dominate with a minimal amount of stroma. Invasiion is either absent or minimal. There are bizarre cell forms present with an increased proliferation of the epithelium.

Grade II
The glandular pattern is less well defined. From 25% to 50% of the cells present mitotic figures, and obvious invasion of the stroma has occurred.

Grade III
There is even less glandular pattern evident. From 50% to 75% of the cells are undifferentiated.

Grade IV
No definite glands are formed. Solid sheets of malignant cells exist.

Acanthomatous changes may be found and are indicated by areas of squamous cells, which apparently arise by metaplasia. The findings of these areas does not seem to be of significance in prognostication.

Clinical classification

Stage 0
The carcinoma is confined to the endometrium (carcinoma in situ).

Stage I
The carcinoma is confined to the corpus of the uterus.

Stage IA
The carcinoma is present in a uterus measuring up to 8 cm in length from the external os to the upper limit of the uterine cavity.

Stage IB
The carcinoma is present in a uterus measuring more than 8 cm in length from the external os to the upper limit of the uterine cavity.

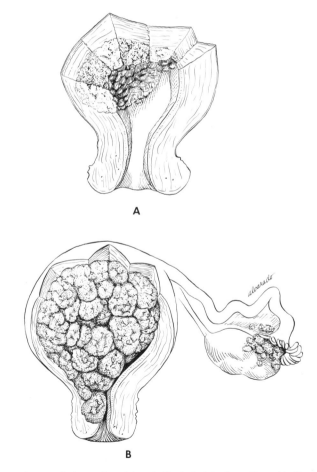

A

B

Fig. 9-5. Adenocarcinoma of the endometrium is illustrated in **A** as Stage IA. **B** reveals an enlarged uterus with extension into the cervix and ovarian metastases, Stage III.

The carcinoma should be subdivided according to the histologic structures in the tissues:

G1—Highly differentiated adenomatous carcinoma

G2—Differentiated adenomatous carcinoma with partly solid areas

G3—Predominantly solid or entirely undifferentiated carcinoma

Stage II

The carcinoma involves the corpus and the cervix but does not extend beyond the uterus.

Stage III

The carcinoma extends beyond the uterus but is confined within the true pelvis.

Stage IV

The carcinoma extends outside the true pelvis or obviously involves the mucosa of the bladder or rectum.

The need for fractional curettage is evident in this classification. Palpation of metastatic lesions outside the uterus may be difficult or impossible in these frequently obese patients. Estimation of uterine size may be particularly difficult.

Therapy

Radiation therapy. There exists a difference of opinion as to the need for radiation in the treatment of Stage I adenocarcinoma of the endometrium. One acknowledged difficulty is the inaccuracy in determining the clinical stage of the cancer. Stage IA lesions with G1 histologic diagnoses have less myometrial invasion and excellent prognosis when treated by surgery alone. All G2 and G3 lesions should received preoperative radiation. Those who would combine radiation with abdominal total hysterectomy and bilateral salpingo-oophoretcomy believe that better results are obtained, since postoperative metastases in the vaginal wall are less common. Similarly preoperative radiation therapy tends to kill cancer cells that may be situated in the pericervical lymphatics. The majority administer radiation preoperatively about the cervix and within the cervix, as well as within the uterine cavity, by application of radium or radioactive cobalt. A few suggest that x-ray therapy may be used for this same purpose.

In patients who are not to have surgical therapy, radiation may be used as the definitive therapy with good results. When hysterctomy will not be done, it is important that the endometrial cavity be thoroughly irradiated. In Stockholm the technique of using multiple radium sources and filling the endometrial cavity with radium containers has been tried with considerable success. The application with colpostats about the cervix is essential to include paracervical extension, as well as vaginal extensions.

Endometrial cancer may be found in patients who have uterine enlargement and distortion of the endometrial cavity caused by myomas. (It has not been shown that myomas predispose to development of adenocarcinoma.) Under these circumstances the proper placement of radiation sources becomes difficult, and necrosis of the myomas is likely to occur as a postradiation complication.

Surgical therapy. Surgical excision must include the cervix for reasons previously detailed. It is particularly important that the ovaries and tubes be removed because of the likelihood of metastasis thereto. Indeed, every uterus removed in which there has not been a preoperative histologic diagnosis of the endometrium should have inspection of the endometrial cavity in the operating room to avoid leaving ovaries that may bear tumor tissues.

The advisability of excision of pelvic lymph nodes is entertained because of the fact that, when the growth has extended into the lower portion of the uterus and the cervix, metastases to those nodes are often found. The majority, however, do not suggest lymphatic resections, believing that, if such metastases are present, the prognosis is not appreciably improved by an attempt at surgical excision. Some suggest that enlarged nodes be removed for purposes of prognostication and also as an indication for more intensive external radiation.

Chemotherapy. In 1961 a synthetic progestogen, 17α-hydroxyprogesterone-17-N-caproate, was reported to benefit some patients with adenocarcinoma of the endometrium. For this agent to be effective it was administered intramuscularly in large dosages of 1250 mg or more each week. Later medroxyprogesterone and megestrol in large doses were given with benefit. The majority of patients improved symptomatically with decrease in pain, increase in appetite, etc. Objective evidence of benefit could be noted by a decrease in the size of palpable or radiologically evident lesions. Histologic changes noted were those of a secretory glandular change, along with acanthomatous conversion of areas of the neoplasm. The use of these agents is not curative but affords some degree of palliation with minimal side effects.

Cyclophosphamide (Cytoxan), 5-fluorouracil (5-FU), and doxorubicin hydrochloride (Adriamycin) have been used with limited success for metastatic endometrial cancer.

Prognosis

In large groups of patients treated in various ways the results have been as follows:

Stage I lesions have been associated with 73% of patients surviving 5 years.

Stage II lesions have yielded a rate of 22% for 5-year survival.

In certain series with earlier stages at diagnosis, the 5-year survival rate has been as high as 86%. The presence of the growth in the cervix and the cervicoisthmic region of the uterus, an increase in the size of the uterus, and deep myometrial invasion indicate less favorable prognoses. After removal of ovaries with metastases and adequate radiation, 5-year survival of 25% has been reported.

SARCOMA OF UTERUS

Sarcoma of the uterus, an uncommon class of malignant growths, may arise from any tissue in the uterus having a mesodermal origin: muscle, connective tissue, blood vessels, myomas, or endometrial stroma. Sarcoma botryoides, a rare pink grapelike growth, occurs almost exclusively in children. Mixed mesodermal tumors have been found most commonly in patients between the ages of 40 and 60. Leiomyosarcomas, the most common type of uterine sarcoma, usually occur at a slightly later age and are likely to arise in an area of a preexisting myoma. Stromal endometriosis, a relatively benign sarcoma, presents wormlike masses of yellow elastic protrusions from veins on cut surface. Stromal sarcomas are typically large soft masses.

Diagnosis

Sarcoma botryoides of the cervix is diagnosed when bleeding occurs during childhood and a mass either is palpated within the vagina or protrudes from the vagina. Sarcoma of mixed mesodermal origin, found later in life, is likely to present as a cause of abnormal bleeding with associated mass formation. Some of these tumors have been diagnosed by obtaining material on curettage when investigating such cases. Any patient with a rapidly enlarging uterus, particularly if the enlargement occurs postmenopausally, should be suspected of having a sarcoma. In some instances the mass protrudes from the cervix and the patient does not seek attention until necrosis with a foul discharge has occurred.

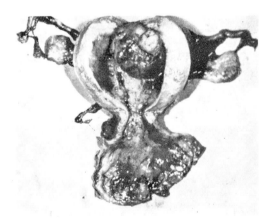

Fig. 9-6. Surgical specimen of a malignant mixed mülerian (mesodermal) neoplasm of the uterus in a 57-year-old patient.

From Krupp, P.J., Jr., and others: Am. J. Obstet. Gynecol. **81**:959, 1961.

The diagnosis of sarcomatous degeneration in a myoma may be somewhat difficult. It is suspected grossly much more often than it occurs since necrosis and liquefaction of the myoma may suggest it.

The spread of sarcoma occurs by direct continuity, by the bloodstream, and by lymph channels. The lungs are the favorite site of metastasis. Next in order of frequency are the liver, intestine, omentum, kidney, pleura, and brain.

Therapy

Radiation has resulted in 5-year survival in a very few cases of sarcoma botryoides. It has not proved effective in other forms of sarcoma. Surgical excision of the tumor-bearing uterus before extension outside the uterus is the only hope for cure. Five-year survival rates may be as high as 50% for leiomyosarcomas, but 30% is more likely. Mixed mesodermal tumors usually offer little chance of 5-year survival.

SELECTED REFERENCES

Acosta-Sison, H.: Statistical study of chorionepithelioma in Philippine General Hospital, Am. J. Obstet. Gynecol. **58:**125, 1949.

Arneson, A.N.: The natural history of uterine cancer, Clin. Obstet. Gynecol. **4:**445, 1961.

Boutselis, J.G., and Ullery, J.C.: Sarcoma of the uterus, Obstet. Gynecol. **20:**23, 1962.

Bricker, E.M., Butcher, H.R., and McAfee, A.: Results of pelvic exenteration, Arch. Surg. **73:**661, 1956.

Briggs, R.M.: Dysplasia and early neoplasia of the uterine cervix, Obstet. Gynecol. Surv. **34:**70, 1979.

Brown, W.E., Meschen, I., Kerekes, E., and Sadler, J.M.: Effect of radiation on metastatic pelvic lymph node involvement in carcinoma of cervix, Am. J. Obstet. Gynecol. **62:**871, 1951.

Brunschwig, A., and Daniel, W.: The surgical treatment of cancer of the cervix, Am. J. Obstet. Gynecol. **82:**60, 1961.

Bunker, M.L.: The terminal findings in endometrial carcinoma, Am. J. Obstet. Gynecol. **77:**530, 1959.

Burns, B.C., Jr., Everett, H.S., and Brack, C.B.: Value of urologic study in the management of carcinoma of the cervix, Am. J. Obstet. Gynecol. **80:**997, 1960.

Carter, B., et al.: The follow-up of patients with cancer of the cervix treated by radical hysterectomy and radical lymphadenectomy, Am. J. Obstet. Gynecol. **76:**1094, 1958.

Chanen, W., and Hollyock, V.E.: Colposcopy and the conservative management of cervical dysplasia in carcinoma in situ, Obstet. Gynecol. **43:**527, 1974.

Charles, E.H., and Savage, E.W.: Cryosurgical treatment of cervical intraepithelial neoplasia, Obstet. Gynecol. Surv. **35:**539, 1980.

Crossen, R.J.: Wide conization of cervix; follow-up on 1,000 cases from 2 to 14 years, Am. J. Obstet. Gynecol. **57:**187, 1949.

Crossen, R.J., and Hobbs, J.E.: Relationship of late menstruation to carcinoma of corpus uteri, J. Missouri Med. Assoc. **32:**361, 1935.

DiSaia, P.J., and Creasman, W.T.: Clinical gynecologic oncology, St. Louis, 1980, The C.V. Mosby Co.

Fox, C.H., Turner, F.G., Johnson, W.L., and Thorton, W.N.: Endometrial cytology, Am. J. Obstet. Gynecol. **83:**1582, 1962.

Gambrell, R.D., Massey, F.M., Casteneda, T.A., et al.: Use of the progestogen challenge test to reduce the risk of endometrial cancer, Obstet. Gynecol. **55:**733, 1980.

Graham, J.A., and Graham, R.M.: The sensitization response in patients with cancer of the uterine cervix, Cancer **13:**5, 1960.

Greiss, F.C., Blake, D.D., amd Lock, F.R.: Treatment of cancer of the cervix by radiation and elective radical hysterectomy, Am. J. Obstet. Gynecol. **82:**1042, 1961.

Gusburg, S.B., and Frick, H.C.: Corscadan's gynecologic cancer, Baltimore, 1978, The Williams & Wilkins Co.

Hay, R.C., Yonezawa, T., and Derrick, W.S.: Control of intractable pain in advanced cancer by subarachnoid alcohol block, J.A.M.A. 169:1315, 1959.

Jones, W.N., and Mahoney, P.L., Jr.: A study in postmenopausal uterine bleeding, Am. J. Surg. 23:58, 1957.

Kaufman, R.H., Abbott, J.P., and Scheihing, W.C.: Use of the refrigerated microtome for rapid diagnosis of cervical conization specimens, Am. J. Obstet. Gynecol. 84:107, 1962.

Kistner, R.W., and Duncan, C.J.: An analysis of one hundred and five radical hysterectomies at the Free Hospital for Women, Surg. Gynecol. Obstet. 104:733, 1957.

Kistner, R.W., Gorbach, A.C., and Smith, G.V.: Cervical cancer in pregnancy: review of the literature with presentation of thirty additional cases, Obstet. Gynecol. 9:554, 1957.

Kottmeier, H.L.: Carcinoma of the corpus uteri: diagnosis and therapy, Am. J. Obstet. Gynecol. 78:1127, 1959.

Latour, J.P.O.: Results in the management of preclinical carcinoma of the cervix, Am. J. Obstet. Gynecol. 81:511, 1961.

Lerner, H.M., Jones, H.W., and Hill, E.C.: Radical surgery for the treatment of early invasive cervical carcinoma (Stage IB): review of 15 years' experience, Obstet. Gynecol. 56:413, 1980.

McCall, M.L.: The radical vaginal operative approach in the treatment of carcinoma of the cervix, Am. J. Obstet. Gynecol. 78:712, 1959.

Meigs, J.V.: Cancer of the cervix, an appraisal, Am. J. Gynecol. 72:467, 1956.

Nolan, James F., and Darden, John S.: Treatment failures in Stage I carcinoma of the uterine corpus, Am. J. Obstet. Gynecol. 83:949, 1962.

Novak, E., and Yui, E.: Relation of endometrial hyperplasia to adenocarcinoma of uterus, Am. J. Obstet. Gynecol. 32:674, 1936.

Parsons, L., and Sommers, S.C.: Gynecology, ed. 2, Philadelphia, 1978, W.B. Saunders Co.

Schewe, E.J., Jr., and Sala, J.M.: Bilateral ureteral obstruction complicating the treatment of carcinoma of the cervix, Am. J. Roentgen. 81:125, 1959.

Shingleton, H.M., and Gore, H.: Third world congress for cervical pathology and colposcopy, Obstet. Gynecol. Surv. 34:783, 1979.

Sweeney, W.J., III, Douglas, R.G.: Treatment of carcinoma of the cervix with combined radiation and extensive surgery, Am. J. Obstet. Gynecol. 84:981, 1962.

Te Linde, R.W., Galvin, G.A., and Jones, H.W., Jr.: Therapy of carcinoma in situ, Am. J. Obstet. Gynecol. 74:792, 1957.

Varga, A., and Henriksen, E.: Clinical and histopathologic evaluation of the effect of 17-alpha-hydroxyprogesterone 17-N-caproate on endometrial carcinoma, Obstet. Gynecol. 18:658, 1961.

Chapter 10

TUMORS OF THE FALLOPIAN TUBE

As noted in Chapter 3, hydatids of Morgagni are common vestigial cystic masses attached to the fimbriae. Salpingitis isthmica nodosa, adenomyosis, and endometriosis may cause masses that are not neoplasms. Primary carcinoma of the salpinx is the least common cancer of the reproductive system. Benign tumors are found even less frequently.

BENIGN TUMORS

Teratomas and leiomyomas of the tube have been reported to produce palpable masses and undergo torsion. Adenomatoid tumors, adenomatous polyps, fibromas, and leiomyomas have usually been asymptomatic and have been diagnosed when surgery for other disease was performed.

MALIGNANT TUMORS

Primary sarcoma is so rare that fewer than 50 cases have been reported. Metastatic carcinoma of the salpinx is more common than primary carcinoma. Ovarian and endometrial cancers are likely to spread to the tube. With involvement of the ovary, tube, and endometrium, at times the origin of the neoplasm cannot be determined. Primary carcinoma of the salpinx comprises 0.1% to 1% of all malignancies of the reproductive structures of women.

Pathology. The gross findings in tubal cancer are variable. It may extend as a friable growth from the fimbriated end of the tube. The fimbriated end may be occluded and the salpinx distended with tumor and fluid. Often the surgeon is of the opinion that chronic hydrosalpinx or pyosalpinx exists. In fact, salpingitis can accompany the neoplasia. The extension of the growth is most often by seeding on various peritoneal surfaces.

Three microscopic grades have been described:

Grade I
Papillary growth is confined to the tube with some areas of normal epithelium and few mitotic figures.

Grade II
Invasion of the muscularis and glandular formation are noted.

Grade III
Invasion of lymphatics, numerous mitoses, and solid sheets of cancer cell are found.

Diagnosis. The preoperative diagnosis is seldom made. The pelvic mass when felt preoperatively is most often suspected to be caused by tubal inflammation or ovarian neoplasia. When a vaginal discharge occurs it is likely to be bloody. The diagnosis can be suspected when malignant calls are found on vaginal smears and no cervical or endometrial neoplasm is found. This situation has been the principal guide to the correct preoperative diagnosis. When a bloody uterine discharge continues after no neoplasm is found on curettage, tubal carcinoma is suspected. A watery discharge followed by temporary relief of abdominal pain has been noted as a sign of salpingeal disease. When this phenomenon is noted postmenopausally, tubal cancer may be the cause.

Therapy. Bilateral salpingo-oophorectomy and hysterectomy should be performed. Except for Grade I lesions limited to the salpinx, external radiation should be used to supplement excision.

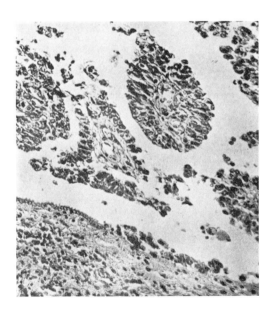

Fig. 10-1. Microscopic section. The tubal lumen contains papillary carcinoma. Note the contiguity of the normal mucosa with a row of tumor cells in the lower right hand corner.

From Schenck, S.B., and Mackles, A.: Am. J. Obstet. Gynecol. **81:**782, 1961.

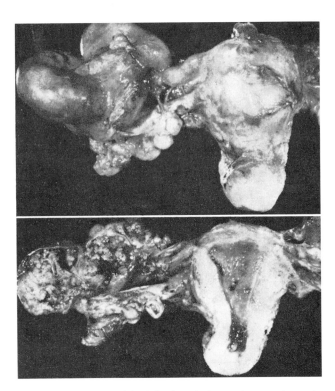

Fig. 10-2. Carcinoma of the left tube. The lower photograph reveals the papillary growth in the lumen.

From Green, T.H., Jr., and Scully, R.E.: In Ingersoll, F.M., editor: Symposium on the fallopian tubes. Clinical obstetrics and gynecology, September, 1962, Hoeber Medical Division, Harper & Row, Publishers.

Prognosis. About 5% to 10% of patients survive 5 years after treatment for tubal cancer. The best outcome occurs when the distal end of the tube has been occluded by salpingitis and a Grade I lesion has been removed.

SELECTED REFERENCES

Abrams, J., Kazal, H.L., and Hobbs, R.E.: Primary sarcoma of the fallopian tube, Am. J. Obstet. Gynecol. **75**:180, 1958.

Brewer, J.I., and Guderian, A.M.: Diagnosis of uterine tube carcinoma by vaginal cytology, Obstet. Gynecol. **8**:664, 1956.

Golden, A., and Ash, J.E.: Adenomatoid tumors of the genital tract, Am. J. Pathol. **21**:63, 1945.

Grimes, H.G., and Kommesser, J.C.: Benign cystic teratoma of the oviduct, Obstet. Gynecol. **16**:85, 1960.

Hershey, D.W., Fennell, R.H., and Major, F.J.: Primary carcinoma of the fallopian tube, Obstet. Gynecol. **57**:367, 1981.

Hu, C.Y., Tazmor, M.L., and Hertig, A.T.: Primary carcinoma of the fallopian tube, Am. J. Obstet. Gynecol. **59**:58, 1950.

Krugman, P.T., and Fisher, J.E.: Primary carcinoma of the fallopian tubes, Am. J. Obstet. Gynecol. **80**:722, 1960.

Roberts, C.L., and Marshall, H.K.: Fibromyoma of the fallopian tube, Am. J. Obstet. Gynecol. **82**:364, 1961.

Sinka, A.C.: Hydrops tubae profluens as a presenting symptom in primary carcinoma of the fallopian tube, Br. Med. J. **2**:996, 1959.

Chapter 11

ENDOMETRIOSIS

In 1921 Sampson first called attention to tissue microscopically resembling endometrium and found ectopically in various locations in or near the pelvic cavity. In the uterus it is designated as internal endometriosis or adenomyosis. When there is distinct tumor formation containing muscle it is termed "adenomyoma." The extrauterine types are sometimes called external endometriosis. In the ovaries it is likely to form a cyst containing material that looks somewhat like chocolate. In addition to the *uterus* and the *ovaries* the many possible locations include *uterine ligaments* (uterosacral, broad, and round); *pelvic peritoneum* covering the uterus, salpinges, rectum, sigmoid, or bladder; *vermiform appendix; vagina; cervix uteri;* laparotomy and cesarotomy *scars; hernial sacs; tubal stumps; umbilicus; vulva; urinary bladder*, and *lymph glands* (Fig. 11-1). It has been reported in the axillae and on the pleura.

Etiology. The three chief theories for the etiology of endometriosis are as follows:

1. Transtubal regurgitation of endometrial tissue at the time of menstruation with its subsequent implantation and growth was propounded by Sampson. Obviously this theory cannot explain all cases of pelvic endometriosis or any of those of the uterine musculature. Some of the latter may be caused by direct invasion.

2. The coelomic metaplasia theory is based on the fact that the lining mucous membrane of nearly all parts of the müllerian canal (tubes, uterus, and vagina), the germinal epithelium covering the ovary, and the pelvic peritoneum are derived from the same tissue. Some of the less highly differentiated portions retain the power of further differentiation in later life when acted upon by unknown stimuli. Experimental metaplastic endometriosis involving glandular growth without stromal growth was demonstrated by Merrill.

3. Halban's theory than endometriosis may reach its destination by way of the lymphatic and venous channels in extrapelvic locations seems to be an acceptable explanation. Endometriosis has been found in pelvic lymph nodes with relative frequency when sought. Endometriosis of lymph nodes, however, does not produce any particular pathologic disturbance.

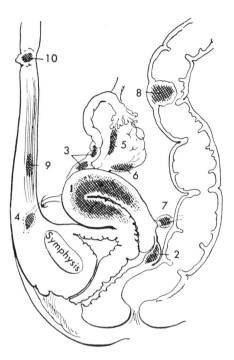

Fig. 11-1. Sites of endometriosis. *1,* Uterus; *2,* rectovaginal septum; *3,* tube; *4,* round ligament; *5,* ovary; *6,* uteroovarian ligament; *7,* uterosacral ligament; *8,* sigmoid colon; *9,* rectus muscle; *10,* umbilicus.

From Cullen, T.S.: Arch. Surg. **1:**217, 1920.

Te Linde and Scott demonstrated that endometrium desquamated from the menstruating uterus of a monkey can be implanted and grown on its peritoneum. Meigs observed that endometriosis is predominantly a disease of private patients and exists with relative infrequency among ward and indigent patients. He has suggested that delayed marriage and delayed childbearing in the upper economic groups may be etiologic factors. He also stated that fewer pregnancies in the private patient category may be a factor; however, recent reviews reveal that many patients with endometriosis have had two or more children. We agree with Stewart Taylor that private patients' demands for relief of symptoms are greater than those of indigent patients and that much endometriosis is diagnosed at laparotomy. He says, "A ward patient with the same preoperative signs and symptoms often is erroneously treated conservatively for chronic salpingo-oophoritis."

Pathology. External endometriosis is occasionally found in patients 18 to 25 years of age; however, the majority of patients are past 30 years. Adenomyosis is usually found in older women (past 35 years). The courses of this disease are vari-

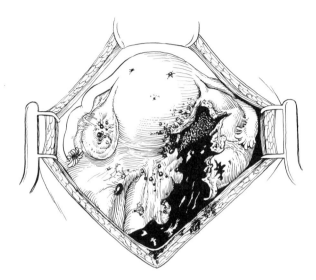

Fig. 11-2. Endometriosis of ovaries, uterus, uterosacral ligaments, and rectum is illustrated with escape of chocolate material from the ruptured endometrial cyst.

able as to rates of progression or regression, symptoms, and objective findings. The cardinal microscopic characteristics are ectopic endometrial glands, endometrial stroma, and subepithelial phagocytes filled with hemosiderin. The gross findings vary from a tiny solitary brownish black spot to densely adherent pelvic organs. Dense fibrous tissue develops around the areas of collection of inspissated blood. The ectopic endometrium tends to infiltrate into the bowel wall, which often adheres to it. One common type of endometrioma is the endometrial ovarian cyst. It is lined or partly lined by endometriumlike tissue. This tissue is hormonally influenced, but it cannot continue to behave as normal endometrium because it is hemmed in and its blood supply is abnormal. Intracystic bleeding somewhat like menstruation occurs, resulting in the distention of the cyst by a dark chocolate-colored material. The accumulating contents, the advancing growth of the endometrial tissue, or both may cause early perforation of the cyst wall and leakage, resulting in implantations and dense adhesions of the affected ovary to adjacent structures. Invasion may occur, as shown by Fig. 11-2. In extensive pelvic endometriosis the pelvis is classified as frozen because the internal genital organs are immobile on palpation.

Endometriosis uteri may exist without external endometriosis and may occur in a diffuse form *(adenomyosis)* or a circumscribed form *(adenomyoma)*. The former may involve the entire corpus uteri, causing a diffuse thickening of the uterine wall. If only one wall is affected, it is usually the posterior. Although the glands surrounded by endometrial stroma may occasionally function with resultant cystlike spaces filled with retained menstrual blood, the endometrium-like tissue is more often of the immature, nonfunctioning type. This is compatible with the idea that the origin of the endometriosis is from the basal portion of the endometrium that does not take part in the physiologic changes involved in the menstrual cycle.

Stromal endometriosis is a rare condition in which it is suggested that only the endometrial stroma invade the uterine muscle. Novak and Novak prefer the designation "stromal adenomyosis" despite the absence of gland elements, stating that it is relatively rare. We agree with them that the term "stomatosis" is very expressive. Their classification of the histologically and clinically malignant type as endometrial sarcoma is logical.

Symptoms and signs. The symptoms in general are similar to those of a low-grade chronic pelvic inflammation, but with special emphasis on the slowly progressive character of the symptoms and findings on examination, on the recurring attacks of pain (caused by distention of the cyst or leakage of contents) without definite fever, on the close association of the exacerbations with menstruation, and on the absence of definite evidences of infection (namely, fever, rapid erythrocyte sedimentation rate, and leukocytosis). Endometriosis may cause sterility because of pelvic adhesions, tubal obstruction, or decreased ovarian function. Although a patient with endometriosis may be asymptomatic, the classic symptomatology includes pain in the form of acquired dysmenorrhea (which may be progressive), localized pain caused by pressure on bowel, bladder, or nerves, and dyspareunia. Colicky pain caused by partial intestinal obstruction may occur. Uterine bleeding may be irregular or in the form of hypermenorrhea or polymenorrhea. If the lesions involve the vagina or cervix, a vaginal discharge or postcoital bleeding may occur. Small firm nodules may be palpable in the uterosacral ligaments or in the rectovaginal septum. The fundus uteri may be in the cul-de-sac of Douglas, but regardless of its location adherent adnexal masses result in the limitation of its mobility, and attempts to move it cause pain. Bleeding from the rectum or urinary bladder associated with the menses is strongly indicative of endometriotic involvement. If the adnexal masses palpated are caused primarily by "chocolate" cysts of the ovary, they are usually less than 7 cm in diameter. Rarely ovarian masses 7 to 15 cm in diameter develop. Since atrophy occurs because of the lack of estrogen stimulation, endometriotic lesions regress after the menopause.

Diagnosis. An accurate history of any of the previously discussed symptoms is important. Since the course of the disease is variable, observation of the patient over a period of several months has been associated with an increase in accuracy of preoperative diagnosis. Pelvic pain and tenderness not explained by infection or tumor should cause consideration of endometriosis. When this diagnosis is thought to be probable, it is well to know, in evaluating abnormal bleeding, that excessive uterine bleeding is often absent in external endometriosis and frequently found in adenomyosis. Finding the typical nodules in the uterosacral ligaments or thereabouts strongly suggest the diagnosis. Laparoscopy allows accurate diagnosis and is employed for cases of unexplained infertility and pelvic pain. Hospital records prove that the diagnosis is most often correctly made during operations, and records of the pathology department show that adenomyosis is usually not diagnosed until the specimen reaches the pathologist. At laparotomy one typically finds ovarian endometrioma containing a thick brown fluid. "Burned-match" areas may be seen on the pelvic peritoneum. Dense adhesions result in adnexal fixation to adjacent structures. In some cases the vermiform appendix is plastered to the endometrioma.

Therapy. Endometriosis is a disease of the reproductive period; consequently therapy should be as conservative as possible. The following should be evaluated: degree of symptoms, age, marital state, desire for progeny, husband's sexual status, fertility rating, presence of other pelvic disease, removability of the endometriosis, and physiologic and psychologic condition of the patient. Since pregnancy has a beneficial effect on endometriosis, it is desirable that younger patients with minimal degrees of endometriosis marry early and reproduce quickly and regularly. Those patients already married should be informed as to the anticipated effects of gestation on endometriosis. If infertility is encountered, thorough investigation of the patient and her husband is indicated to determine its cause before laparotomy is considered. Surgical therapy has been reported to yield higher pregnancy rates than hormonal therapy. To properly evaluate improved fertility the physician must scrutinize the size of lesions, density of adhesions, and involvement of peritoneum, ovary, and tube. Where possible, all areas of endometriosis should be resected or fulgurated. Normal ovarian, tubal, and peritoneal tissue should be conserved. Ovarian and tubal adhesions should be lysed. Gentle meticulous technique, precise hemostasis, and careful peritonization aid in avoiding postoperative adhesions. Prophylactic antibiotics—dexamethasone and promethazine parenterally and dextran solution intraperitoneally—are advocated to prevent adhesions.

Treatment includes (1) observation and analgesia, (2) hormonal therapy, and (3) operation. The first category includes patients with minimal symptoms. Examinations at intervals of 6 months are necessary. Reassurance and mild analgesics should prove helpful in many cases.

Therapy for endometriosis was suggested by the observation that during pregnancy endometriotic lesions decreased in size and often became asymptomatic. The first efforts at endocrine therapy utilized large doses of estrogens—diethylstilbestrol was given in a manner to prevent menstruation for at least 6 months. Because of nausea, fluid retention, increased weight, and inability to prevent endometrial bleeding at times, this method was not widely accepted. When orally effective progestogens became available, they were combined with oral estrogens in large doses to mimic the changes of pregnancy. Norethynodrel with mestranol was started in a dosage of 2.5 mg daily and increased to 20 mg daily. For those who decided upon a parenteral method, medroxyprogesterone acetate was given in a dosage of 200 mg every 2 weeks. Estradiol valerate was given in a 10 mg dose to avoid breakthrough bleeding. An improvement rate of 83% and a pregnancy rate of 47% were reported in one large series.

In recent years it has been found that large doses of estrogens and progestogens are not necessary, so that many use a combined oral contraceptive—type medication, which is given daily, and increase doses only in case of endometrial bleeding. Complications with this therapy are infrequent, and amenorrhea can be maintained over 6 to 18 months.

Danazol, a derivative of 17α-ethinyl testosterone, has an antigonadotropic action; it can reduce FSH and LH levels. It is mildly androgenic and exhibits no estrogenic, progestational, antiestrogenic, antiprogestational, or antiandrogenic activity. It has been used alone to produce a postmenopausal-like state resulting in improvement in symptomatology and objective improvement as determined by laparoscopic observation in patients with endometriosis. As with combined estrogen-progestogen therapy, the areas of endometriosis are decreased but not entirely eliminated and there is a recurrence after discontinuation of this therapy. An increase in acne and a degree of hirsutism, along with irregular uterine bleeding in some patients, are the main drawbacks for use of this particular agent.

Surgical treatment is indicated if the degree of disability is pronounced despite nonoperative measures or if masses in the pelvis suggest the likelihood of neoplasia. Partial intestinal obstruction is a rare indication. In some cases troublesome bleeding necessitates dilation and curettage and careful examination under anesthesia. Ovarian endometrial cysts over 5 to 6 cm are considered an indication for operation because endometriosis can destroy functioning ovarian tissue and the possibility of ovarian neoplasia is to be considered. Conservatism should be the rule. It may be possible to resect an endometrioma from the ovary and conserve valuable ovarian tissue. Areas of endometriotic tissue may be excised or fulgurated in some cases. Hysteropexy is indicated at the time of laparotomy if the uterus is in a retroposition. Presacral neurectomy should be performed when dysmenorrhea and/or dyspareunia are prominent in the preoperative history. Removal of the target organ (the uterus), with conservation of ovarian tissue, has proved to be the surgical treatment of choice for some patients. When hilar involvement of the ovary precludes resection that will allow adequate ovarian blood supply, the ovary is better removed. Total hysterectomy and bilateral salpingo-oophorectomy prove advantageous when preservation of ovarian function is not necessary or when extensive involvement of the bowel precludes complete excision. Previously external radiation was used for patients with extensive involvement. It is now seldom employed, however, since the technical ability of properly trained gynecologic surgeons allows safe excision in the more extensively involved cases. The inherent disadvantages of radiation for endometriosis are the loss of childbearing ability and the possibility of overlooking an associated neoplasm of the adnexa or uterus.

Endometrioid carcinoma has been reported to be accompanied by endometriosis in 11% to 28% of cases; clear cell carcinoma is accompanied by endometriosis in about 50% of cases. In large series of surgical specimens of endometriosis less than 1% have associated malignancy.

SELECTED REFERENCES

Acosta, A.A., Buttram, V.C., Besch, P.K., et. al.: A proposed classification of pelvic endometriosis, Obstet. Gynecol. **142:**19, 1973.

Beecham, C.T., and McCrae, L.E.: Endometriosis of the urinary tract, Urol. Surv. **7:**2, 1957.

Benson, R.C., and Sneeden, V.D.: Adenomyosis: a reappraisal of symptomatology, Am. J. Obstet. Gynecol. **76:**1044, 1958.

Brewer, J.I., and Maher, F.M.: Conservatism in endometriosis, Am. J. Obstet. Gynecol. **68:**549, 1954.

Cooke, W.R.: Observations on the massive stilbestrol therapy of endometriosis, Am. J. Obstet. Gynecol. **71:**569, 1956.

Counseller, V.S., and Crenshaw, J.L., Jr.: A clinical and surgical review of endometriosis, Am. J. Obstet. Gynecol. **62:**930, 1951.

Dmowksi, W.P., and Cohen, M.R.: Treatment of endometriosis with an antigonadotropin, danazol, Obstet. Gynecol. **46:**147, 1975.

Gainey, H.L., Keeler, J.E., and Nicolay, K.S.: Endometriosis in pregnancy, Am. J. Obstet. Gynecol. **63:**511, 1952.

Gardner, H.L.: Cervical endometriosis, Am. J. Obstet. Gynecol. **84:**170, 1962.

Javert, C.T.: The spread of benign and malignant endometrium in the lymphatic system with a note on coexisting vascular involvement, Am. J. Obstet. Gynecol. **64:**780, 1952.

Karnaky, K.J.: The use of stilbestrol for endometriosis, South. Med. J. **41:**1109, 1948.

Kistner, R.W.: Conservative treatment of endometriosis, Postgrad. Med. **25:**505, 1958.

Meigs, J.V.: Medical treatment of endometriosis and the significance of endometriosis, Surg. Gynecol. Obstet. **89:**317, 1949.

Merrill, J.A.: Endometrial induction of endometriosis across millipore filters, Am. J. Obstet. Gynecol. **94:**780, 1966.

Ranney, B.: Endometriosis. III. Complete operation, Am. J. Obstet. Gynecol. **109:**1137, 1971.

Ranney, B.: Endometriosis, Clin. Obstet. Gynecol. **23:**863, 1980.

Ridley, J.H., and Edwards, I.K.: Experimental endometriosis in the human, Am. J. Obstet. Gynecol. **76:**783, 1958.

Sampson, J.A.: Perforating hemorrhagic (chocolate) cysts of the ovary, Arch. Surg. **3:**245, 1921.

Scott, R.B., and Wharton, L.B., Jr.: The effect of estrone and progesterone on the growth of experimental endometriosis in rhesus monkeys, Am. J. Obstet. Gynecol. **74:**852, 1957.

Stearns, H.C.: A study of stromal endometriosis, Am. J. Obstet. Gynecol. **75:**663, 1958.

Taylor, E.S.: Essentials of gynecology, ed. 2, Philadelphia, 1962, Lea & Febiger.

Te Linde, R.W., and Scott, R.B.: Experimental endometriosis, Am. J. Obstet. Gynecol. **60:**1147, 1950.

Chapter 12

OVARIAN TUMORS AND CYSTS

The ovary's normal size varies with growth during childhood, follicle maturation, corpus luteum formation, and climacteric atrophy. Appreciation of the variation in size and knowledge of the appearance of the normal ovarian structures such as the corpus hemorrhagicum, corpus luteum, and follicles are important lest ovarian section or removal be erroneously performed. If palpation during the years of menstruation reveals a mass estimated to exceed 5 cm in diameter, the possibility of an ovarian neoplasm should be entertained and repeated examinations are in order.

NONNEOPLASTIC CYSTS
Follicle cysts

With failure of ovulation a follicle can persist and enlarge. It may be associated with abnormal bleeding and usually subsides in 1 to 3 months; however, if it persists for 3 months with a diameter of 5 cm or more, excision is advisable.

Corpus luteum cysts

Corpus luteum cysts may be associated with normal menstruation or pregnancy. Conversely they can cause amenorrhea or irregular bleeding. Management is similar to that of follicle cysts.

Theca-lutein cysts

Theca-lutein cysts are associated with hydatidiform mole and choriocarcinoma in about 10% of patients. They disappear after the trophoblastic source of gonadotropin is eliminated.

Polycystic ovaries

The majority of polycystic ovaries are associated with dysfunctional bleeding and should not be resected or excised. Combined estrogen-progestogen therapy will usually result in regular endometrial bleeding and decreased ovarian size. All functional cysts will regress with adequate FSH-LH suppression.

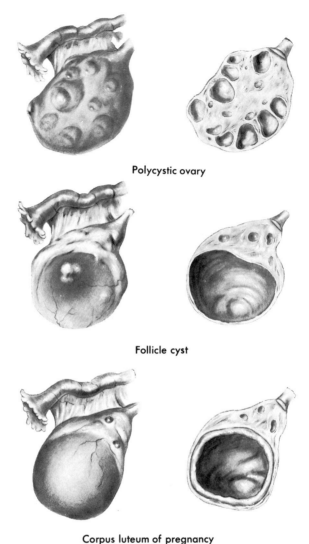

Polycystic ovary

Follicle cyst

Corpus luteum of pregnancy

Fig. 12-1. Ovarian enlargement without neoplasia.

NEOPLASTIC CYSTS

The various types of ovarian tumors are discussed below (see Table 12-1).

Serous cystadenomas

Serous cystadenomas may not abnormally enlarge the ovary, or they may cause it to fill the abdomen. Their origin is the germinal epithelium of the ovary. They may be unilocular or multilocular, papillary or nonpapillary, and they are found

Table 12-1   OVARIAN NEOPLASMS

Tissue origin	Principal structure	Endocrine produced
Coelomic epithelium		
Serous	Cystic	None
Mucinous	Cystic	None
Endometrioid	Cystic	None
Mesonephroid	Cystic	None
Brenner	Solid	None
Undifferentiated carcinoma	Solid	None
Mixed mesodermal	Solid	None
Germ cell		
Mature teratoma		
Dermoid cyst	Cystic	None
Solid adult	Solid	None
Struma ovarii	Cystic	Thyroxine
Squamous carcinoma	Cystic	None
Immature teratoma	Cystic	None
Dysgerminoma	Solid	None
Embryonal carcinoma	Solid	HCG
Choriocarcinoma	Solid	HCG*
Gonadoblastoma	Solid	Androgens and estrogens
Specialized stroma		
Granulosa-theca		
Granulosal	Solid	Estrogen
Thecoma	Solid	Estrogen
Sertoli−Leydig cell		
Arrhenoblastoma	Solid	Androgens
Sertoli cell	Solid	Androgens
Gynandroblastoma	Solid	Androgens and estrogens
Lipid-cell	Solid	Androgens
Nonspecific mesenchyme		
Fibroma, hemangioma, and	Solid	None
lipoma	Solid	None
Lymphoma	Solid	None
Sarcoma		
Metastatic		
Gastrointestinal tract (Krukenberg's)	Solid	None
Breast	Solid	None
Endometrium	Solid	None
Lymphoma	Solid	None

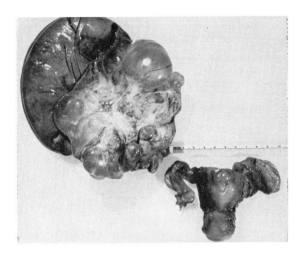

Fig. 12-2. Multilocular, serous cystadenoma.

From Willson, J.R., Beecham, C.T., Forman, I., and Carrington, E.R.: Obstetrics and gynecology, St. Louis, The C.V. Mosby Co.

most frequently in patients between the ages of 20 and 50 years. About 18% are bilateral. They are filled with a thin, pale yellow fluid. A variation of this tumor is the serous adenofibroma, which is more solid than cystic. The epithelial lining is cuboidal, with variations as to architecture in papillary and malignant types of this tumor. When papillary projections are found within the cysts, malignancy is more likely. When papillary portions are seen on the surface of the ovary, the possibility of peritoneal spread is strong. The prediction of the rate of spread is best based on the microscopic grading of the tumor.

Serous cystadenocarcinomas

Serous cystadenocarcinomas are malignant cysts that occur bilaterally in 47% (Pemberton) to 71% (Taylor) of cases. It is the most common type of ovarian malignancy. Malignant areas may develop in its benign counterpart, or the malignancy may have been present from the onset of growth.

Mucinous cystadenomas

Mucinous cystadenomas are slightly more common than serous cystadenomas. Unilocular are less common than multilocular types. About 10% of these cysts in their benign form occur bilaterally. The histologic diagnosis reveals tall columnar epithelium and goblet cells. The fluid is characteristically thick and viscid, but it may be thin, so that grossly the growth cannot be differentiated from the serous

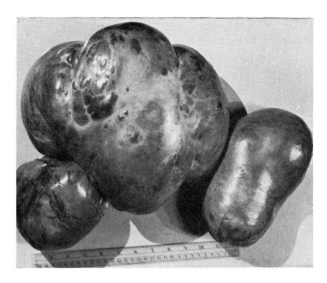

Fig. 12-3. Bilateral, multilocular pseudomucinous cystadenoma.

From Willson, J.R., Beecham, C.T., Forman, I., and Carrington, E.R.: Obstetrics and gynecology, St. Louis, The C.V. Mosby Co.

variety. Papillary areas are found in about 10% of these tumors, and about 5% are thought to undergo malignant changes. Rupture of the benign variety can occur to allow peritoneal implantation and the development of pseudomyxoma peritonei with formation of large amounts of gelatinous material in the abdomen.

Mucinous cystadenocarcinomas

Mucinous cystadencarcinomas are found about one third as often and tend to be larger than serous cystadenocarcinomas. Pseudomyxoma peritonei is more likely to occur with them than with their benign counterpart.

Endometrioid adenocarcinomas

Endometrioid adenocarcinomas may be associated with ovarian endometriosis. These tumors are usually cystic and may have areas of "chocolate" accumulation and acanthomatous change. The cure rate and prognosis are about twice as favorable as with papillary serous cystadenocarcinoma.

Mesonephroid tumors

Mesonephroid tumors are believed to arise from mesonephronic remnants in the ovary. The tubular arrangement of peglike cells with some tufts is characteristic.

Brenner tumors

Brenner tumors are often found as a component of mucinous tumors. They may occur as separate, principally solid tumors that are white with yellow streaks and small hemorrhagic areas. Grossly they are like fibromas.

Undifferentiated carcinomas

Undifferentiated carcinomas are often grayish, friable, and necrotic. Hemorrhagic areas are common. Although they have more solid than cystic areas, most exhibit some cystic areas. At least half are bilateral when discovered. Primary solid ovarian carcinomas are described as adenocarcinoma, papillary carcinoma, medullary carcinoma, carcinoma simplex, scirrhous carcinoma, alveolar carcinoma, and plexiform carcinoma, depending on such histologic characteristics as the arrangement of epithelial cells and the amount of connective tissue.

Mixed mesodermal tumors

Mixed mesodermal ovarian tumors are highly malignant and extremely rare, with carcinomatous and sarcomatous portions.

GERM CELL TUMORS
Benign teratomas

Benign teratomas are common (20% of benign ovarian neoplasms) with bilateral occurrence in about 20% of patients. A benign teratoma is the most common ovarian neoplasm in girls. Most benign teratomas are termed "dermoid cysts" and can usually be identified grossly because they contain hair and sebaceous material that solidifies at room temperature. Areas of calcification are common, and the tumors may contain teeth. Histologic study reveals adult-type structures of the skin and may include osseous, cartilaginous, intestinal, neural, or thyroid elements—all adult-type tissues. Carcinoma, which has been found in 1% to 3% of dermoid cysts, is squamous cell in type. Benign teratomas are rarely principally solid. Destruction of normal tissue occurs by tumor expansion. Since dermoid cysts can be identified grossly, they may be shelled out to leave normal tissue in situ.

Struma ovarii

The term "struma ovarii" is applied when thyroid tissue predominates in teratomas, benign or malignant. In a few patients hyperthyroidism has resulted.

Immature teratomas

The amount and degree of immaturity of tissues found in about 1% of teratomas is related to their malignant potential. Physicians must search for areas of embryonal carcinoma or choriocarcinoma. Children and young women develop im-

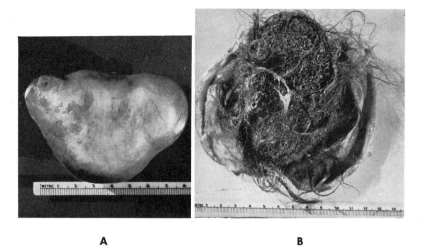

Fig. 12-4. A, Dermoid cyst. **B,** Dermoid cyst opened.

From Willson, J.R., Beecham, C.T., Forman, I., and Carrington, E.R.: Obstetrics and gynecology, St. Louis, The C.V. Mosby Co.

mature teratomas; however, their bilateral occurrence and high mortality usually justify bilateral oophorectomy.

Dysgerminomas

Dysgerminomas are rare ovarian tumors identical with seminomas of the testis. Most have been found in children of young women. Principally a solid rubbery growth, the tumor is grayish pink on cut section. Although one third are malignant, unilateral oophorectomy is sufficient if the tumor has not infiltrated the ovarian capsule. External radiation may be a valuable adjunct to surgery if removal is incomplete.

Embryonal carcinoma

This rare, highly malignant neoplasm, also referred to as endodermal sinus or "yolk-sac" tumor, appears in children and young women. α-Fetoprotein may be detected in the patient's serum. Elevated chorionic gonadotropin indicates some choriocarcinoma components. High mortality and bilateral occurrence justify removal of both adnexauteri and the uterus. Triple chemotherapy is used for this radioresistant neoplasm.

Choriocarcinoma

Unlike the choriocarcinoma that occurs during gestation, choriocarcinoma occurring in a nonpregnant patient does not respond to the antineoplastic drugs used for trophoblastic tumors. Usually part of a mixed germ cell tumor, choriocarcinoma is very rare (see Chapter 13).

Gonadoblastomas

Gonadoblastomas are rare ovarian tumors apt to be found in intersexual patients of female habitus with a 46 XY or XO/XY chromosomal pattern. Gonad removal is in order, since malignancy is high and reproduction impossible.

SPECIALIZED GONADAL STROMAL TUMORS
Granulosa cell tumors

Granulosa cell tumors usually produce estrogen, are yellow on cut surface, vary from less than 1 cm to 15 cm or more in diameter, may be cystic, occur bilaterally in about 27% of reported cases (Allan and Hertig), exhibit malignancy in about 25% of patients, and require detailed study of fixed sections for identification. Before the menarche and after the menopause, evidences of intrinsic estrogenic stimulation suggest the possibility of their presence. In young women unilateral oophorectomy is advised; however, in older women bilateral excision is recommended despite the normal appearance of the other ovary.

Thecomas

Thecomas are less common and less malignant than the uncommon granulosa cell tumors. Estrogen production causes similar clinical manifestations. A solid tumor with cystic areas, it may appear grossly like a fibroma.

Estrogen-producing tumors cause proliferative or hyperplastic endometria. Ingraham and Novak suggest that endometrial cancer is associated with these tumors.

Luteomas

Luteomas are yellow ovarian tumors that may be luteinized granulosa cell tumors. Some luteomas found during pregnancy appear to be physiologic changes, since they regress spontaneously. Estrogenic or progestational effects may be noted in the endometrium.

Sertoli–Leydig cell neoplasms

Most Sertoli–Leydig cell tumors have been termed "arrhenoblastomas"; however, some do not produce androgens. Typically defeminization (amenorrhea and decreased size of breasts and hips) is followed by masculization (enlarged clitoris, hirsutism, and deeper voice). The malignant potential of and therapy for these rare tumors are the same as for granulosal cell tumors.

Gynandroblastomas

Gynandroblastomas are very rare and exhibit typical areas of arrhenoblastoma together with granulosa or theca cell areas. If hormonally active, masculinization is likely to predominate.

Lipid-cell neoplasms

Lipid-cell tumors have parenchymas of polygonal cells containing a lipid, which usually makes them yellow. Adrenal rest tumors, Leydig cell tumors, or masculin-ovablastomas are included in this group and are often unilateral. They are rare tumors that may produce androgens; many are malignant.

Nonspecific mesenchymal tumors

The nonspecific connective tissues of the ovary may give rise to malignant sarcomas or benign hemangiomas, lymphomas, leiomyomas, or fibromas. Large benign fibromas may by transudation produce ascites and hydrothorax (Meigs' syndrome). Removal of the benign tumor cures the problems; however, malignant ovarian tumors can also cause Meigs' syndrome with tumor spread to the pleura.

METASTATIC OVARIAN CANCER

Of endometrial cancers, 7% involve the ovary. Rarely does cancer of the cervix or uterine sarcoma spread to the ovary. Salpingeal cancer often extends to the ovary. Cancer from the opposite ovary may be the source of spread. Digestive tract malignancy and breast cancer may metastasize to one or both ovaries. Krukenberg's tumors exhibit signet-ring (mucoid) cells. When these tumors are found, a search of the digestive tract for the primary lesion is indicated.

CLINICAL DIAGNOSIS OF NONFUNCTIONING OVARIAN TUMORS

Benign and malignant ovarian neoplasms are asymptomatic in their beginning. Ideally they should be found in pelvic palpation during routine examination. (Early detection of ovarian malignancy is a principal reason for annual or semiannual examinations of women of 35 years and older.) When an adnexal mass estimated to be 5 cm or more is found to persist for 3 months in regularly menstruating women, diagnostic laparotomy is indicated. Ovarian tumors can be 15 cm or more before the patient is conscious of any enlargement. Large ovarian cysts must be differentiated from ascites and pregnancy. At times large pancreatic cysts cause confusion.

Pedicled ovarian tumors (dermoid cyst, for example) may lie anterior or posterior to the uterus. If nonadherent, they may rise out of the pelvis and be moved about during palpation. A full urinary bladder or rectum, subserous myomas, par-

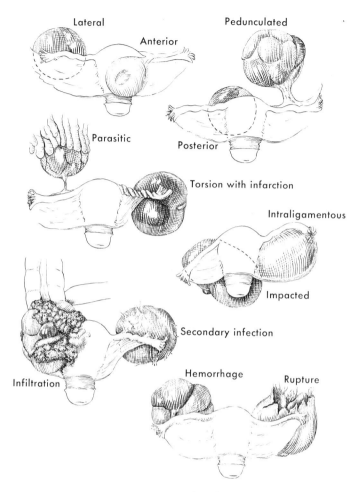

Fig. 12-5. Diagnosis of ovarian tumors.

ovarian cysts, hydrosalpinx, sigmoid colon, tubal pregnancy mass, pelvic kidney, retroverted uterus, intestinal and omental adhesions, and marked obesity may obscure or cause confusion in palpating ovarian tumors. Inadequate relaxation caused by fear or pelvic tenderness may prevent adequate examination.

Torsion of ovarian (adnexal) masses initially causes pain referred to the flanks. When circulatory impairment leads to infarction and hemorrhage into the mass, the adjacent parietal peritoneum is painfully irritated. Low-grade fever and leukocytosis result. Nausea and vomiting often follow the pain.

Rupture of ovarian cysts, the contents of which may irritate the peritoneum,

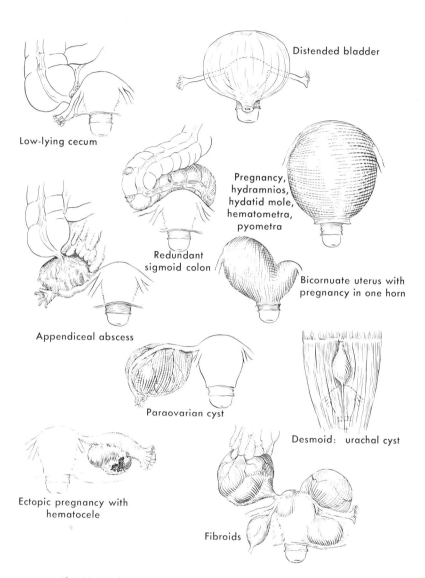

Fig. 12-6. Pelvic masses that may be confused with ovarian tumors.

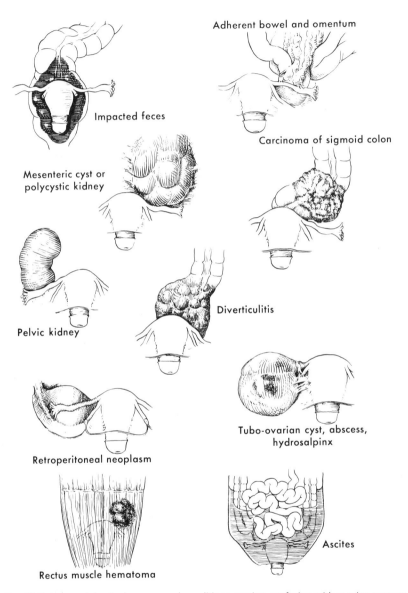

Fig. 12-7. Lower abdominal masses and conditions causing confusion with ovarian tumors.

often causes abdominal pain. The sebaceous material from benign teratomas, when in contact with the peritoneum for several days, causes a marked reaction.

Hemorrhage may occur into an ovarian tumor with resulting pain. Intra-abdominal bleeding with rupture of vessels is unlikely but may produce shock if extensive. Intra-abdominal bleeding from areas of endometriosis is usually slight but painful.

Infection of ovarian cysts usually indicates continuity with the intestine or spreading of intestinal, tubal, or bladder infection.

In the absence of torsion, rupture, infection, or hemorrhage, pain is absent or is aching in type. A sensation of pressure with a feeling of bearing down may occur.

Ascites, large tumors, and partial intestinal obstruction lead to anorexia, constipation, and weakness. Ascitic fluid should be studied for malignant cells.

Changes in menstrual cycles seldom occur unless an endocrine-producing tumor is present. Endometrial ovarian cysts are an exception. Postmenopausal bleeding can occur with ovarian cancer because of uterine metastases or possibly because of changes in pelvic circulation.

Metastases of ovarian cancer may be felt in the cul-de-sac. ("Rectal shelf" is the lower edge of the cul-de-sac filled with cancer.) Inguinal nodes may be found enlarged or containing metastatic cancer on biopsy. Ascites is too often the first symptomatic manifestation of ovarian cancer. The possibility of specific tumor antigens allowing immunodiagnosis allows hope for future earlier diagnosis.

X-ray examination may reveal calcification in dermoid cysts and soft tissue masses in the pelvis and may identify renal shadows to rule out pelvic kidney. Urography and cystoscopy may be indicated. If ovarian cancer is suspected, proctoscopy, a barium enema, and a gastrointestinal series are in order to rule out the gastrointestinal tract as the primary source.

Ultrasonographic visualization offers additional diagnostic information when palpation is limited and may suggest whether a mass is solid or filled with fluid. Pathognomonic findings are not expected.

CT scanning does not reveal masses less than 3 cm and usually adds scant information in the diagnosis of pelvic masses.

Therapy

Removal is the treatment for all ovarian neoplasms. If the benign nature of dermoid cysts, fibromas, and unilocular smooth-walled cysts is grossly evident, the tumor may be resected to leave remaining normal tissue. If the tumor is multilocular or presents papillary areas, oophorectomy is indicated. Excision of the other ovary (and total hysterectomy with bilateral salpingectomy) is decided on only after considering the tumor's malignant potential and the patient's age and desire for

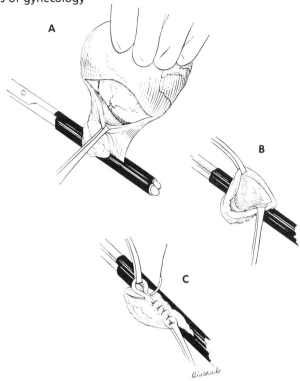

Fig. 12-8. Large ovarian dermoid cysts and endometriomas can be "shelled-out" to leave most of the ovary in place.

childbearing. With peritoneal spread, omentectomy is done. Large malignant masses may often be removed for palliation. Should metastases to bladder or bowel by extensive, biopsy may be employed and then chemotherapy or external radiation used with the hope that the masses' size may decrease and that improved mobility may allow for more complete excision later.

To evaluate the effectiveness of therapy for ovarian cancer the stage of involvement at the time of beginning treatment, as well as the histologic classification of these epithelial tumors, must be evaluated. The staging of carcinoma of the ovary should be based on clinical examination as well as observation at laparotomy. Proper staging requires exploration of the entire abdominal cavity, cytologic sampling of the abdominal cavity, omentectomy, retroperitoneal node sampling, and liver inspection and biopsy if involvement is detected. Germ cell tumors, hormone-producing neoplasms, and metastatic carcinomas should be excluded from therapeutic statistical reporting on ovarian epithelial tumors.

Stage I
The carcinoma is confined to the ovaries.

Stage IA
The carcinoma is confined to one ovary without ascites:
(1) capsule ruptured; (2) capsule not ruptured.

Stage IB
The carcinoma is confined to both ovaries without ascites:
(1) capsule ruptured; (2) capsule not ruptured.

Stage IC
The carcinoma is confined to one or both ovaries with ascites and the presence of malignant cells in the fluid:
(1) capsule ruptured; (2) capsule not ruptured.

Stage II
The carcinoma involves one or both ovaries with pelvic extension.

Stage IIA
The carcinoma extends and/or metastasizes to the uterus and/or fallopian tubes only.

Stage IIB
The carcinoma extends to other pelvic tissues.

Stage III
The carcinoma involves one or both ovaries with widespread intraperitoneal metastasis to the abdomen (the omentum, the small intestine, and its mesentery).

Stage IV
The carcinoma involves one or both ovaries with distant metastasis outside the peritoneal cavity.

Stage I cancer of the ovary may be associated with presence of malignant cells in peritoneal fluid. It has been advised that cytologic studies be made from washings obtained at laparotomy. If malignant cells are present, radioactive isotopes may be used intraperitoneally after the wound is healed. Since about 70% of the patients with Stage I growths survive 5 years or more with surgical excision alone, it is difficult to evaluate the additional effects of the prophylactic use of intraperitoneal radioactive isotopes. For anaplastic tumors and when there is doubt as to local extension, external radiation of the pelvis is in order.

For ascites or pleural effusion associated with ovarian metastatic cancer, radioactive isotopes or alkylating agents have been injected. They appear effective in about 50% of patients in reducing ascites. Ascites may be decreased by oral or intravenous administration of alkylating agents.

Most therapists agree on the advisability of external radiation for small residual tumor masses. More intense radiation is given in the pelvic area, and the total abdominal cavity is irradiated commonly by the strip technique. For larger residual metastases alkylating agents are tried. In general a 50% chance of response is anticipated. The most suitable agents are melphalan (Alkeran), which is used orally; cyclophosphamide (Cytoxan), which can be used orally or intravenously; chlorambucil (Leukeran), which is used orally; and thiotepa, which is given intravenously. When alkylating agents do not produce response, a combination of actinomycin D, 5-fluorouracil, and cyclophosphamide may be effective. A combination of drugs may be the best choice for primary chemotherapy for the more anaplastic papillary cancers.

The radioactive isotopes for intraperitoneal use are Au 198, radioactive gold, which has a half-life of 2.69 days and emits beta and gamma radiation, and P 32, radioactive phosphorus, which has a half-life of 14.3 days and emits only beta radiation. Problems concerning lack of distribution of these agents throughout the cavity and their limited effectiveness has decreased enthusiasm for using isotopes.

Some cancer treatment centers have discontinued the use of radiation in treating metastatic epithelial ovarian carcinoma. In some cases the use of melphalan has been supplanted by a combination of doxorubicin, cis-platinum, and hexamethylmelamine. Experience has shown that there are no suitable biologic markers with which to follow epithelial ovarian cancers. Similarly, attempts at use of ultrasound visualization are frequently inaccurate. A second laparotomy appears to have a place in the overall management of patients who are apparently responding to therapy.

PREVENTION OF OVARIAN CARCINOMA

Because of the insidious onset of ovarian carcinoma with its lack of definitive symptoms, the patient is not led to seek treatment until the condition has advanced far beyond the chance of cure. Because of these facts H. S. Crossen in 1942 advised as a preventive measure the removal of the ovaries in women at or near the menopause (43 years of age) while the abdomen was open for other necessary pelvic work. This suggestion was criticized by Randall because of the low incidence of ovarian carcinoma and also because he felt that ovarian function continued and was important during the menopause and for some years afterward.

There exists much difference of opinion as to the advisability of prophylactic oophorectomy, which is the only means of prevention of ovarian cancer. Since 80% or more of ovarian malignancies are found in women past 50 years of age, it would appear that removal of atrophic postmenopausal ovaries at the time of hysterectomy is desirable and does not deprive the patient of significant estrogenic support. Oophorectomy before the menopause must be evaluated with due regard for the loss of intrinsic estrogens, which not only are a stimulus for maintenance of the secondary sexual characteristics of femininity but also are probably associated with less atherosclerotic change of the arterial system. Consideration of the psychologic effects of oophorectomy on the woman and on her husband is important.

SELECTED REFERENCES

Allan, M.S., and Hertig, A.T.: Carcinoma of the ovary, Am. J. Obstet. Gynecol. **58**:640, 1949.

Banner, E.A., and Dockerty, M.B.: Theca cell tumors of the ovary, Surg. Gynecol. Obstet. **81**:234, 1945.

Barber, H.R.K.: Ovarian tumors, Clin. Obstet. Gynecol. **12**:929, 1969.

Blackwell, W.J., Dockerty, M.B., Masson, J.C., and Mussey, R.D.: Dermoid cysts of ovary, Am. J. Obstet. Gynecol. **51**:151, 1946.

Bulbrook, R.D., and Greenwood, F.C.: Persistence of urinary oestrogen excretion after oophorectomy and adrenalectomy, Br. Med. J. **1**:662, 1957.

Crossen, H.S.: Menace of "silent" ovarian carcinoma, J.A.M.A. **119**:1485, 1942.

Dockerty, M.B., and Mussey, E.: Malignant lesions of the uterus associated with estrogen-producing ovarian tumors, Am. J. Obstet. Gynecol. **61**:147, 1951

Emge, L.A.: Functional and growth characteristics of struma ovarii, Am. J. Obstet. Gynecol. **40**:738, 1940.

Fagan, G.E., Alan, E.D., and Klawans, A.H.: Ovarian neoplasms and repeat pelvic surgery, Obstet. Gynecol. **7**:418, 1956.

Frawco, J., Hall, B.E., and Hales, D.R.: Effect of prednisone in the treatment of malignant effusions, J.A.M.A. **168**:1645, 1958.

Gardiner, G.A., and Slate, J.: Malignant tumors of the ovary, Am. J. Obstet. Gynecol. **70**:554, 1955.

Hreshchyshyn, M.M., et al.: The role of adjuvant therapy in Stage I ovarian cancer, Am. J. Obstet. Gynecol. **138**:139, 1980.

Ingraham, C.B., Black, W.C., and Rutledge, E.K.: The relationship of granulosa cell tumors of the ovary to endometrial carcinoma, Am. J. Obstet. Gynecol. **48**:760, 1944.

Ireland, K., and Woodruff, J.D.: Masculinizing ovarian tumors, Obstet. Gynecol. Surv. **31**:83, 1976.

Jones, G.E., and Te Linde, R.W.: The curability of granulosal cell tumors, Am. J. Obstet. Gynecol. **50**:691, 1945.

Karsh, J.: Secondary malignant diseases of ovary, Am. J. Obstet. Gynecol. **61**:154, 1951.

Levi, A.A.: Ovarian conservation during surgery with reference to bilateral dermoids and endometriosis, N. Engl. J. Med. **238**:83, 1948.

Meigs, J.V.: Fibroma of the ovary with ascites and hydrothorax—Meigs's syndrome, Am. J. Obstet. Gynecol. **67**:962, 1954.

Mengert, W.F.: Physiologic approach to the problem of oophorectomy, Texas J. Med. **41**:465, 1946.

Miller, N.F., and Willson, J.R.: Surgery of the ovary, New York J. Med. **42**:1851, 1942.

Mueller, C.W., Topkins, P., and Laff, W.A.: Dysgerminoma of ovary. An analysis of 427 cases, Am. J. Obstet. Gynecol. **60**:153, 1950.

Novak, E.R., and Woodruff, J.D.: Mesonephroma of the ovary, Am. J. Obstet. Gynecol. **77**:632, 1959.

Novak, E.R., and Woodruff, J.D.: Novak's gynecologic and obstetric pathology, Philadelphia, 1979, W.B. Saunders Co.

Pedowitz, P., Felmus, L.B., and Grayzel, D.M.: Dysgerminoma of the ovary, Am. J. Obstet. Gynecol. **70**:1284, 1955.

Peterson, W.F.: Malignant degeneration of benign cystic teratomas of the ovary, Obstet. Gynecol. Surv. **12**:793, 1957.

Randall, C.L.: Ovarian carcinoma, Obstet. Gynecol. **3**:491, 1954.

Randall, C.L.: Ovarian preservation, Obstet. Gynecol. **20**:880, 1962.

Randall, C.L., and Hall, D.W.: Clinical consideration of benign ovarian cystomas, Am. J. Obstet. Gynecol. **62**:806, 1951.

Rawson, A.J., and Helman, M.R.: Malignant Brenner tumors, Am. J. Obstet. Gynecol. **69**:429, 1956.

Rosenshein, N.B., Leichner, P.K., and Volgensang, G.: Radiocolloids in the treatment of ovarian cancer, Obstet. Gynecol. Surv. **34**:708, 1979.

Schueller, E.F., and Kirol, P.M.: Prognosis in endometrioid carcinoma of the ovary, Obstet. Gynecol. **27**:850, 1966.

Schwartz, P.E., and Smith, J.P.: Second look operations in ovarian cancer, Am. J. Obstet. Gynecol. **138**:1124, 1980.

Smith, J.P., and Day, T.G.: Review of ovarian cancer at the University of Texas Systems Cancer Center, M.D. Anderson Hospital and Tumor Institute, Am. J. Obstet. Gynecol. **135**:984, 1979.

Smith, J.P., and Rutledge, F.: Chemotherapy in the treatment of cancer of the ovary, Am. J. Obstet. Gynecol. **107**:691, 1970.

Sommers, S.C., and Wadman, P.J.: Pathogenesis of polycystic ovaries, Am. J. Obstet. Gynecol. **72:**160, 1956.

Sternberg, W.H.: The morphology, androgenic function, hyperplasia, and tumors of the human ovarian hilus cells, Am. J. Pathol. **25:**493, 1949.

Tate, M.A.: Metastasis of ovarian carcinoma, Am. J. Obstet. Gynecol. **19:**285, 1930.

Teilum, G.: Carcinoma arising from ovarian endometriosis, Acta Obstet. Gynecol. Scand. **25:**377, 1945.

Willson, J.R., and Carrington, E.R.: Obstetrics and gynecology, St. Louis, 1980, The C.V. Mosby Co.

Wolfe, S.A.: Metastatic carcinoid tumor of the ovary, Am. J. Obstet. Gynecol. **70:**563, 1955.

Young, R.C., Chabner, B.A., Hubbard, S.P., et al.: Advanced ovarian adenocarcinoma: a prospective clinical trial of melphalen versus combination chemotherapy, N. Engl. J. Med. **299:**1261, 1978.

Chapter 13

COMPLICATIONS OF PREGNANCY

ABORTION

Abortion is defined as the expulsion of the products of conception before the fetus is sufficiently mature to survive. The term "miscarriage" is used by the laity, to whom the word "abortion" implies an intentional procedure. "Termination of pregnancy" is the term often used by the medical profession instead of induced abortion.

Since the manifestations of abortion such as abnormal bleeding or pain account for many of the reasons why patients consult physicians and since the reproductive organs may have disease that existed before pregnancy, thorough knowledge of this subject is essential for gynecic therapy.

Definitions. Classification requires the use of the following terms.

Spontaneous abortion is abortion occurring naturally, i.e., without outside intervention.

Induced abortion is abortion brought on intentionally. It is considered therapeutic if induced to safeguard the health of the mother. It is criminal if performed without legal sanction. Legal elective abortions for social reasons are performed in many countries.

Threatening abortion exists when the patient has uterine bleeding and/or pain.

Threatened abortion is one in which the bleeding and pain have subsided.

Incomplete abortion applies if only a portion of the products of gestation has been expelled from the uterus.

Complete abortion means that all of the products of conception have been expelled.

Missed abortion is said to exist when the embryo or fetus is dead and the uterus fails to expel it within 4 weeks thereafter.

Habitual abortion implies that three or more successive pregnancies have been spontaneously aborted.

Etiology. In the United States it is estimated that at least 10% of all conceptions result in spontaneous abortion. Of these, more than 50% occur because of embry-

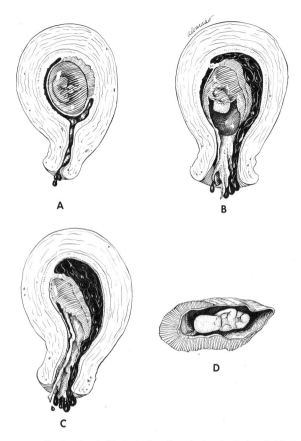

Fig. 13-1. Spontaneous early abortion is illustrated as threatening in **A,** inevitable in **B,** and incomplete in **C.** Complete abortion is indicated by the intact expelled products of pregnancy in **D.**

onic defects. Mall found defective development in 80% of the embryos when abortion occurred during the first 2 months of gestation. Hertig found in his study of 1000 spontaneous abortions that defects of the conceptus existed in 61.7% and emphasized that hydatidiform mole changes were often present. Other causes of spontaneous abortion include uterine myomas, congenital anomalies of the uterus, incompetent internal cervical os, previously amputated cervix, endometrial polyps, tuberculous endometritis, disseminated lupus erythematosus, diabetes mellitus, nephritis, severe febrile illnesses, severe malnutrition, syphilis, cervical implantation, rupture of membranes, and torsion or compression of the umbilical cord. The roles of possible hormonal imbalance, psychic disturbances, and poorly developed endometrium may be of etiologic significance in some pregnancies. Many abortions occur in which routine methods of investigation do not reveal the cause. The frequency of chromosomal abnormalities noted in association with spontaneous abortion and found when large numbers of specimens from legal abortions are evaluated suggests the importance of genetic material as a cause of abortion. There is some evidence to substantiate the theory that fertilization of overripe human oocytes is an important cause of abortion.

Abortion may be induced by placing foreign bodies such as catheters, metal or wooden objects, or gauze in the uterine cavity. Administration of oxytocics orally or parenterally usually will not disturb a normal early pregnancy. (Prostaglandins stimulate sufficient uterine contractions to cause termination.) Similarly, if a pregnancy is entirely normal, vigorous exercises will not cause abortion to occur. Radiation applied to the embryo or to the fetus during its early development, if in sufficient concentration, will stop growth, and abortion may soon follow. The use of agents for the treatment of leukemia and other malignancies can result in abortion for similar reasons. Operations performed on the uterus during pregnancy increase myometrial irritability and may cause abortion; however, cervical biopsy and cauterization of the cervix seldom disturb cyesis.

Pathology. Bleeding and infection are the principal pathologic processes. The amount of bleeding that occurs varies greatly and at times can result in lethal exsanguination. Bleeding may occur from the site of implantation or from shedding of the decidua. Hemorrhage and necrosis of the decidua, degeneration of the fetus, anomalies of the cord, deformities of the fetus, early hydramnios, and hydatidiform changes of the trophoblast may be found. Bleeding ceases when separation of the trophoblasts is complete and the decidua is expelled. Should some trophoblasts remain attached, continued bleeding is anticipated.

The infection that can occur may be limited to the products of conception and the decidua; however, when the uterus has been inoculated with virulent organisms such as streptococci, staphylococci, and the coliform group, particularly when criminal abortion is attempted, the lining of the uterus that has been traumatized serves as a wound for the spread of infection. Lymphatic involvement can lead to parametritis and extensive cellulitis at times. Invasion of the bloodstream with the development of suppurative pelvic thrombophlebitis can be the forerunner of abscesses occurring particulary in the lungs and ultimately in organs throughout the body. Should infection spread into the salpinges, severe salpingitis and peritonitis are anticipated. Deaths that occur from infection following abortion are generally caused by overwhelming peritonitis, severely toxic bacteremia, or metastatic abscesses in other portions of the body.

When a missed abortion of a gestation of over 14 weeks occurs, the possibility of the development of hypofibrinogenemia is entertained. If severe hemorrhage and shock occur or should infection be overwhelming, a lower nephron nephrosis may ensue.

In about 5% of Rh_0-negative women who suffer abortion with gestations exceeding 6 weeks, isoimmunization occurs. The likelihood of transfer of Rh_0 antigen from the fetus to the mother is increased when the abortion is induced or when curettage is necessary.

Diagnosis. Because of irregularity in menstrual cycles and the common occurrence of uterine bleeding during the first few weeks after conception, clinically evident amenorrhea may or may not be present in patients threatening to abort. In any patient who could be pregnant, irregularities in uterine bleeding should lead one to suspect the possibility of abortion. When profuse uterine bleeding occurs without other obvious cause, abortion is the most likely explanation. If nausea, mastalgia, and frequency of urination together with some degree of amenorrhea have been present, the diagnosis becomes more likely. Typically the pain associated with abortion is cramplike. Pelvic examination may reveal softening and enlargement of the uterus if the pregnancy has progressed sufficiently. Mild tenderness is common. Expulsion of any tissue from the uterus should be adequately investigated. Once some decidua has been passed, the abortion becomes inevitable. The finding of an intact amniotic sac or a complete cast of the uterus is the most reliable evidence that the abortion is complete.

Pregnancy tests may not become positive if failure of growth of the trophoblast occurs sufficiently early. If there has been sufficient production of chorionic gonadotropins to render the test positive, it may remain positive for 1 or more weeks, even though the fetus is no longer developing. When a previously positive pregnancy test becomes negative before the uterus attains the size of a 16-week gestation, abortion is suspected.

Management. When threatening spontaneous abortion is diagnosed, the patient should be advised to restrict physical activities and should be given mild analgesics and sedatives. Examination is essential to determine the cause of her symptoms, which may mimic other conditions such as functional uterine bleeding, bleeding from neoplasia, and ectopic pregnancy with little or no hemoperitoneum. Since the majority of early abortions do not have causes for which the administration of hormones would be effective, hormonal therapy is not indicated for the majority of patients. The patient should be instructed to avoid douching and intercourse and to save any "possible" tissue passed. Repeated examinations will be necessary to determine the progress of the pregnancy. If bleeding is recurrent and the uterus is enlarging, progesterone given intramuscularly or a synthetic progestogen administered orally may be of value. With failure of enlargement of the uterus, the diagnosis of missed abortion may be made if the size of the uterus has been sufficient to diagnose pregnancy in the first place.

Missed abortion can be diagnosed by repeated examinations of the patient. At times a soft uterine myoma may cause symmetric enlargement of the uterus, and at times obesity and position of the uterus may interfere with estimation of its size;

consequently missed abortion may be difficult to determine. Ultrasound β-scans allow visualization of the uterine contents to aid diagnosis. This type of abortion is best managed by waiting for the forces of Nature to intervene. As long as the uterine cavity is not invaded, there is no danger of infection.

The danger of hypofibrinogenemia developing with a late abortion should be of concern although its occurrence is rare. A high dose of oxytocin (40 to 60 U in 1000 ml) administered intravenously is usually effective; however, water intoxication can occur because of the antidiuretic effects of oxytocin. Amniocentesis and instillation of hypertonic (20%) glucose or saline solution after about 15 hours will increase myometrial response to oxytocics; however, gas bacillus and other infections have occurred with glucose, and maternal death has resulted from hypertonic saline injection. These infrequent tragedies, along with the possibility of Rh sensitization, have decreased the usage of instillation of hypertonic solutions into the amniotic fluid. Prostaglandin $F_{2\alpha}$ by intra-amniotic or vaginal administration can cause effective uterine contractions.

An abortion is said to be *inevitable* when dilation of the cervix has progressed, even though no part of the conceptus or decidua has been passed. The escape of a gush of amniotic fluid in early pregnancy is diagnostic. A determination of inevitability based on the rate of blood loss alone may be erroneous. Administration of oxytocics, particularly oxytocin intravenously by infusion, will expedite the inevitable outcome. When the pregnancy is of 12 weeks' duration or less, curettage after evacuation of the uterus with sponge forceps may be in order to stop the bleeding. When the pregnancy is of more than 12 weeks' duration, because of the size of the fetus and placenta to be passed, it is better to manage the patient without early operative interference.

Most patients with early incomplete abortion will continue to have vaginal bleeding and cramps. The symptoms may stop and recur several days later. To prevent further blood loss and debility most patients with incomplete abortion should be given the benefit of curettage.

When a patient admits to or is thought to have had an unskilled abortion, infection is anticipated. Broad-spectrum antibacterial agents should be administered, along with serum containing antibodies against the tetanus and gas gangrene bacteria. When septic abortion is present, the patient usually has chills and high fever. Palpation may reveal induration of the parametrial areas along with marked tenderness. A mild degree of tenderness may be found without infection of the uterus in other types of abortion. Oxytocics may be administered; however, gentle evacuation of the uterus may be required to remove the necrotic infected placental tissue. The patient should be observed for evidences of septic emboli by chest x-ray films. Cultures of material from the uterus and blood should be made. Septic shock caused by the effects of endotoxins of gram-negative bacilli demands exacting management, as detailed in Chapter 7. If the infection does not respond to antibacterial therapy within a reasonable period, in some patients ligations of the vena cava and ovarian veins are lifesaving.

After repeated abortions have occurred, diagnosis of anatomic, genetic, endocrine, or infectious states must be evaluated. Hysterosalpingography should first be performed, thus enabling the physician to diagnosis subseptate and septate uterine deformities. Submucous myomas and incompetence of the cervix may be identified, and Asherman's syndrome may be found. Incompetence should be suspected when there has been a rapid relatively painless abortion after 14 weeks. It may be suspected when a No. 10 Hegar dilator can be passed without resistance. One should search for inadequate luteal phase. This is suspected when the basal temperature rise lasts 10 days or less, when progesterone determinations on the seventh postovulatory day are less than 6 ng/ml, and when the endometrum's histologic changes are inadequate for the time of progesterone stimulation.

Once habitual abortion has occurred, approximately 10% of the parents will exhibit chromosomal changes. When there have been repeated neural tube defects, evaluation during pregnancy of the amniotic fluid for α-fetoprotein and by ultrasound can be diagnostic even though chromosomal studies will be normal. Karyotypic analysis of the products of a failed conception, although expensive, may aid in explaining the abortion and, in the majority of instances, will inform the physician if the patient can expect, when next pregnant, to carry the fetus to full term.

Anatomic causes producing abortion can usually be corrected. For cervical incompetence Shirodkar or MacDonald procedures can be instituted in a future pregnancy after ultrasonography has determined the fetus's normalcy. A deformed uterus can usually be adequately repaired by various techniques. Myomas can be removed. When doubt exists as to the nature of synechiae in Asherman's syndrome, visualization with a contact hysteroscope is ideal.

The administration of progesterone just before implantation and during the first few weeks of pregnancy is justified by the results that have been obtained after a deficient luteal phase has been demonstrated. When no prepregnancy evidence of luteal phase deficiency exists, progesterone is of doubtful value. Since recent reports reveal an increase in anomalies with the use of estrogens and progestogens in early pregnancy, these should be avoided whenever possible.

The time-honored measures of prolonged bed rest and sedation in an attempt to avoid abortion, particularly late abortion and premature labor, apparently still have a place in the management of this difficult problem. Suggestion and reassurance as psychotherapeutic methods to aid the woman are important and may aid in maintaining pregnancy.

Proper management of severe renal infections and diabetes may add much to the patient's ability to maintain a pregnancy. Other conditions such as disseminated lupus erythematosus and pelvic tuberculosis continue to offer a poor prognosis in the patient with recurring abortion.

Induced abortion

Abortion may be induced to eliminate a known or suspected defective fetus. Rubella virus infecting the fetus at the time of organogenesis during early gestation may cause cataracts, heart deformity, or CNS damage. Genetically transmitted malformations or metabolic disorder can be predicted as to probability and may be diagnosed by study of the amniotic fluid and the cells therein. Changes in the laws of the various states of the United States and in various countries throughout the world have allowed increased legal abortion. In addition to protecting the mother's health and life, abortions may be performed to remove a defective fetus, in instances of rape, or on request of the pregnant woman. Of a total of 1,157,776 legal abortions reported in the United States in 1978, the death rate, excluding ectopic pregnancies, was 0.6 per 100,000 abortions. Four of 11 deaths resulted from ectopic pregnancy. Perforation of the uterus, hemorrhage, infection, and cervical damage to cause cervical incompetence are the more common complications of induced abortion. The longer the duration of gestation, the more likely are the complications of induced abortion.

The uterine contents may be removed without anesthesia or with paracervically injected anesthetics in ambulatory patients. For patients pregnant for 4 weeks or less, special cannulas with syringe suction allow removal of the trophoblastic tissue in 98% of the patients. Since some are not pregnant, the term "menstrual extraction" is used.

For gestations under 12 weeks, dilation of the cervix can be sufficient to allow curettage or suction evacuation to remove the embryo, placental tissue, and decidua. When fetal development exceeds 12 weeks, the amount of tissue to be removed, the increased vascularity of the uterus, and the small diameter to which the cervix can be safely stretched with metal dilators render the curettage less effective and more dangerous. For patients with gestations of 14 weeks or more, hypertonic saline solution (20% to 30%) has been injected into amniotic sacs and after 12 to 15 hours oxytocin stimulation is usually effective. Hysterotomy can be performed as a major surgical procedure to remove the products of pregnancy with advanced pregnancy.

To accomplish gradual dilation of the cervix and thereby avoid tears, the Japanese use the little roots of kelp, which are termed "laminaria tents." These will afford sufficient dilation of the cervix to allow suction or curet evacuation of the uterus in early pregnancies. When pregnancy is past 12 weeks, the laminaria tents may be followed by curet and forceps evacuation.

Prostaglandins, which are 20-carbon fatty acids with a carboxyl in the side chain and a five-membered ring, will cause abortion by bringing about contractions of the uterus. Prostaglandin F_{2a} is available for intra-amniotic or intravaginal administration.

When abortion is induced in Rh_o-negative women or when abortion occurs spontaneously after 6 weeks' gestation, the mother should receive the immune anti-D globulin (Rh_oGAM) to prevent sensitization.

ECTOPIC GESTATION

Eccyesis is pregnancy out of place. It is usually extrauterine and most commonly is tubal. Fig. 13-2 depicts varieties of the tubal type and indicates that the developing fertilized oocyte may lodge in any part of the salpinx. Other possible ectopic sites include (1) uterine cornu, (2) ovary, (3) broad ligament, (4) abdomen, and (5) cervix uteri. The third and fourth sites are usually secondary in origin. The fifth site has been reported very rarely.

Incidence. The incidence of ectopic pregnancy is estimated to be about 1 per 250 pregnancies. The ratio of eccyesis to deliveries at Charity Hospital in New Orleans, La., before 1969 was 1:108. The ratio in patients treated by the Southern California Permanente Medical Group from 1966 to 1975 was 1:116. This same group found an incidence of 1:54 in 1974 to 1975. Increased use of IUDs and increased rate of salpingitis were associated.

Oral contraception prevents tubal pregnancy, as well as uterine pregnancy, whereas IUDs decrease the likelihood but do not prevent tubal implantations. The incidence of tubal pregnancy is 1 per 1000 woman years use. The ratio of tubal to intrauterine pregnancies in patients with IUDs is reported as 1 to 20.

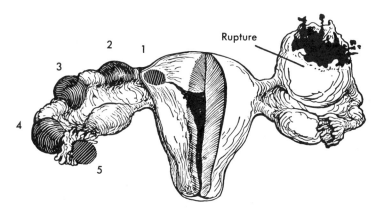

Fig. 13-2. Various sites of tubal pregnancy. *1,* Intramural; *2,* isthmic; *3,* ampullar; *4,* infundibular; *5,* ostial.

From Crossen, R.J.: Diseases of women, St. Louis, The C.V. Mosby Co.

Etiology. Normally the spermatozoon impregnates the oocyte in the fallopian tube, and by the time the trophoblastic stage has been reached it has progressed into the uterine cavity where implantation occurs. If the fertilized oocyte cannot complete its tubal course before then, ectopic pregnancy may result. Interference with its downward progress is usually caused by some obstruction, which may be situated anywhere between the ovary and the uterine cavity. *Tubal causes* include the following:

1. *Salpingitis* results in the destruction of tubal cilia, adhesions producing pockets, and strictures causing traps.
2. *Perisalpingitis* may cause constriction of the tubal lumen by adhesions or kinks and may impair tubal peristalsis.
3. *Congenital malformations* include diverticula, tortuosity, accessory ostia forming cul-de-sacs, and malformed lumina.
4. *Endometrium-like foci in the tubal mucosa* may favor tubal implantation by chemotaxis of the oocyte.
5. *Tumors* can cause tubal obstruction.
6. *Tubal surgery* results in fibrosis and some impairment of tubal function.

Ovular causes of tubal pregnancy result in an oversized oocyte that cannot transverse the salpinx because of (1) rapid cell division, (2) growth during migration from the opposite ovary, or (3) adhering membrana granulosa.

Pathology. The principal pathologic process is bleeding. The trophoblasts soon grow through the endosalpinx and invade the tubal wall and its blood vessels. Some of the stromal cells of the endosalpinx exhibit decidual changes, but Nitabuch's membrane as ordinarily formed in the endometrium is lacking. Extravasation of blood occurs first subepithelially and separates some trophoblasts from an active blood supply.

As indicated in Fig. 13-3, with continued bleeding, blood distends the capsularis and separates it from the chorion. When the capsularis consisting of tubal epithelium, fibrin, and some decidual cells ruptures, blood escapes into and further distends the lumen of the tube. If there has not been any escape of blood from the salpinx into the peritoneal cavity or broad ligament, the term "unruptured tubal pregnancy" is commonly used. As the tube is rapidly distended and attempts to expel its contents, cramping pain occurs. Cramping pain can likewise occur from uterine contractions at this stage. After intraluminal rupture, blood leaks from the fimbriated end of the tube into the peritoneal cavity. Bleeding from the site of implantation does not enter the endometrial cavity except in intramural pregnancies. If complete separation of the chorionic villi occurs, the products of pregnancy and associated blood clots may escape into the abdomen as a tubal abortion; however, seldom is a tubal abortion complete (Fig. 13-4).

The erosive action of trophoblasts may cause penetration through the tubal sero-

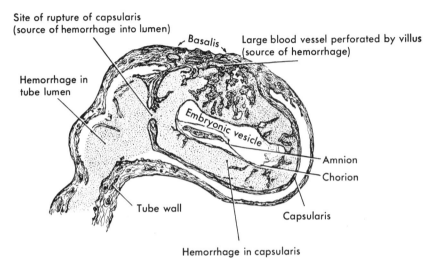

Site of rupture of capsularis
(source of hemorrhage into lumen)

Basalis

Large blood vessel perforated by villus
(source of hemorrhage)

Hemorrhage in
tube lumen

Embryonic vesicle

Amnion

Chorion

Tube wall

Capsularis

Hemorrhage in capsularis

Fig. 13-3. Schematic drawing of bleeding into lumen in tubal pregnancy.

After J.C. Litzenberg.

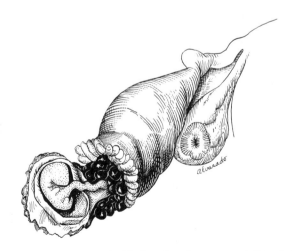

Fig. 13-4. Tubal abortion illustrated with the tube edematous and distended with blood.

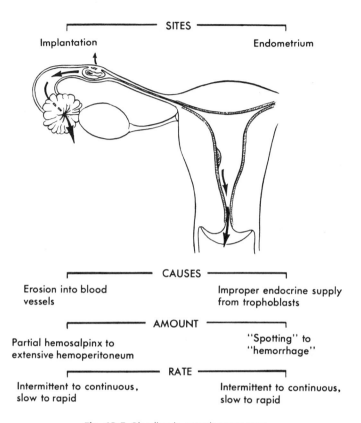

Fig. 13-5. Bleeding in ectopic pregnancy.

sa with bleeding directly into the abdominal cavity. With sufficient erosion of the tubal wall, arterial pressure may cause actual rupture to occur.

The rate and time of bleeding at the site of implantation are variable (Fig. 13-5). When pregnancy is in the intramural portion of the salpinx, the surrounding myometrium may allow gestation to continue for 3 months or more until erosion through uterine peritoneum occurs with sudden extensive hemorrhage. The isthmic portion of the oviduct is not easily distended, and erosion through the tube usually occurs in 6 weeks or less, with marked hemorrhage intraperitoneally. The ampullary portion of the tube is distensible, and pregnancy may continue longer than in the isthmic portion; however, on occasion an artery of sufficient size may rupture to cause rapid bleeding. Since the extent and rate of bleeding at the implantation site are variable, the pain caused by tubal distention or peritoneal irritation of extravasated blood is variable. As more blood escapes into the abdomen, pain may occur in the upper abdomen, or irritation of the diaphragm may cause referred pain in the shoulder.

The hormonal production of the trophoblast is interfered with when separation from an active blood supply occurs. If sufficient estrogens and progesterone are not produced, the endometrium will be shed. Usually the decrease in hormonal production is gradual or intermittent, so that bleeding from the endometrium is intermittent and small in amount. Infrequently, with an abrupt endocrine decrease, the uterine decidua may be expelled as a partial or complete cast of the uterus. After uterine bleeding has continued for several days, the portion of the endometrium exhibiting decidual change has usually been shed, and the study of the remaining uterine lining will reveal no evidence of pregnancy.

Breast changes and nausea depend upon sufficient endocrine production and accordingly may be absent or of short duration in eccyesis. The assay of chorionic gonadotropin (pregnancy tests) similarly may be negative in this variable condition. β-Subunit radioimmune assay or radioreceptor assay on serum or a β-subunit tube test on urine should be used as a pregnancy test to reveal lower HCG levels.

Pelvic masses develop in varying fashions. The salpinx may be markedly distended in sausagelike fashion by intraluminal bleeding. The fetus, amniotic sac, and placenta may continue to grow to form a mass that is intratubal or extratubal in location. The collection of blood clots and liquid blood may become pseudoencysted by adhering bowel, omentum, and adjacent genital organs. Edema with induration of these structures soon occurs as reabsorption of the blood begins. If of long standing, collections of blood invite infection.

Should complete separation of the trophoblast from an active maternal blood supply occur, necrosis begins and spontaneous cure can result by absorption of the products of gestation, which by then are most likely to have been aborted into the abdomen.

In rare cases, as erosion through the tube occurs, there is not sufficient bleeding to separate enough of the chorionic villi from their sources of sustenance and the embryonic mass gradually escapes into the abdominal cavity as the trophoblasts find new areas of attachment on adjacent structures. An abdominal pregnancy then exists and may progress to term.

Ovarian pregnancy results when implantation in a ruptured follicle or on the ovarian surface takes place. This is a very rare occurrence. As mentioned in Chapter 3, rudimentary uterine horns may be inadequate sites for placentation and constitute another type of eccyesis.

Death from ectopic pregnancy is usually a result of extensive intra-abdominal hemorrhage.

Symptoms and diagnosis. The symptoms depend on many factors, including the site, type, status, and duration of the eccyesis and the patient's pain threshold and general condition. Basically the physician must recognize hemoperitoneum and search for an abnormal mass.

1. In the rarely diagnosed *intact early* (so-called unruptured) *tubal pregnancy* the patient may consult a physician because of amenorrhea. She may or may not have nausea, breast consciousness, and urinary frequency without burning. If present, cervical softening and vaginal discoloration are compatible with pregnancy. Slight uterine enlargement may be detectable if the examiner has seen the patient previously. Pain upon movement of the cervix should cause one to consider the possibility of eccyesis. One should palpate the adnexa gingerly, attempting to find a very small tender mass but being careful not to rupture a corpus luteum of pregnancy or a gravid salpinx. If a pregnancy test is requested, the report should be evaluated with due consideration of the fact that a negative report does not rule out eccyesis or very early uterine pregnancy and that a positive one simply indicates that there are living chorionic villi in contact with the maternal circulation. In a doubtful case free of abnormal symptoms, the patient should be examined at intervals of 1 to 2 weeks until a definite diagnosis has been made. If spotting occurs, one may suspect ovular unrest, and, if lower abdominal pain develops, one may perform a culdocentesis, being mindful that a negative result does not rule out intact tubal pregnancy. The services of an expert culdoscopist or laparoscopist prove valuable in some cases. If examinations disclose a tender tubal mass and the uterus fails to enlarge progressively as a pregnant uterus should, culdotomy or laparotomy is indicated. Obviously the blood group and Rh-Hr status of every patient should be known as a precautionary measure.

2. In cases of *tubal abortion* or *rupture without acute symptoms* the history is ordinarily not spectacular. Included may be the following: pregnancy symptoms, slight to moderate pelvic pain, spotting to moderate bleeding through the vagina, and constitutional manifestations as weakness, malaise, headache, or dizziness. The differential diagnosis will include, such possibilities as abortion (threatening, threatened, incomplete, or missed), ruptured corpus hemorrhagicum or luteum, salpingo-oophoritis, appendicitis, and ovarian cyst. Lower abdominal tenderness is usually elicitable. An abnormal mass may or may not be felt. Manipulation of the uterus proves painful, and positive culdocentesis clinches the diagnosis. In patients suspected of having incomplete abortion, cervical dilation and uterine curettement reveal what is in the uterus and prove curative if the suspected diagnosis is correct. Romney and associates have proved that endometrial studies in eccyesis are unreliable because the endometrium may vary from an early proliferative to a late secretory or decidual stage, depending on the individual case. The presence of chorionic villi in the scrapings indicates that the patient had an intrauterine gestation, but it does not rule out an extrauterine one. The terms "combined" or "heterotopic" are applied to such pregnancies occurring simultaneously.

3. The *acute ruptured type* of eccyesis presents a classic picture following a period of amenorrhea and bleeding that varies from spotting to profuse. Severe

pelvic pain is followed by weakness, syncope, and shock. The physical findings include falling blood pressure, rising pulse rate, subnormal temperature unless the patient has a febrile condition, pallor, abdominal tenderness, very rarely Cullen's sign (bluish discoloration of the umbilicus seen in some patients having a large quantity of blood in the peritoneal cavity), pain upon motion of the cervix uteri, bloody uterine discharge, and slight enlargement of the uterus unless it harbors a tumor or pregnancy; an adnexal or cul-de-sac mass may be palpable, depending upon the patient. Culdocentesis proves positive if there should be any doubt as to the presence of hemoperitoneum; in this procedure aspirated blood should be observed for at least 6 minutes. If it is from hemoperitoneum it will not clot, but it is from a blood vessel it will clot within that interval except in some blood dyscrasias. The aspiration of fragments of old blood is interpreted as positive (Fig. 13-6).

4. The fourth type, labeled *pelvic hematocele* or *old ruptured ectopic pregnancy*, is diagnosable, provided one obtains a history compatible with recent tubal rupture or abortion. This may have occurred several weeks before admittance. Because of recurrent lower abdominal pain, recurrent uterine bleeding, pain upon cervical motion, limited uterine mobility, tender pelvic mass, and perhaps such factors as accelerated erythrocyte sedimentation rate and fever, the following deserve consideration: salpingo-oophoritis PID, tubo-ovarian abscess, uterine myomas, endometriosis, incomplete abortion in a "fixed" uterus, ovarian cyst, and malignancy. Some patients are found to have one or more of these disturbances plus a pelvic hematocele. If an abscess is suspected, culdotomy is indicated and will allow the correct diagnosis to be made.

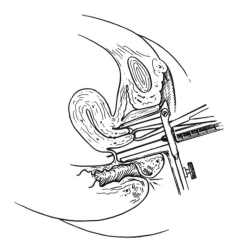

Fig. 13-6. Culdocentesis. The instruments used are a speculum, a volsella, an 18-gauge spinal needle, and a syringe.

Therapy. Ectopic pregnancy should be treated surgically without delay. The bleeding vessels should be ligated promptly. The matter of anesthesia should be determined by the condition of the patient. Spinal anesthesia is often used in good-risk patients with little or no blood in the peritoneal cavity. Blood should be available for any patient suspected of having eccyesis, but it should be administered for replacement of acute blood loss and not for the treatment of chronic anemia. In cases of shock the patient's abdomen can be opened while she is receiving oxygen by mask, and enough blood can be given intra-arterially (common or internal iliac) to raise the systolic blood pressure to 90 mm Hg, which results in palpable radial pulse. Further administration should be continued intravenously as indicated. In patients with acute rupture with massive bleeding the operation should be limited to the involved adnexum. The ipsilateral ovary should be saved if possible. The opposite tube and ovary should be examined to be sure that there is no pregnancy, neoplasm, or reparable condition of the tube. Provided the patient's condition is good, the liberation of adhesions at the ostium and pertubation or other indicated procedures may restore tubal patency, thus permitting future pregnancy. If the patient has lost the contralateral salpinx or it is beyond repair, the products of conception may be removed from the gravid tube to allow its salvage in some instances. The incidence of repetition of eccyesis is thought to be between 3% and 5% of all such patients operated upon. It is higher among patients in whom tuboplasty has been done.

Unusual types of eccyesis. The physician who is conscious of eccyesis must also keep in mind the possibility of the occurrence of the following uncommon varieties.

Intramural (interstitial) pregnancy. Bleeding caused by rupture is classically profuse. In some cases salpingectomy and resection of the involved portion of the uterus can be done. In others the uterus must be sacrificed too.

Ovarian pregnancy. Although rarely seen, the symptoms of ovarian pregnancy are like those of tubal pregnancy. One must consider the possibility of a ruptured corpus luteum cyst, torsion, and endometriosis.

Abdominal pregnancy. A few well-documented cases have proved the possibility of the very rare primary type. In the secondary variety there is the history of a tubal abortion or rupture. Transverse or other abnormal positions of the fetus should arouse suspicion. Fetal movements are painful as a rule. The fetal heart tones may be louder than in a normal pregnancy. Fetal parts may be palpable directly under the abdominal wall or next to the posterior vaginal fornix. If the corpus uteri is displaced upward and forward by the pregnancy mass, the cervix is situated near the symphysis and its location may require a search. If the corpus can be outlined, the diagnosis is clinched. The oxytocic test may reveal the absence of the uterus around the fetus. The placenta may be visualized by arteriography. Ultrasonography may reveal absence of the uterine wall and abnormal contours of the amniotic sac. In some patients a Simpson sound may be used to ascertain the depth of the uterine cavity, but this should not be employed if there is a possibility of a uterine gestation. Generally speaking, patients with abdominal cyesis should be operated on promptly because there is slight possibility of obtaining a normal baby by letting it get closer to maturity. Placental management deserves individualization following the dictum that it should be removed only if its blood supply can be controlled. The quantity of blood available for the patient should be adequate. Lithopedions very rarely occur in the United States.

DISEASES OF THE TROPHOBLAST
Hydatidiform mole

A small portion of all of the chorionic villi formed during a pregnancy may undergo hydropic degeneration to become cystic structures. Slight degrees of cystic change occur frequently in spontaneous early abortion. It is very unusual that an appreciable degree of cystic change exists in the placenta of a term pregnancy. When most of the chorionic villi become small cystic structures, the entire mass has the appearance of a grapelike accumulation (Fig. 13-7). When this is marked, the embryo or fetus is seldom found; certainly, if the cystic change is of sufficient degree, there is not sufficient nutrition for embryonic development. Hydatidiform moles are estimated to occur in from 1 in 500 to 1 in 2500 pregnancies. On microscopic examination the villi are very large, with the absence of capillaries, and the trophoblast may be more proliferative than that found in a normal pregnancy. According to Hertig, 73.5% of hydatidiform moles run a benign course; i.e., they do not abnormally invade the uterine wall or spread to other portions of the body. Recent studies indicate that about 3% of hydatidiform moles are followed by choriocarcinoma.

Signs, symptoms, and diagnosis. A pregnancy that is destined to become a molar one is similar at its onset to a normal pregnancy. The first disturbance noted is spotting and, at times, there is brisk bleeding. When enlargement of the uterus is more than that expected in normal pregnancy, a mole should be suspected. When the uterus is of an 8- to 10-weeks size, ultrasonographic visualization will allow the diagnosis of the mole and should be employed. This method has replaced amniography as the best for diagnosis. When the uterus is the size of an 18- to 24-week pregnancy, examination by x-ray and auscultation or ultrasound search for fetal circulation may reveal no evidence of a fetus. With larger moles albuminuria, hypertension, and edema may develop. If the molar pregnancy has not been diagnosed previously, the diagnosis may be made when there is the passage of hydatids. When pregnancy tests are employed with molar pregnancy, the results should be positive. One would expect the molar pregnancy to produce higher levels of chorionic gonadotropin than a normal pregnancy; however, since in the case of normal

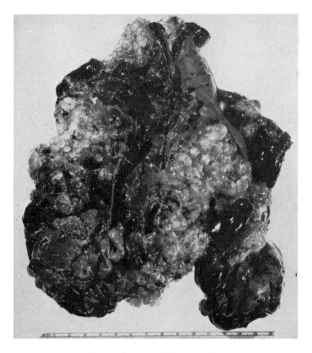

Fig. 13-7. Hydatidiform mole.

From Willson, J.R., Beecham, C.T., Forman, I., and Carrington, E.R.: Obstetrics and gynecology, St. Louis, The C.V. Mosby Co.

pregnancy high levels are attained 60 to 80 days after the last normal menstrual period, gonadotropic determinations play little part in the original diagnosis of hydatidiform mole. If any importance is to be given to the assays, they must be done repeatedly over a period of several weeks. Since anemia is common and coagulopathy may occur, platelet counts and clotting function studies should be performed in addition to a complete blood count (CBC). Chest x-ray films are in order because of the possibility of pulmonary metastasis and congestion. Since both normal and neoplastic trophoblasts produce thyrotropic hormone, thyroid studies are in order.

Management. Once the diagnosis of hydatidiform mole has been made, therapy calls for the evacuation of the molar tissue from the uterus. The uterine wall may be partially invaded and somewhat thin; consequently care must be taken. Suction evacuation is the preferred method, particularly for large moles when the cervix is not appreciably dilated. When the cervix is sufficiently dilated, the fingers and sponge forceps may be used and followed with a sharp curettement.

In approximately 10% of moles, palpation of the adnexa will reveal ovaries larger than average. This is caused by lutein cysts that form following gonadotropic stimulation. In the absence of gross cysts, histologic study would reveal marked luteinization. These ovarian changes will regress once the trophoblastic tissue has been adequately removed; consequently no surgical therapy for the ovarian masses is indicated.

The patient must be observed for evidences of intra-abdominal bleeding, which may be caused by an invasive mole that has penetrated through the uterine serosa or by bleeding into or from the lutein cysts of the ovaries. Laparotomy is then indicated for the arrest of hemorrhage. If further childbearing is not desired, total abdominal hysterectomy before removal of the mole may be in order. Hysterectomy may avoid the blood loss in the removal of the mole, may allow for a more accurate diagnosis by examination of the myometrium for the possibility of choriocarcinoma, and may possibly be a factor in reduction of choriocarcinoma. If bleeding continues too long or increases after removal of a mole, secondary curettage may be required for the removal of the remaining fragments. Uncontrolled hemorrhage may require hysterectomy.

It is imperative that follow-up examinations be made for at least a year to determine the possibility of choriocarcinoma following a mole. Pregnancy should be avoided during this period, since there may be confusion between a new gestation and residual functioning trophoblasts. Sensitive gonadotropic assays (not pregnancy tests) should be performed every 2 weeks until the result indicates only the levels expected from pituitary secretion. If the HCG are not down after 8 weeks, invasive mole or choriocarcinoma is likely. When there is a rise in chorionic gonadotropin and a new pregnancy can be excluded, the likelihood of choriocarcinoma is great. Oral contraceptives will have no effect in decreasing chorionic gonadotropins.

Choriocarcinoma

Choriocarcinoma, a highly malignant cancer of trophoblastic cells, is fortunately very rare. Its occurrence is approximately 1 in 25,000 pregnancies. Of the choriocarcinomas that have been found, about 50% have followed hydatidiform moles, 25% have followed abortions, and 25% have followed term pregnancies. The diagnosis of this condition depends on finding the tissue, which must be examined histologically. Clinically the disorder may first manifest itself by a metastatic lesion in the lungs, bone, brain, liver, vagina, or gastrointestinal tract. These lesions may result in pain and/or bleeding. An enlarged uterus that does not involute and cease bleeding after a normal pregnancy or abortion should be suspected of this disorder. As indicated in the discussion of follow-up examinations of patients with hydatidiform moles, curettage of the uterus is in order. With the development of choriocarcinoma, which may occur weeks or years after a pregnancy, none of the cancerous tissue may be found on curettage. In fact, when trophoblastic cells are obtained by curettage, the pathologist may have difficulty in determining the exact nature of the condition.

Syncytioma is a strictly benign, self-limiting condition that may be associated with vaginal bleeding and subinvolution of the uterus. It is characterized by persistent trophoblastic tissue found at the placental site on curettage. The highly trained gynecologic pathologist is not likely to make a mistake in diagnosing this condition as a malignancy. The differentiation of chorioadenoma destruens from choriocarcinoma may be more difficult. This condition is a locally invasive hydatidiform mole associated at times with metastatic lesions, particularly in the lung. In this condition the uterus is more likely to be markedly enlarged than it is with choriocarcinoma. On examination some hydropic villi will be found buried within the deep layers of the myometrium. After removal of the pelvic lesions by hysterectomy, the lung lesions sometimes disappear.

Most choriocarcinomas cause the blood serum to have high titers of gonadotropins. Certainly, when there is a question as to the presence of choriocarcinoma, serial quantitative determinations of gonadotropins should be done using a sensitive radioimmune assay.

The treatment of these unusual, often fatal neoplasms should be accomplished in centers so that benefit of experience and excellent bioassays may be utilized. Methotrexate and actinomycin D are highly toxic preparations that have been effective in the majority of patients. Experience indicates that hysterectomy usually is not required as a part of treatment; however, often without hysterectomy the diagnosis must be probable choriocarcinoma or invasive mole. In areas of the Orient where there is a high incidence of trophoblastic disease, prophylactic methotrexate administration is used.

Prognosis

Death rarely occurs from benign hydatidiform mole and, when it happens, it is usually because of hemorrhage from the uterus. Death is more likely from an invasive mole in which the bleeding may be not only by way of the vagina but also into the pertoneal cavity after penetration through the uterine wall. Choriocarcinoma usually kills by hemorrhage and necrosis in vital organs of the body.

When metastases from gestational trophoblastic neoplasms have been identified, poor prognosis is indicated by an initial urinary HCG titer greater than 1000 IU every 24 hours or a serum HCG titer greater than 40,000 IU per milliliter. Other indications of poor prognosis are symptoms lasting over 4 months, liver or brain metastases identified on scan, attempts at previous chemotherapy, and occurrence after a term pregnancy.

SELECTED REFERENCES
Abortion

Barnes, A.C.: Conization and scarification as a treatment for cervical incompetency, Am. J. Obstet. Gynecol. **82:**920, 1961.

Barter, R.H., Dusbabek, J.A., Riva, H.L., and Parks, J.: Closure of the incompetent cervix during pregnancy, Am. J. Obstet. Gynecol. **75:**511, 1958.

Brown, W.E., and Hanisch, E.C.: A review of the aggressive management of abortion, Am. J. Obstet. Gynecol. **76:**716, 1958.

Carr, B.H.: Genetic factors in pregnancy wastage, Med. Clin. N. Am. **53:**1039, 1969.

Colvin, E.D., Bartholomew, R.A., Grimes, W.H., and Fish, J.S.: Salvage possibilities in threatened abortions, Am. J. Obstet. Gynecol. **59:**1208, 1950.

Eriksen, P.S., and Philipsen, T.: Prognosis in threatening abortion evaluated by hormone assays and ultrasound scanning, Obstet. Gynecol. **55:**435, 1980.

Grimes, D.A., and Cates, W.: Complications of legally-induced abortion: a review, Obstet. Gynecol. Surv. **34:**177, 1979.

Gruenberger, W., Leodolter, S., and Spona, J.: The LH/HCG test, a valuable aid in the diagnosis of tubal pregnancy, Gynecol. Obstet. Envest. **9:**150, 1978.

Hertig, A.T., and Livingstone, R.C.: Spontaneous, threatened, and habitual abortion: their pathogenesis and treatment, N. Engl. J. Med. **230:**797, 1944.

Hodgkinson, C.P., Igna, E.J., and Bukeovich, A.P.: High potency progesterone drugs and threatened abortion, Am. J. Obstet. Gynecol. **76:**279, 1958.

Hughes, E.C., Lloyd, C.W., Van Ness, A.W., and Ellis, W.T.: The role of the endometrium in implantation and fetal growth. Pregnancy wastage, Springfield, Ill., 1953, Charles C Thomas, Publisher.

Irani, K.R., Henriques, E.S., Friedlander, R.L., Berlin, L.E., and Swartz, D.P.: Menstrual induction: its place in clinical practice, Am. J. Obstet. Gynecol. **46:**596, 1975.

Javert, C.T.: Spontaneous and habitual abortion, New York, 1957, McGraw-Hill Book Co., Inc.

Jones, H.W., Jr., Delfs, E., and Jones, G.E.: Reproductive difficulties in double uterus: the pace of plastic reconstruction, Am. J. Obstet. Gynecol. **72:**865, 1956.

Lash, A.F., and Lash, S.R.: Habitual abortion: the incompetent internal os of the cervix, Am. J. Obstet. Gynecol. **59:**68, 1950.

Lubin, S., and Waltman, R.: Missed abortion: evaluation of conservative management, Am. J. Surg. **77:**202, 1949.

Mall, F.P., and Meyer, A.W.: Studies on abortions: a survey of pathologic ova in the Carnegie Embryological Collection, Contrib. Embryol., No. 56, 1921, Carnegie Institute, Washington, D.C.

Manabe, Y.: Artificial abortion at midpregnancy by mechanical stimulation of the uterus, Am. J. Obstet. Gynecol. **105:**132, 1969.

Mann, E.C., McLarn, M.D., and Hyat, D.B.: The physiology and clinical significance of the uterine isthmus, Am. J. Obstet. Gynecol. **81:**209, 1961.

Marrs, R.P., Kletzky, O.A., Howard, W.F., and Mishell, D.R.: Disappearance of human chorionic gonadotropin and the resumption of ovulation following abortion, Am. J. Obstet. Gynecol. **135:**731, 1979.

Moghissi, K.S., and Murray, C.P.: The function of prostaglandins in reproduction, Obstet. Gynecol. Surv. **25:**281, 1970.

Nesbitt, R.E.L., Jr.: Pathology of abortion (in uterus, placenta, appendages and ovofetus). In Novak, E.R., and Woodruff, J.D., editors: Novak's gynecologic and obstetric pathology, ed. 5, Philadelphia, 1962, W.B. Saunders Co., p. 545.

Pritchard, J.A., and MacDonald, P.C.: Williams obstetrics, New York City, 1980, Appleton-Century-Crofts.

Spraitz, A.F., Jr., Welch, J.S., and Wilson, R.B.: Missed abortions, Am. J. Obstet. Gynecol. **87:**877, 1963.

Ectopic gestation

Beacham, W.D., Hernquist, W.C., Beacham, D.W., and Webster, H.D.: Abdominal pregnancy at Charity Hospital in New Orleans, Am. J. Obstet. Gynecol. **84:**1257, 1962.

Beacham, W.D., Webster, H.D., and Beacham, D.W.: Ectopic pregnancy at New Orleans Charity Hospital, Am. J. Obstet. Gynecol. **72:**830, 1956.

Breen, J.L.: A 21 year survey of 654 ectopic pregnancies, Am. J. Obstet. Gynecol. **106:**1004, 1970.

Hallatt, J.G.: Ectopic pregnancy associated with the intrauterine device: a study of seventy cases, Am. J. Obstet. Gynecol. **175:**754, 1976.

Litzenberg, J.C.: Microscopical studies of tubal pregnancy, Am. J. Obstet. Gynecol. **1:**223, 1920.

Romney, S.L., Hertig, A.T., and Reid, D.E.: The endometria associated with ectopic pregnancy, Surg. Gynecol. Obstet. **91:**605, 1951.

Schumann, E.A.: Extra-uterine pregnancy, New York, 1921, D. Appleton & Co.

Stromme, W.B., McKelvey, J.L., and Adkins, C.D.: Conservative surgery for ectopic pregnancy, Obstet. Gynecol. **19:**294, 1962.

Winer, A.E., Bergman, W.D., and Fields, C., Combined intra- and extrauterine pregnancy, Am. J. Obstet. Gynecol. **74:**170, 1957.

Diseases of the trophoblast

Acosta-Sison, H.: Diagnosis of hydatidiform mole, Obstet. Gynecol. **12:**205, 1958.

Coppleson, M.: Hydatidiform mole and its complications, J. Obstet. Gynaec. Br. Emp. **65:**238, 1958.

Delfs, E.: Quantitative chorionic gonadotrophin; prognostic value in hydatidiform mole and chorionepithelioma, Obstet. Gynecol. **9:**1, 1957.

Hammond, C.B., et al.: Management of gestational trophoblastic neoplasia, ACOG Tech. Bull. 59, December 1980.

Hertig, A.T., and Mansell, H.: Tumors of the female sex organs. I. Hydatidiform mole and choriocarcinoma, Washington, D.C., 1956, Armed Forces Institute of Pathology.

Hertz, R., Lewis, J., Jr., and Lipsett, M.B.: Five years' experience with the chemotherapy of metastatic choriocarcinoma and related trophoblastic tumors in women, Am. J. Obstet. Gynecol. **82:**631, 1961.

Li, M.C., Hertz, R., and Spencer, D.B.: Effect of Methotrexate therapy upon choriocarcinoma and chorioadrenoma, Proc. Soc. Exp. Biol. Med. **93:**361, 1956.

Chapter 14

DISTURBANCES OF FUNCTION

The normal endocrine control of the uterus (of the endometrium in particular) has been presented in Chapter 1. Some known endocrine changes and other factors causing disturbances of function, not presented in other portions of this book, are discussed in this chapter.

AMENORRHEA

Amenorrhea can be classified as (1) *primary*, in which no menses have occurred, and (2) *secondary*, in which there is absence of menses after the menarche.

Congenital abnormalities as cause. Discussions of the absence of the uterus or ovaries, gynatresia, and intersexuality are presented in Chapter 3. Extra X chromosomes may be associated with mental deficiency and late menarche. Kallman's syndrome of olfactory lobe absence and hypogonadism and the Laurence-Moon-Biedl syndrome of mental deficiency, polydactylism, and adiposogenital dystrophy are congenital.

Hypothalamic and pituitary causes. *Late hypothalamic maturation* is diagnosed by exclusion of other causes of primary amenorrhea and by the prediction of a delayed menarche, which is preceded by breast and sexual hair development. These "late bloomers" comprise the largest group with primary amenorrhea under 18 years of age.

Anorexia nervosa is an emotional disorder with inadequate nutrition causing emaciation. LH levels are low. Menstruation returns with proper nutrition and with improvement of mental functions. Amenorrhea that is, at times, associated with severe weight reduction diets appears to be similar to the amenorrhea associated with anorexia nervosa although it occurs less severely. When the patient regains a normal amount of subcutaneous fat, the extraovarian production of estrogen is apt to increase; a better metabolic balance is thus obtained. Conversely, with onset of marked obesity extraovarian estrogens are at times produced in excess and amenorrhea may result; however, it is more likely that dysfunctional irregular bleeding will occur.

Pituitary neoplasms. About 50% of hypophyseal growths are chromophobic and have varying degrees of secretory activity. When they are of limited activity and when the active portions of the gland are compressed, childhood dwarfism results; in adults amenorrhea, genital atrophy, and obesity are likely. Basophilic tumors cause Cushing's disease. (See adrenal causes.) Acidophilic tumors may produce gigantism, if the tumors are active before epiphyseal closure, or acromegaly in adults. Amenorrhea, weight gain, hyperhidrosis, asthenia, hypertrichosis, cutaneous pigmentation, and glycosuria are typical symptoms.

Craniopharyngiomas are nonsecretory neoplasms and decrease pituitary function. Metastatic carcinoma may also damage the pituitary.

Pituitary adenomas and carcinomas are rare. When amenorrhea persists for prolonged periods repeated radiographic views of the sella turcica and visual field determinations should be done. Unexplained galactorrhea likewise indicates investigation. High prolactin levels unrelated to medication may be produced by microadenomas, which can only be diagnosed by polytomography, since routine views of the sella turcica are normal. Since considerable radiation is used in polytomography, repetition should be limited to avoid radiation injury.

Pituitary injury. Infarction may occur with obstetric shock (Sheehan's syndrome), resulting in the loss of trophic hormones that affect the ovaries, thyroid gland, adrenal glands, and growth. Loss of functioning tissue may be caused by sarcoidosis, tuberculosis, or syphilis. Survival of head injury with pituitary trauma is rare. With improved care infarction and infection have become rare. Irradiation and surgical destruction or removal are expected to cause a decrease or cessation of pituitary function.

Inappropriate lactation. As indicated previously, neoplasms or disease may damage the hypothalamus and decrease the prolactin-inhibiting factor, or prolactin may be produced in larger amounts by acidophilic pituitary tumors. The most common reasons for excess prolactin are drugs, which decrease the level of catecholamines in brain tissue (phenothiazines, the tricyclic antidepressants, reserpine, and methyldopa), and frequent nipple stimulation during sexual activities. Increased lactogenic hormone is associated with decreased levels of LH and FSH. If the cause for hyperprolactinemia is eliminated or if bromocriptin is administered, the lactogenic hormone decreases and menses return.

Galactorrhea and amenorrhea following pregnancy are symptoms of the Chiari-Frommel syndrome. Without pregnancy the syndrome is termed Ahumada–del Castillo syndrome.

Thyroid causes. *Hypothyroidism* or *hyperthyroidism* may cause amenorrhea or excessive uterine bleeding. After the thyroid disorder is corrected, regular endometrial behavior usually returns. (See p. 38.)

Adrenal causes. Hyperadrenalism causes amenorrhea by excessive androgenic effects. In congenital adrenal hyperplasia there is one or more enzymatic defects, so that hydrocortisone is not formed. The resulting high levels of ACTH cause increased production of testosterone, dehydroepiandrosterone, and androstanedione. Adequate daily dosage of prednisone, methylprednisolone, or dexamethasone will decrease ACTH stimulation and lower the abnormal levels of androgens that are reflected by increased levels of 17-KS in the urine. For some patients with Cushing's syndrome in which the major manifestations are those of excessive cortisol, there may also be increases in androgens. When there is proper treatment either by decreasing abnormal ACTH secretion from the pituitary or by bilateral adrenalectomy with proper replacement of glucocorticoids, the moderate excess of androgens is removed and normal pituitary function should allow for the return of menstruation and ovulation. In some patients there appears to be an excess production of androgenic substances by the adrenal glands and no abnormal increase in cortisol levels. It has been found that the androgenic production by the adrenal glands in these patients can be decreased through the administration of small amounts of dexamethasone; for some there is a return of menstruation and ovulation.

Hypoadrenalism (Addison's disease), when present for some time, has amenorrhea as a typical symptom.

Ovarian causes. *Massive destruction of ovarian tissue* by infection, tumors, radiation, or surgical attack may so decrease estrogen production as to cause amenorrhea.

Ovarian masculinizing tumors are considered in Chapter 12.

Polycystic ovary syndrome. In 1935, Stein and Leventhal described the classic syndrome of oligomenorrhea, hirsutism, obesity, and palpably enlarged ovaries. Wedge resection resulted in a 95% return of ovulatory cycles and an 85% conception rate. The syndrome was thought to be a precise entity. However, improved knowledge of hypothalamic, pituitary, adrenal, ovarian, and nonglandular endocrine changes, together with knowledge of induction of ovulation by the administration of clomiphene and extrinsic gonadotropins, has changed the understanding and management of anovulatory polycystic ovaries.

When the normal cyclic variations in hypothalamic-pituitary-ovarian function do not occur over several months, amenorrhea and, at times, dysfunctional endometrial bleeding occur. The ovarian capsule thickens, and subcapsular cysts develop with hyperplasia of the theca interna and often luteinization. Abnormal steroidogenesis occurs as indicated by increased production of androstenedione, dehydroepiandrosterone, and testosterone. Usually LH levels are increased, but the surge of LH required for ovulation does not occur.

Hirsutism is present in approximately 50% of the patients with polycystic ovary syndrome. Virilism is not expected. Many patients are obese. Enlargement of both

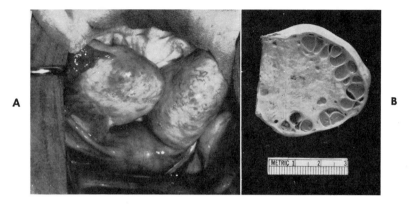

Fig. 14-1. A, Stein-Leventhal ovary. Note the ovaries are enlarged, their surface is white, and small cysts are in the cortex near the surface. **B,** Wedge resection specimen depicting the typical thick cortical rind, the immediately subjacent ring of closely crowded small follicular cysts, the absence of corpora lutea, and the wide central cyst-free expanse of fibrous ovarian stroma.

From Jackson, R.L., and Dockerty, M.D.: Am. J. Obstet. Gynecol. **73:**161, 1957.

ovaries usually occurs and may be determined by palpation. Estrogen levels are adequate as evidence by vaginal cells and endometrium; however, estrogen levels found in urine do not have the two peaks typical of ovulatory cycles.

Mild adrenal hyperfunction can cause obesity, mild hirsutism, dysfunctional uterine bleeding, and amenorrhea. Since dehydroepiandrosterone, androstenedione, and testosterone can be of adrenal origin, the question of adrenal involvement in the polycystic ovary syndrome is expected. The conversion of androstenedione and dehydroepiandrosterone to testosterone or estrone outside the ovaries and adrenal glands is another variable that complicates the understanding of anovulation and hirsutism.

Although gross and microscopic changes are found in the polycystic ovary syndrome, these changes are not permanent. After ovulation has been induced by the administration of clomiphene or menopausal gonadotropins with chorionic gonadotropins, the appearance of the ovary changes to that during ovulatory cyclic menstruation. This reversion to normalcy leads one to judge that the primary disturbance may be hypothalamic-pituitary rather than ovarian.

It is difficult to delineate criteria for the clinical diagnosis of the polycystic ovary syndrome. Patients may exhibit short periods of anovulation and amenorrhea associated with periods of anxiety or depression. In general, it is only for those patients who have prolonged periods of amenorrhea and anovulation that one uses the term "polycystic ovary syndrome."

Spontaneous premature ovarian failure is diagnosed with (1) the absence of ovarian disease, (2) the endometrium responsive to stimulation, and (3) normal or high FSH levels. It may be noted in women in their early thirties. Inability of the ovary to respond is the primary disturbance. Premature spontaneous menopause is similar to normal menopause symptomatically.

Physiologic causes. The physiologic causes of amenorrhea include (1) pregnancy, (2) menopause, (3) adolescent skipping (not indicative of disease), (4) premenopausal skipping (not indicative of disease), (5) lactation, (6) temporary emotional disturbances (fear, anxiety, pseudocyesis), (7) changes in climate and altitude, and (8) marked increase in exercise.

Therapeutic causes. Amenorrhea may be the result of previous therapeutic measures. Surgical excision is self-explanatory. The application of small doses of roentgen radiation to ovaries may temporarily result in amenorrhea, whereas larger doses as used in cancer therapy result in the permanent amenorrhea of ovarian atrophy. Radium applications to the endometrium in sufficient amounts cause complete atrophy. When applications are made to eradicate malignancy, ovarian atrophy results. Chemotherapeutic agents used for cytotoxic effects on cancer may impair ovarian function. Phenothiazines, tricyclic amines, reserpine, and methyldopa may increase prolactin levels and cause amenorrhea. Prolonged administration of estrogens in large doses can produce amenorrhea for 3 months or more. Combinations of estrogens and progestogens can produce longer periods of amenorrhea.

Debilitating diseases. Tuberculosis, lymphomas, severe liver or renal failure, and severe malnutrition are possible causes of amenorrhea.

ABNORMAL UTERINE BLEEDING

Definitions. The terms used to indicate the principal types of abnormal bleeding are as follows:

Hypermenorrhea: Excessive menstrual bleeding ("flooding").

Hypomenorrhea: Scanty menstrual bleeding.

Polymenorrhea: Too frequent menstruation.

Intermenstrual bleeding: Bleeding other than at the time of menstruation. (Ovulatory bleeding is of this type and usually occurs for only 1 or 2 days at the time of ovulation as a result of a decrease in estrogens.)

Causes. Following is a list of causes of abnormal uterine bleeding:

Uterine lesions: Cervical laceration, ulcerations, polyps, and cancer; endometrial cancer, polyps, tuberculosis, endometritis, and submucous myoma.

Pregnancy disorders: Abortion, eccyesis, placental separation, hydatidiform mole, and choriocarcinoma.

Endometriosis: Uterine or ovarian.

Ovarian lesions: Tumors and inflammation.

Constitutional diseases: Purpura, pseudohemophilia, severe malnutrition, etc.

Exogenous estrogens: Too often this is the cause in premenopausal as well as postmenopausal years.

Exogenous progestogens: (Long-acting medroxyprogesterone given intramuscularly inhibits ovulation for months. Low-dose oral progestogens allow breakthrough bleeding.)

Intrinsic endocrine malfunction: (See discussion under amenorrhea and dysfunctional bleeding.)

Concepts of endometrial bleeding

Two terms are in common usage to describe endometrial bleeding as related to endocrines. "Breakthrough" bleeding is a term used to indicate that the bleeding occurs from the endometrium when the estrogen or estrogen-progestogen level remains relatively constant or increases. This term implies that the bleeding occurs in spite of sustained steroid stimulation. The second term, "withdrawal" bleeding, is applied when there is either a significant decrease in estrogen levels, which results in a lack of support for the endometrium, or a decrease in progestogen levels with similar endometrium breakdown.

In Fig. 14-2 the concept of a threshold of estrogen levels necessary for bleeding to occur is indicated. When total urinary estrogens for 24 hours are less than 10 μg, endometrial stimulation is not sufficient, so that neither withdrawal nor breakthrough bleeding can occur. Ten micrograms per 24 hours is then taken as the minimum threshold for bleeding to occur. Although breakthrough bleeding is possible if the urinary estrogens are in the range of 10 to 20 μg per 24 hours, it is uncommon. When an output of over 20 μg in 24 hours is present, then either breakthrough or withdrawal bleeding becomes likely. Fig. 14-3 illustrates the occurrence of bleeding when estrogens are administered in constant daily dosages. The bleeding may occur because of variations in ovarian estrogens that are pro-

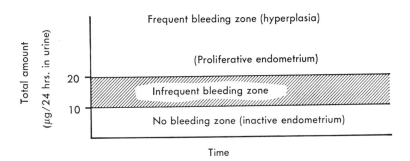

Fig. 14-2. Estrogen threshold of uterine bleeding.

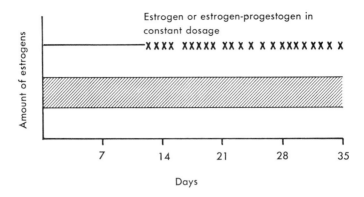

Fig. 14-3. Breakthrough bleeding.

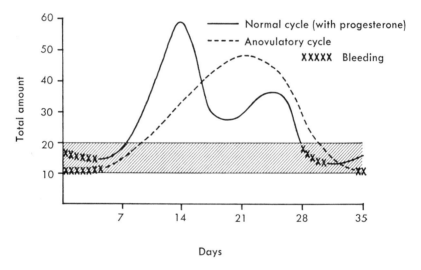

Fig. 14-4. Cyclic estrogen withdrawal bleeding.

duced in small amounts. As higher levels are reached, hyperplasia of the endometrium and increase in vascularity are anticipated. In Fig. 14-4, which depicts a normal ovulatory cycle, estrogen production begins in the early part of the cycle at a level near the threshold of bleeding and then gradually rises and gradually decreases until withdrawal bleeding occurs. The sequence in the typical anovulatory cycle is somewhat similar.

In Fig. 14-5 progestogen withdrawal bleeding is shown. It should be emphasized that this type of bleeding will occur in spite of sustained level of estrogens.

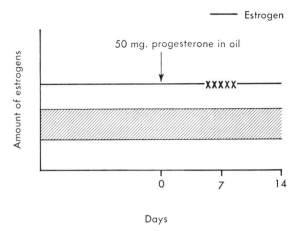

Fig. 14-5. Progestogen withdrawal bleeding.

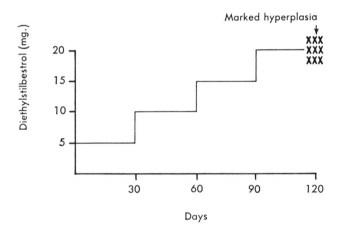

Fig. 14-6. Increasing extrinsic estrogens to delay withdrawal bleeding.

This will explain in part why progestogens are effective when used to produce bleeding in patients with sustained estrogen levels, as may occur in the climacteric.

If a patient is experiencing breakthrough bleeding, estrogen levels may be increased to cause regeneration of the endometrium and stop the bleeding (Fig. 14-6). However, if higher levels of estrogen are continued over a sufficient time, marked vascularity and thickness associated with hyperplasia result, so that when ultimate shedding of the endometrium does occur the bleeding is apt to be more profuse.

Dysfunctional uterine bleeding

Use of the term "dysfunctional" implies that the variations in hormonal stimulation of the endometrium are occurring in an abnormal manner. Dysfunctional uterine bleeding is caused by improper endocrine control. Difficulty in establishing the diagnosis as dysfunctional is in part because of the impracticality and inaccuracy of chemical determinations of estrogen and progestogen levels and because of the expense and impracticality of frequent determinations of FSH and LH. In the majority of cases, to gain some knowledge of the proper production of these hormones one must make gross and microscopic evaluations of the tissues that respond to the hormones. Changes in vaginal cells, cervical mucus, basal temperature, and endometrial components indicate recent estrogen and/or progestogen influence. Since abnormal bleeding can be caused by other conditions, it is important that neoplasia, infection, pregnancy, trauma, blood dyscrasia, or endocrine administration be ruled out. Not only are adequate history and physical examination required, but also endometrial biopsy or dilatation and curettage and laboratory studies are commonly required. After the diagnosis is made, repeated observations over a period of months may add information to indicate that the original opinion was in error (e.g., fixation and masses caused by endometriosis).

The levels of the ovarian steroids and their patterns of secretion as related to endometrial growth and shedding must be understood. As indicated in Fig. 14-4, estrogens cause proliferation of the endometrium. The extent of the proliferation is directly related to the level of estrogens and the length of time that this level exists. If the level drops sufficiently low (20 μg per 24 hours in urine or lower) and remains low for a few days, shedding of the endometrium will be adequate. If the level does not drop sufficiently low or does not remain low for a sufficient period of time, shedding will be incomplete and bleeding will continue.

Progesterone does not cause growth (proliferation). It causes cellular changes of the glandular and stromal portions of the endometrium. Once these cellular changes have been effected, the cells cannot revert back to the proliferative stage, so that when progesterone support is withdrawn, cellular disintegration and menstruation are inevitable. If there is a rapid decrease in the progesterone level, the shedding of the previously changed portions of the endometrium is complete and precise. To reiterate, if the progesterone production has been adequate over a sufficient number of days, the cellular changes of the secretory endometrium occur properly and, with a rapid decrease in progesterone secretion from the corpus luteum, normal menstrual bleeding is anticipated. Progesterone opposes the proliferative effects of estrogens. This action leads to less endometrial bleeding and is particularly important in understanding the use of synthetic progestogens in controlling excessive uterine bleeding.

For ovulation to occur and for corpus luteum formation to follow, the FSH and

LH levels must be essentially normal. This would indicate why ovulatory menstrual cycles are usually more normal than anovulatory cycles. Once a corpus luteum has been formed, shedding of the endometrium will occur unless pregnancy follows. This is explained by the fact that once the secretory changes have occurred the endometrium will be shed when progesterone support decreases. If this phenomenon is true, in nonpregnant patients amenorrhea indicates lack of ovulation. The life of a corpus luteum is relatively predictable. Progesterone secretion from the corpus luteum, as indicated through progesterone levels in blood, usually is very low (2 pg or less) 12 to 13 days after ovulation. If stimulation of the corpus luteum by LH is inadequate, progesterone production is apt to be inadequate, so that premenstrual bleeding occurs or the luteal phase is shortened. If the corpus luteum function persists too long, progesterone and estrogen are produced in low amounts, so that endometrial shedding is not complete and increased or prolonged menstrual bleeding can occur.

Since the life of the corpus luteum is relatively constant, the length of cycles is related more to the proliferative phase. This means that most short cycles have a short proliferative phase and most long cycles have a long proliferative phase. When bleeding occurs every 2 weeks the two most likely explanations are ovulatory bleeding, which can be as profuse as menstrual bleeding, or anovulatory cycles, which have short periods of adequate estrogen stimulation.

In understanding variations in endometrial bleeding, one must consider the levels of estrogens and progestogens in regard to not only whether sufficient time is allowed for proliferation or secretory change but also whether the lower levels of estrogens and progestogens exist over a sufficient number of days to allow complete shedding. If the levels of estrogens do not decrease sufficiently and remain so for a few days or if they are slow to increase after they have been low, the number of days of bleeding is increased.

Some of the mechanisms that influence the length and extent of bleeding deserve discussion. Light bleeding indicates less estrogenic proliferation. This proliferation may have been inhibited by the secretion of a relatively high level of progesterone resulting in good secretory change in the endometrium and then by a rapid drop in progesterone; as a result the shedding is more precise and the bleeding less. Light bleeding indicates less vascularity of the endometrium and, at times, of the uterus. Light bleeding may occur because the total endometrial surface is less. Heavy bleeding is associated with increased endometrial proliferation caused by increased levels of estrogens over longer periods of time. It may indicate lack of progesterone opposition to estrogenic proliferation or lack of adequate progesterone change, so that the shedding is less precise. The vascularity of the uterus or the total endometrial surface may be increased, thus causing the heavy bleeding. Prolonged bleeding is related more to a lack of precise shedding. It may indicate that the estrogens were slow in decreasing or slow in increasing. It may indicate inadequate progesterone influence or, more particularly, lack of a rapid drop in the progesterone level.

From the foregoing discussion it should be apparent that dysfunctional bleeding is commonly associated with lack of ovulation. Anovulatory cycles are considered normal at the onset of reproductive life and occur often before menopause. These are the times during which dysfunctional bleeding is more common. Abnormal bleeding can occur from atrophic, hyperplastic, proliferative, or secretory endometrium. It has been estimated that at least 10% of gynecologic patients have dysfunctional bleeding. Practically all women have some degree of dysfunctional bleeding at some time.

The abnormal patterns of estrogen and progestogen production may be caused by disturbances at the hypothalamic, pituitary, or ovarian sites. There may be combinations of causes. Our present knowledge suggests that the hypothalamic level is the most commonly affected area. In some women dysfunctional bleeding is correlated with periods of psychic disturbance. In other women marked mental disturbance has little or no effect on the regularity of endometrial shedding. In the management of dysfunctional bleeding proper attention must be directed to all the areas involved in steroid metabolism in somewhat the same manner that it is directed in understanding amenorrhea. The control of the endometrium can usually be affected by administration of extrinsic estrogens and progestogens, but this administration should be done with due regard for the adequate evaluation of the patient.

Anovulation may be determined by review of basal temperature records, repeated observation of the cervical mucus and of vaginal cells, or biopsy of the endometrium. Remember that if bleeding has occurred for more than 2 or 3 days then the endometrium obtained at biopsy is apt to be the basal portion and the portion that had been previously affected by progesterone may have been shed. Biopsy immediately before the onset of bleeding or during the first day of bleeding is apt to be more correctly correlated with ovulation. When biopsy is performed 5 days or more after the onset of the increased or prolonged bleeding and when secretory areas are found, the term "irregular shedding of the endometrium" is used. This is apt to be caused by prolonged activity of the corpus luteum.

When hyperplasia of the endometrium is diagnosed by biopsy or curettage, it is correlated with prolonged estrogen stimulation. This stimulation may have been associated with estrogen-producing ovarian tumors; it may have been associated with the polycystic ovary syndrome; it may have been caused by extrinsic estrogens. Hyperplasia indicates the lack of progestogen influence, and its future development may be prevented by producing progestogen withdrawal bleeding at proper intervals.

Normal secretory endometrium can be obtained in patients with excessive uterine bleeding. Excessive bleeding occurring in a cyclic regular manner suggests the lack of any endocrine problem. There is a likelihood of uterine changes such as increased vascularity or increased size after repeated pregnancy or both or abnormalities of the uterus. The total amount of endometrial surface is related to the amount of bleeding. Increased regular bleeding that occurs with myomas is thought to be caused by the increased surface of the endometrium, as well as the vascular changes associated with the myomas. It is important to remember that submucous myomas may not be detected by pelvic palpation.

Therapeutic measures. The following are the most commonly employed methods of treating dysfunctional uterine bleeding.

Dilation and curettage. If bleeding is extensive, mechanical removal of the endometrium offers the most rapid means of control. Abnormal bleeding may not return, at least for several months, after dilation and curettage.

Estrogens and progestogens. The administration of estrogens alone such as 0.05 mg ethinyl estradiol given for 21 days will usually inhibit ovulation and be followed in 2 to 10 days by withdrawal bleeding. On the fifth day after the onset of bleeding estrogen administration is started again for 21 days. This method of controlling cyclic bleeding was formerly used; however, a better control of bleeding is accomplished by using estrogens together with progestogens. The combined pills used for oral contraception are effective. Those tablets containing 50 μg of ethinyl estradiol or 80 μg of mestranol combined with small amounts of progestogens are usually effective. It is important that the dose be adequate to suppress the production of FSH and LH, be sufficient to avoid breakthrough bleeding, and be of sufficient progestogen-estrogen ratio to provide an endometrium of limited vascularity to avoid excessive bleeding.

The estrogens and progestogens used in oral contraceptive tablets are rapidly eliminated, so that withdrawal bleeding is more precise. When combinations of estrogens and progestogens are given parenterally, the duration of their action is less precise and their action decreases more gradually, so that the bleeding that results may be more prolonged. Hydroxy-progesterone caproate usually results in withdrawal bleeding 12 to 14 days after intramuscular injection. Estradiol valerate given intramuscularly has an effect over a period of 12 to 18 days. These two substances can be given in combination and, at times, are used as a substitute for oral estrogen-progestogen combinations, particularly when nausea results from the oral administration of estrogens. When cyclic bleeding about every 28 days is desired, the first injection is given on the fifth day of bleeding and is followed in 10 days by another injection so that the withdrawal bleeding is likely to occur approximately 28 to 30 days from the onset of the original bleeding.

Short-acting progestogens (50 to 100 mg of progesterone in oil given as a single injection or medroxyprogesterone given orally in a dosage of 10 mg daily for 5 days) cause withdrawal bleeding about 7 days after the initial administration. They may be used as means of treating or avoiding the hypermenorrhea of hyperplasia associated with prolonged estrogen stimulation. When bleeding has been profuse or prolonged, it is important to use a short-acting progestogen to cause more rapid shedding.

When intolerance to combined estrogen-progestogen preparations exists, progestogens may be used either cyclically or on a prolonged basis to avoid abnormal endometrial bleeding. Norethindrone acetate, 5 mg daily, may be given for 21 days to decrease withdrawal bleeding, and it may be used in increasing doses continuously to avoid any bleeding for several months. Should it be ineffective, 40 mg of the potent progestogen megestrol acetate may be given daily for several months. Similarly 100 to 200 mg of danazol may be given daily morning and night to decrease bleeding. When danazol is given in larger doses prolonged amenorrhea results. In choosing methods of therapy the physician must consider the cost of medication, any side effects, and the regimen's effectiveness.

In certain situations in which dysfunctional bleeding is associated with other pathologic states such as myomas or endometriosis, combined estrogens and progestogens can be used in a continuous manner over a period of several weeks to avoid any bleeding. This would allow for correction of anemia.

Control of endometrial shedding can be accomplished by the administration of extrinsic estrogens and progestogens. Usually the drugs are applied as a temporary means of cure with the hope that the psychic disturbances will subside and that after the drugs are discontinued normal cyclic bleeding will return. If the disturbances are caused by a pituitary lesion, thyroid disease, or adrenal disease that can be corrected, temporary control may be followed by cure.

If no further childbearing is desired or if sterility has been persistent in spite of adequate investigation and therapy, hysterectomy is suggested. The decision should be based on the severity of the abnormal bleeding, lest these women so frequently plagued by psychosomatic disorders prove to be only mildly improved after the hysterectomy. When dysfunctional bleeding occurs near the menopause, hysterectomy for abnormal bleeding can be avoided by use of cyclic therapy. To decide whether or not to use cyclic therapy for premenopausal bleeding, one should conduct a thorough investigation. Endometrial biopsy is imperative, and the potential dangers of estrogen must be balanced against the potential dangers of surgery and anesthesia

To properly use endocrine therapy, the physician must be knowledgeable of endocrinology. The production of endogenous ovarian hormones must be considered and an effort made to correlate cyclic changes if regularity of endometrial shedding is desired. If irregularity of ovarian activity is marked and if responsiveness of the endometrium is impaired, it is little wonder that attempts at psychotherapy alone are often not successful. The use of adequate strength cyclic estrogen-progestogen combinations causes inhibition of gonadotropins and thereby decreases the intrinsic ovarian hormones, so that cyclic therapy is more effective.

If it is impractical to perform a curettage immediately in patients with marked amounts of bleeding, the bleeding may be temporarily arrested by large doses of estrogens; however, it should be realized that the thickness of the endometrium will be markedly increased and the withdrawal bleeding after cessation of treatment is apt to be quite heavy. However, in special situations a few precious days may be saved.

In certain patients it may be desirable to promote prolonged periods of amenorrhea in an effort to allow the patient to replenish her iron stores and correct the anemia that exists. These long periods of amenorrhea can be accomplished with the use of estrogen-progestogen combinations orally or parenterally. Increasing doses may be needed to prevent break-through bleeding.

Consideration of abnormal uterine bleeding in various age groups. The patient's age can be correlated with causes of bleeding.

From birth to 10 years of age. Neonatal uterine bleeding is caused by the withdrawal of maternal estrogens and subsides in a few days without treatment. Trauma or ulceration from foreign bodies placed in the vagina becomes more likely as a cause of bleeding from the vagina or vulva as the child grows older.

Uterine bleeding may occur with *precocious puberty*. This condition is associated with early maturation of the ovaries. With follicular growth, estrogen stimulation causes premature development of the breast and pubic hair. Endometrial bleeding occurs and may be preceded by ovulation. No neoplasia is found. The child will develop normally but at an accelerated rate. The parents and child must be prepared to cope with the problems of early sexual development. *Granulosa cell* or *theca cell tumors* are rare causes of uterine bleeding in children. If an ovarian mass is palpable, and since the tumors may be malignant, laparotomy is in order to allow accurate diagnosis and oophorectomy if an estrogen-producing neoplasm is present.

Neoplasms of the uterus are rare in children. Sarcoma botryoides is an extremely rare mixed mesodermal tumor that may appear as a mass in the introitus or may be found on vaginal inspection. Pelvic exenteration or radiation is now advocated for this otherwise fatal disease; however, seldom does the victim survive more than 1 year. If a carcinoma is found in a child's cervix, it is usually adenocarcinoma.

From 10 to 18 years of age. All the causes listed for abnormal bleeding must be considered. Thorough history taking and adequate physical and laboratory examinations are imperative. Hereditary disorders of blood clotting are likely to be found in this age group. Rectal examination is done if the hymen will not admit one finger. The use of anesthesia may be necessary to prevent psychic distress and to allow satisfactory examination. After pregnancy, trauma, and organic causes have been ruled out, dysfunction is the working diagnosis. Iron for anemia, proper diet, vitamin supplementation, and proper weight control are stressed as needed. If bleeding is heavy or prolonged, estrogens may be given to temporarily stop bleeding. If bleeding ceases, progestogens such as norethindrone acetate (Norlutate) may be used to provide prolonged periods of amenorrhea. Should they prove ineffective, curettage under anesthesia is required. This is often therapeutic and may reveal an unsuspected condition. Cyclic combined estrogen-progestogen therapy is usually effective. As a rule, with maturation of the hypothalamus, pituitary, and ovaries the abnormal bleeding ceases.

From 18 to 40 years of age. Pregnancy and its complications are the most common causes of abnormal bleeding during this period. Invasion of the uterus is avoided if viable pregnancy is suspected until observation over a few weeks settles the question. Of course, with a small uterus and hemorrhage, curettage may be imperative. Pelvic infections, endometriosis, uterine myomas, ovarian tumors, and blood dyscrasias require thorough interrogation and physical assessment with indicated laboratory studies. A search for cancer must be made (cytosmears and biopsy). Diagnostic curettage becomes more important with the increased age of the patient. Dysfunctional bleeding is a common problem in this age group.

Over 40 years of age. The possibility of malignancy must be constantly entertained. Since reproduction is seldom desired by the patient, hysterectomy is more often used if abnormal bleeding is recurrent. Diagnosis must be as accurate as possible to avoid an improper method of therapy and particularly to avoid procrastination in definitive treatment of cancer.

Radiation therapy, once popular for control of endometrial bleeding of benign cause, has been replaced in the United States by hysterectomy, which (1) allows more accurate diagnosis, (2) permits preservation of ovarian function, and (3) eliminates the possibility of uterine cancer development.

Postmenopausal. If 1 year or more after the last menses any bleeding occurs, a thorough search for cancer should be done. Cytologic examination, cervical biopsy, and endometrial study are indicated. Endometrial polyps, senile endometrium with endometritis, senile vaginitis, and particularly trichomoniasis are among nonmalignant causes.

DYSMENORRHEA

When painful menstruation has occurred from the menarche, it is termed *primary* or *intrinsic*. Usually no anatomic cause can be found. *Secondary* dysmenorrhea develops months or years after the onset of menstruation, and gross pathologic changes may be found. The pain may be (1) intermittent cramping in type, which is thought to be associated with uterine contractions, or (2) constant aching in type, which is considered to be caused by "vascular congestion." Weakness, anorexia, nausea, vomiting, sweats, fainting, and headache may be associated, one or all, particularly with primary dysmenorrhea. Most women have, at times, some discomfort during menstruation. A minority require therapy.

Etiology. Dysmenorrhea may have one or more causes.

Psychogenic causes. Ignorance of the significance and hygiene of menstruation or association with women experiencing dysmenorrhea may condition the individual to have somatic symptoms if the psyche is disturbed. Education, reconditioning, and reassurance are in order. Advice to continue most of the patient's routine activities and, at times, the use of special exercises may be of aid.

Anatomic variations. Very rarely a separate uterine horn is the cause. Cervical stenosis, congenital or acquired, is rarely the cause. With intrauterine clotting or shedding of large fragments of the endometrium, interference with the outflow may be important. Anteflexion or third-degree retroplacement of congenital origin is not likely to be significant. Pain reception from the cervix is more acute in some women. (Perhaps this represents a variation in the nerve structures.)

Pathologic conditions. Endometriosis, pelvic inflammation, and uterine or ovarian neoplasms may cause painful menstruation. Complications of pregnancy with bleeding must not be confused with dysmenorrhea. Pain of peritoneal, bladder, ureteral, intestinal, or joint origin may occur simultaneously with the menses.

Prostaglandins. Prostaglandins are produced by the endometrium in increasing amounts under progesterone influence. The subjective changes after administration of prostaglandins are similar to those changes noted with menstruation. Perhaps inhibition of ovulation, which prevents the prostaglandin increase that is caused by progesterone, is effective because the prostaglandins are at fault.

Therapy. Since dysmenorrhea is a subjective symptom rather than a specific diagnosis, relief may be effected in the proper therapy for the disease condition that has caused painful menstruation.

When no organic cause exists, the functional disturbance may be corrected by various means.

1. Endocrine therapy is highly effective. Inhibition of ovulation can be accomplished by administration of ethinylestradiol in a dosage of 50 μg daily for 21 days to allow crampless withdrawal bleeding. More precise bleeding follows the administration of combined estrogen-progestogen tablets as used for contraception.

Dydrogesterone is a rapidly excreted synthetic progestogen that does not inhibit ovulation and gives good results when administered three times daily for 21 days. Low-dose progestogens used as "minipills" oppose endometrial proliferation and perhaps lower prostaglandin levels.

2. Prostaglandin antagonists administered 3 days before and during the first 2

days of menstruation relieve many patients. Mefenamic acid, indomethacin, ibu-profen, and naproxen have been effective, but these anti-inflammatory agents may cause gastrointestinal irritation and bleeding in susceptible patients.

3. Analgesics may offer sufficient relief of pain. Potent narcotics should seldom be used. Codeine, $\frac{1}{2}$ grain, with aspirin, 5 grains, has not been found to cause habituation.

4. Cervical dilation may give relief.

5. Pregnancy usually causes marked improvement.

6. Marriage may result in improvement by psychic change and coital benefits.

7. Resection of the sensory nerves from the uterus at the presacral or uterosacral areas is used only in women with severe pain for whom other methods of therapy are not practical or sufficient.

PREMENSTRUAL TENSION

Premenstrually, the psychoneurotic patient is likely to be most symptomatic and the happier woman less happy. Manifestations of this cyclic syndrome include depression, irritability, abdominal distention, headache, backache, nausea, and slight edema. Changes in the electrolyte balance with an increase in sodium may occur. This leads to water retention and weight gain, which subsides with the onset of endometrial shedding.

The restriction of salt intake and the use of diuretics will aid some women. Tranquilizing drugs may offer symptomatic relief. Analgesics may be added if pain is a problem. Combined estrogen-progestogen administration reduces or eliminates symptoms in some patients. Severe symptoms and social disability deserve psychiatric evaluation and are not likely to respond to "airing" problems, reassurance, suggestion, and symptomatic therapy, which usually benefit the less disturbed patient.

DYSPAREUNIA

Difficulty or pain of coitus may be slight and temporary, or it may be so severe that intercourse is unbearable.

Causes. Causes of dyspareunia include the following:

1. Anomalies—imperforate hymen and absence of the vagina are very uncommon. Vaginal septa (double vagina) usually cause no obstruction but may obstruct and be torn during coitus.

2. A persistent thick resistant hymen may cause pain in unsuccessful attempts at intercourse. If office dilation is too painful, incision of the hymen and, at times, of a resistant perineum may give great relief.

3. Vulvitis, vaginitis, bartholinitis, skenitis, and urethritis can render vaginal penetration painful.

4. Scars of episiotomy or perineorrhaphy sometimes remain painful and require incision for liberation. Improperly performed perineorrhaphy can decrease the size of the introitus abnormally. Similarly colporrhaphy may excessively reduce vaginal size.

5. Intrapelvic disease caused by infection, endometriosis, or neoplasia may cause pain on deep penetration.

6. In third-degree retroplacement of the uterus the ovaries are in the cul-de-sac and are vulnerable if penetration is sufficiently deep.

7. Senile atrophy, postradiation atrophy, or vulvar dystrophy may decrease the vaginal size to the degree that coitus is painful.

Psychogenic type. When the vulva or the vagina is tender, women reflexly constrict the muscles about the vagina so as to protect it. This constriction (vaginismus) may increase the degree of pain. When no organic cause for dyspareunia exists, vaginismus can most often be explained as a manifestation of fear. This may be of such degree that the patient refuses to introduce a douche nozzle or allow the physician to place one finger in the vagina. Reassurance by the physician as to the normalcy of the genitals and gentle examination may allow the institution of gradual dilation of the introitus. Some patients can overcome their fear of vaginal penetration by using vaginal dilators (Young's).

Instruction as to the contraction and relaxation of the vaginal constrictors may aid the patient in solving her problem.

At times vaginismus is a manifestation of severe psychoneurosis or psychosis and is best handled in consultation with a psychiatrist.

SEXUAL FRIGIDITY

Although dyspareunia may interfere with or preclude satisfactory sexual response, patients without disease of the reproductive organs may exhibit frigidity or orgasmic failure. Frigidity may be primary or secondary. In the primary situation the woman has never experienced or anticipated the pleasures of erotic stimulation, whereas in secondary frigidity the desire previously felt has been lost. Similarly lack of orgasm may be primary in that the patient has never experienced the acme of sexual exhilaration or secondary in that she can no longer reach this high level of response. For a physician to assist patients with sexual malfunction, physical examination is not sufficient and psychologic inquiry and understanding, together with knowledge of the training and experience of the patient and her consort, are essential. The sexual mores of the patient and her associates, along with the practices that she has learned, are as important as her knowledge of anatomy, physiology, and sexual psychology.

Mild frigidity is apt to be overcome by improvement in sexual response, which occurs with experience. Once erotic stimulation has resulted in pleasant sensations the patient's desire improves. In secondary frigidity, psychologic phenomena are usually involved and the relationship of the patient to her consort must be more thoroughly understood. Similarly investigation of disturbances of emotional and other mental functions must be made.

Orgasmic failure may be caused either by improper or poor techniques of sexual stimulation or by psychologic problems that interfere with desire and performance. As indicated in the section on physiology of the vulva and vagina, physical changes occur that are associated with increased erotic stimulation. In women the time required for these responses is longer than it is in men. It is important that the patient and her consort understand this fact. Similarly, for lubrication of the vagina and vulva to occur, reponse must be adequate; otherwise pain because of friction occurs. Women must know that active participation is essential for maximum excitation and response. They must learn through trial and experience the proper techniques and timing so essential for their enjoyment and the enjoyment of their partner. The problems may be primarily caused by the man. Not only must he be capable in sexual performance as regards his response, but also he must understand and desire response of his consort. Impotence, premature ejaculation, and retarded ejaculation often respond to satisfactory treatment and training. It is usually necessary that both the man and the woman be assisted by the therapist for proper evaluation to occur, for communication to be adequate, and for instruction in training to be more effective.

Physicians vary in their ability and desire to treat women with sexual malfunction. They should recognize sexual malfunction, treat sexual malfunction according to their capabilities, and assist those patients whom they cannot help to find other physicians or sources of relief. In some instances, sexual malfunction is but one part of major mental disorders and the patient should be referred to a psychiatrist for care.

SELECTED REFERENCES

de Alvarez, R.R., and Smith, E.K.: Physiological basis for hormone therapy in the female, J.A.M.A. **168**:489, 1958.

Backer, M.H.: Isopregnenone (Duphaston), a new progestational agent, Obstet. Gynecol. **19**:724, 1962

Chan, W.Y., Dawood, M.Y., and Fuchs, F.: The relief of dysmenorrhea with the prostaglandin synthetase inhibitor ibuprofen: effect on prostaglandin levels in menstrual fluid, Am. J. Obstet. Gynecol. **135**:102, 1979.

Cook, H.H., Gamble, C.J., and Satterwaite, A.P.: Oral contraception by norethynodrel, Am. J. Obstet. Gynecol. **82**:437, 1961.

Cushing, H.: Papers relating to the pituitary body, hypothalamus, and parasympathetic nervous system, Springfield, Ill., 1932, Charles C Thomas, Publisher.

Dignam, W.J., Wortham, J.T., and Hamblen, E.C.:Estrogen therapy of functional dysmenorrhea, Am. J. Obstet. Gynecol. **59**:1124, 1950.

Domingue, J.N., Richmond, I.L., and Wilson, C.B.: The results of surgery in 114 patients with prolactin-secreting pituitary adenomas, Am. J. Obstet. Gynecol. **137**:102, 1980.

Gemzell, C.A.: Induction of ovulation with human pituitary gonadotropins, Fertil. Steril. **13**:153, 1962.

Gold, J.J., and Josimovich, J.B.: Gynecologic endocrinology, Philadelphia, 1980, J.B. Lippincott Co.

Golub, L.J., Long, W.R., Menduke, H., and Gordon, H.C.: Teenage dysmenorrhea, Am. J. Obstet. Gynecol. **74:**591, 1957.

Greenblatt, R.B., and Barfield, W.E.: The progestational activity of 6-methyl-17-acetoxyprogesterone, South. Med. J. **52:**345, 1959.

Greenblatt, R.B., Roy, S., and Mahes, V.B.: Induction of ovulation, Am. J. Obstet. Gynecol. **84:**900, 1962.

Greene, R., and Dalton, K.: The premenstrual syndrome, Br. Med. J. **1:**1007, 1953.

Halbert, D.R., Demers, L.M., and Jones, D.E.D.: Dysmenorrhea and prostaglandins, Obstet. Gynecol. Surv. **31:**77, 1976.

Henriksen, E., and Horn, P.: Causes and treatment of secondary dyspareunia, Am. J. Obstet. Gynecol. **43:**671, 1942.

Ingersoll, F.M., and Meigg, J.V.: Presacral neurectomy for dysmenorrhea, N. Engl. J. Med. **238:**357, 1948.

Jackson, R.L., and Dockerty, M.B.: The Stein-Leventhal syndrome: analysis of 43 cases with special reference to association with endometrial carcinoma, Am. J. Obstet. Gynecol. **73:**161, 1957.

Keetel, W.C., Bradbury, J.T., and Stoddard, F.J.: Observations on the polycystic ovary syndrome, Am. J. Obstet. Gynecol. **73:**954, 1957.

Keizer, H.A., Poortman, J., and Bunnic, G.H.: Influence of physical exercise on sex hormone metabolism, J. Appl. Physiol. **48:**765, 1980.

Kistner, R.W.: Use of clomiphene citrate, human chorionic gonadotropin and human menopausal gonadotropin for induction of ovulation in the human female, Fertil. Steril. **17:**569, 1966.

Kupperman, H.S., Epstein, J.E., Blatt, M.H., and Stone, A.: Induction of ovulation in the human: therapeutic and diagnostic importance, Am. J. Obstet. Gynecol. **75:**301, 1958.

Leventhal, M.: The Stein-Leventhal syndrome, Am. J. Obstet. Gynecol. **76:**825, 1958.

Mann, E.C.: Frigidity, Clin. Obstet. Gynecol. **3:**739, 1960.

Masters, W.H., and Johnson, V.E.: Human sexual response, Boston, 1966, Little, Brown & Co.

McKelvey, J.L., and Samuels, L.T.: Irregular shedding of the endometrium, Am. J. Obstet. Gynecol. **53:**627. 1947.

Nora J.J., Nora, A.H., Blu, J., et al.: Exogenous progestogen and estrogen implicated in birth defects, J.A.M.A. **240:**837, 1978.

Perloff, W.H., and Channick, B.J.: Effect of prednisone on abnormal menstrual function, Am. J. Obstet. Gynecol. **77:**138, 1959.

Ramcharan, S., Pellegrin, F.A., Roy, R.M., et al.: The Walnut Creek contraceptive drug study. A prospective study of the side effects of oral contraceptives, J. Reprod. Med. **25:**347, 1980.

Sheehan, H.L., and Murdock, R.: Postpartum necrosis of the anterior pituitary; pathological and clinical aspects, J. Obstet. Gynaec. Br. Emp. **45:**456, 1938.

Shewchuk, A.B., Adamson, G.D., Lessard, P., and Ezrin, C.: The effect of pregnancy on suspected pituitary adenomas with conservative management of ovulation defects associated with galactorrhea, Am. J. Obstet. Gynecol. **136:**659, 1980.

Shewchuk, A.B., Corenblum, B., Pairudeau, N., et al.: Predicted ovulatory response to brom-alpha-ergocryptin in amenorrhea-galactorrhea syndromes, Am. J. Obstet. Gynecol. **136:**652, 1980.

Short, R.V., and London, D.R.: Defective biosynthesis of ovarian steroids in Stein-Leventhal syndrome, Br. Med. J. **1:**1724, 1961.

Sturgis, S.H., et al.: The gynecologic patient; a psycho-endocrine study, New York, 1962, Grune & Stratton, Inc.

Taylor, E.S., and Lombardi, J.C.: The value of endometrial curettage in the diagnosis and treatment of functional uterine bleeding, New York J. Med. **51:**2488, 1951.

Ullery, J.C., Livingston, N., and Abou-Shabanah, E.: The mucus fern phenomenon in the cervical and nasal smears, Obstet. Gynecol. Surv. **14:**1, 1959.

Chapter 15

INFERTILITY

Determination of the causes for barrenness requires a knowledge of all the aspects of gynecology and serves as a test of gynecic ability. The information in this chapter is presented to emphasize important aspects in management.

Definitions. The types of infertility and their definitions are as follows:

1. Primary infertility—conception has never occurred.
2. Secondary infertility—at least one pregnancy has occurred.
3. Relative infertility—the infertility is caused by various factors that may delay or hinder conception.
4. Absolute infertility—conception is impossible (sterility).

The average time for fertile couples to conceive is 3 months. As a general rule thorough investigation is deferred until after 6 months of trying. Complete investigation or continuing treatment of either person is proper only when the spouse's status can justify it.

Causes. Large studies indicate that the man is responsible in 40% and the woman in 60% of cases of infertility. Factors are outlined below:

I. Male factors
   A. Decreased production of spermatozoa
      1. Varicocele
      2. Testicular atrophy or anomaly
      3. Endocrine disease
      4. Heat, systemic infection, severe malnutrition
   B. Ductal obstruction
      1. Epididymitis
      2. Vasectomy
      3. Absence of vas deferens
      4. Infection of ejaculatory duct
   C. Failure of vaginal deposition
      1. Ejaculatory disturbances, too frequent ejaculation
      2. Impotence and other sexual problems
      3. Hypospadias

    D. Abnormal semen
       1. Volume problems
       2. High viscosity
       3. Necrospermia and agglutination
II. Female factors
    A. Vaginal
       1. Vaginismus
       2. Absence of vagina
       3. Intact hymen
       4. Vaginitis
    B. Cervical
       1. Endocervicitis
       2. Obstruction (posttherapy, tumor)
       3. Inadequate endocervix (surgical or functional)
    C. Uterine
       1. Anomalies
       2. Synechiae
       3. Polyps
       4. Myomas
       5. Chronic endometritis (tuberculosis)
    D. Tubal obstruction or dysfunction
       1. Salpingitis (sexually transmitted disease, puerperal infection, tuberculosis)
       2. Peritonitis (surgery, ruptured appendix or viscus)
       3. Previous tubal or ovarian surgery
       4. Endometriosis
       5. Congenital
    E. Ovulatory
       1. Anovulation
          a. Premature menopause
          b. Polycystic ovarian syndrome
          c. Hyperprolactinemia
          d. Pituitary insufficiency
          e. Hypothyroidism
          f. Functional ovarian or adrenal tumors
          g. Excess or insufficient fatty tissue
          h. Severe liver or renal failure
          i. Diabetes
    F. Immunologic
       1. Sperm immobilization or agglutination

Multiple factors may be involved in couples. The physician must evaluate each factor for severity and correctability in order to determine how to proceed with investigation and therapy.

Investigation

Initial examination. Usually the woman is seen alone; she is apt to be free of symptoms or exhibits only minor symptoms. The history should emphasize previous reproductive history; assessment of uterine bleeding must be detailed, and direct questioning to elicit any evidence of functional, infectious, or operative causes for infertility as indicated in the outline above must be included. An assessment of the patient's knowledge of ovulation and timing of intercourse is essential. Similarly one must inquire as to specifics of coital technique, particulary as regards to the foreign materials placed on the vulva or in the vagina.

The woman should be asked to give as much history as possible about her consort. During this discussion the physician must emphasize that detailed evaluation of sperm analysis and competent examination of the male are essential.

Examination of the woman must be complete, as with most gynecologic disorders. Particular interest during examination should be focused on developmental and endocrinologic assessments. The initial abdominal and pelvic examination should follow a routine for thoroughness; usually a uterine sound should be introduced to determine degree of cervical patency and estimate adequacy of the endometrial cavity.

After the historical and physical examination data have been evaluated, the physician must determine a plan for future investigation. If the patient's menstrual cycle and duration have been regular, it is likely that ovulation has been occurring regularly. Conversely, with amenorrhea or variation in cycles, anovulation is expected and investigation is instituted. Most patients should be instructed on how to determine basal body temperature. Written instructions and graphic forms are used. The reader is referred to the sections in this book on amenorrhea and dysfunctional uterine bleeding for discussions on the evaluation of these disorders. The logical application of endocrine studies, whether they be pregnancy test or thyroxin or TSH, FSH, testosterone, cortisol, or prolactin determination are decided on after proper evaluation of the initial findings.

Any decision to investigate the endometrial cavity for distortion and the tubes for blockage or impairment of function may be, in part, guided by the patient's history as well as findings on palpation. Similarly, the need for endometrial biopsy to assess luteal function or the possibility of intrauterine infection may be suggested. However, one usually must observe the basal temperature curve to suggest the possibility of luteal inadequacy. The majority of patients will need some type of tubal patency studies. All tubal patency studies should be done in the early proliferative phase, soon after the cessation of endometrial bleeding. The type of procedure is chosen after evaluation of available data. If there is a question of infection or other factors, this decision may not be made until a second examination.

During the initial examination the patient should be informed of the orderly procedure required for adequate investigation; she must understand in order to cooperate. The physician at this time may be able to assess the ability of the patient to cooperate; he should be mindful of such factors as lack of education and training that may preclude obtaining adequate basal temperature records and other data from some patients. He must also remember that some of the endocrine interrelationships are complex to physicians and even more confusing to patients, lest his efforts to educate cause additional patient frustration.

It is usually in order at the initial visit to discuss with the patient timing of ovulation, coital technique, foreign substances (including douches), and frequency of intercourse. The physician should emphasize the need for evaluation of the man. Investigation by a urologist should be done.

Plan of investigation. As indicated above the exact procedures will vary with different couples. Most women at least desire the assurance that they are ovulating and that there is no obstruction to the passage of spermatozoa or the ova. This would mean that the ovulatory factors as evidenced by basal temperature curves and any laboratory data must be discussed. Tubal patency tests are usually required. Tubal insufflation can be performed without anesthesia or with cervical anesthesia in the office at minimal cost. Its accuracy requires careful technique and will vary with different patients. The passage of carbon dioxide is ascertained by pressure evaluation, auscultation of the abdomen, and the occurrence of shoulder pain when the patient is erect. Failure of passage may be due to poor technique or tubal spasm. In these situations future attempts at insufflation or other methods of determination of tubal patency are in order. The occurrence of pregnancy after tubal insufflation suggests that it has a therapeutic value possibly by relieving minor tubal obstruction. Some physicians would repeat a tubal test with evidence of patency at least once because of this association of improvement.

Hysterosalpingography offers more information on the endometrial cavity and tubal patency. It should be performed with observation on an image intensifier and with x-ray film recording the tubes and uterus. When the flow of a colored fluid through the tube is observed at laparoscopy, patency can be observed and the physician can view tubal distortions due to adhesions (either after infection or with associated endometriosis). However, the uterine cavity is not adequately evaluated. From this short discussion it can be seen that the techniques of evaluation of the tube give varying information. Methods must be chosen after proper considerations of risks, cost, time, and so on.

Postcoital tests are essential for complete evaluation of couples. These tests not only allow evaluation of the adequacy of the cervical mucus but permit assessment of the sperm's degree of penetration. It should be emphasized that if the test is performed after ovulation the mucus has an increased viscosity and cellularity and is highly resistant to sperm penetration. An adequate Huhner test demands that timing consider the menstrual cycle: it is best done 2 or 3 days before ovulation in the absence of vaginitis or endocervicitis. Most investigators advocate its performance within 2 to 4 hours after coitus, and the technique of obtaining the endocervical mucus must be adequate. It is not a substitute for complete sperm analysis of the man. It may suggest inadequate coital technique or sperm deficiencies as well as the possibility that sperm agglutination and immobilization should be determined.

All infertility investigations require several encounters with the patient and/or her husband. Initially they are for investigation, and later they are principally for evaluation of therapeutic efforts. It must be acknowledged that thorough investigation reveals no obvious cause of infertility in either partner in approximately 25% of cases.

Prognosis of the man. The most important examination is that of the sperm; however, one should not rest with one analysis of the sperm because many factors (such as frequency of ejaculation) may have a marked effect on fertility. Physical examination of the man is essential lest one miss such an obvious finding as marked hypospadia.

Various factors inhibiting fertility are as follows:

Varicocele. Varicocele is a common cause of infertility among men; fortunately, response to surgical correction is good.

Low sperm volume. Although low sperm volume may be associated with other abnormalities, when the sperm present appear normal as to form and motility with adequate liquefaction, intracervical insemination may be tried; however, most clinicians have not had great success. If the volume is high intracervical inseminination of the split ejaculate or withdrawal after the first part of ejaculation may help. Endocrine problems as a cause of men's infertility are not common. When the problem is correctible response is good. Hypothyroidism is a rare cause.

Sexual problems. Failure of ejaculation and problems of timing of intercourse are due to various causes that may at times require psychiatric treatment or, on some occasions that involve diabetes mellitus, previous surgery, or certain drugs. Once the problem is corrected, improvement can be expected.

Ductal obstructions. Obstruction is suggested with a history of infection or surgery and is confirmed on physical examination. Evidence of severe epididymitis may be a bad prognostic sign. Absence or surgical blockage of the vas deferens must be evaluated before determining an attempt at anastomosis of the injured vas. Pregnancy rates have been low, possibly because of a subsequent autoimmune mechanism.

Retrograde ejaculation. The most common cause of this phenomenon is prostatic surgery; however, it may be an indication of a nervous system disorder.

Testicular atrophy or anomaly. This is usually indicated by azospermia or oligospermia. Barr chromatin patterns and chromosomal analyses may be in order. An atrophic testis may suggest the disorder. In some patients a history of orchitis may be elicited. The prognosis is very poor.

Therapy of the woman

Treatment of ovulatory failure. The most common type of anovulation is intermittent and may be classified as a form of polycystic ovary syndrome. If there is any question as to the presence of premature ovarian failure, FSH determination should be done to more properly diagnose this nonresponding syndrome. Infrequent ovulation usually responds to clomiphene when the pituitary gland has not been damaged. Clomiphene is commonly given daily as a 50 mg tablet from the fifth through the ninth days after uterine bleeding begins. If amenorrhea has been present progesterone should be administered to cause withdrawal bleeding before clomiphene administration. Ovulation usually occurs 8 to 10 days after the last clomiphene tablet. When 50 mg daily is not effective, the dose may be gradually increased up to 200 mg per day. For some patients who do not ovulate with clomiphene therapy, HCG can be added to induce ovulation.

When there has been damage to the pituitary and/or hypothalmus, clomiphene will not be effective and human menopausal gonadotropin can be administered along with HCG to cause ovulation. The use of gonadotropins in this manner is expensive and demands careful observation lest excessive stimulation of the ovary occur which may result in the formation of large, friable cysts that can rupture and cause intraperitoneal bleeding. These agents should be used only by experienced gynecologists.

When anovulation is associated with hyperprolactinemia, the physician must evaluate the duration of the problem, the height of prolactin blood levels, and the size of the pituitary tumor if present to decide on a proper course of treatment. With polytomographic evidence of a microadenoma, experience has shown that ovulation will occur after the administration of bromocryptine and that with subsequent pregnancies seldom does the pituitary enlarge enough to damage the optic nerve tracts. Some patients with moderate increases in prolactin have responded with more regular ovulation after the administration of bromocryptine in the absence of any evidence of pituitary structural change.

Most hypothyroid states are diagnosed before the patients come for infertility investigation; however, some minor hypothyroid states may be found that will respond to thyroxin preparations. A few of these patients may be found to have increased levels of prolactin due to excess TRH.

Therapy for other causes of anovulation is given in Chapter 14.

Uterine disease

Destruction or removal of a considerable portion of the endocervix may impair production of endocervical mucus and also cause stenosis of the cervix. Dilatations may offer some relief from the stenosis but there is no way to reproduce the destroyed endocervix. Fortunately, this is not an absolute cause of infertility. Changes in the endometrial cavity due to anomalies usually do not prevent pregnancy but impair the uterus's ability to carry the pregnancy to term. Surgical correction affords good results.

When adhesions obliterate a portion of the uterine cavity they can usually be surgically released; however, successful pregnancy is limited. When feasible, removal of myomas or polyps that impinge on the endometrial cavity offers a good prognosis.

Myomectomy for large tumors and for tumors causing malposition of the ovary or tube should be done with meticulous care to preserve blood supply and avoid adhesions.

Tubal surgery

When tubal obstruction is found the physician must classify the extent of tubal distortion. The finding of extensive tubal adhesions and ovarian adhesions is usually indicative of marked change in the endosalpinx and the tubal musculature, making surgical correction unfeasible. The best prognosis is found in those patients who have had a tubal sterilizing operation done with a band or clip. (Patients who have had destruction of the tube by electrosurgical means usually have so much tubal destruction that operation is much less successful.) The best prognosis seems to be for those patients with minimal tubal loss and with frimbrial adhesion.

Tubal patency cannot be equated with tubal function; many patients with patent tubes after surgical correction have impaired function and pregnancy does not result. Similarly the possibility of tubal pregnancy occurring is much increased. Microsurgical techniques have allowed more meticulous and accurate anastomosis of tubal structures and more precise hemostasis. Some recent results indicate a higher rate of successful pregnancies after microsurgery in properly selected patients.

Endometriosis

The reader is referred to Chapter 11.

Sperm antibodies

Sperm antibodies cause agglutination or immobilization when present in the serum or endocervical mucus. If Condoms are used for 6 months, antigenic stimulation by sperm or seminal fluid will be avoided.

The use of artificial insemination with donor sperm is usually successful within three cycles for fertile women. When the husband is absolutely infertile, has relative infertility that does not respond to therapy, or has a genetically transmissable disorder, the couple after proper consideration may request artificial insemination. Legal counsel is essential to provide legal security for all concerned, including the child.

If conception does not occur for several years, although no reason for sterility is determined after thorough investigation, adoption is advised. Many couples remain childless when no definitive cause can be ascertained. Functional infertility appears to be psychogenic at times.

SELECTED REFERENCES

Annos, T., Thompson, I.E., and Taymor, M.L.: Luteal phase deficiency and infertility: difficulties encountered in diagnosis and treatment, Obstet. Gynecol. **55**:705, 1980.

Asherman, J.G.: Uterine synechiae, J. Obstet. Gynecol. Brit. Emp. **55**:23, 1948.

Black, T.L., Cox, R.I., and Cox, L.W.: Ovulation induction for the treatment of infertility, Aust. N.Z.J. Obstet. Gynaec. **9**:209, 1969.

Bonney, V.: The fruits of conservatism, J. Obstet. Gynaec. Br. Emp. **44**:1, 1937.

Franklin, R.R., and Dukes, C.D.: Antispermatozoal antibody and unexplained infertility, Am. J. Obstet. Gynecol. **89**:6, 1964.

Holloway, A.: Some legal aspects of artificial insemination, Obstet. Gynecol. **7**:621, 1956.

Holman, A.W.: Hysterosalpingography in the study of sterility, West. J. Surg. **64**:971, 1952.

MacLeod, J.: Human male infertility, Obstet. Gynecol. Surv. **26**:335, 1971.

Mishell, D.R., and Davajan, V.: Reproductive endocrinology, infertility and contraception, Philadelphia, 1979, F.A. Davis Co.

Moghissi, K.S., Sacco, A.G., and Borin, K.: Immunologic infertility, cervical mucus antibodies and post-coital tests, Am. J. Obstet. Gynecol. **136**:941, 1980.

Rock, J., Mulligan, W.J., and Easterday, C.L.: Polyethylene in tuboplasty, Obstet. Gynecol. **3**:21, 1954.

Rubin, I.C.: Myomectomy in the interest of fertility, Tr. New Jersey Obstet. Gynecol. Soc. **2**:7, 1957.

Rubin, I.C.: Therapeutic aspects of uterotubal insufflation in sterility, Am. J. Obstet. Gynecol. **50**:621, 1945.

Valle, R.F.: Hysteroscopy in the evaluation of female infertility, Am. J. Obstet. Gynecol. **137**:425, 1980.

Wallach, E.E., and Kempers, R.D.: AFS modern trends in infertility and conception control, Baltimore 1979, The Williams & Wilkins Co.

Wilson, R.B., Overton, D.H., Jr., and Decker, D.G.:Minimal versus intensive therapy of infertility, Int. J. Fertil. **4**:220, 1959.

Woltz, J.H., Bradford, W.Z., Bradford, W.B., and McCoy, J.B.: Complications of hysterosalpingography, Am. J. Obstet. Gynecol. **76**:736, 1958.

Chapter 16

CONTRACEPTION

Contraceptive advice should be routinely offered at the time of premarital examination and during postpartum visits. Patients may come at other times to ask advice and instruction when they have gained information from friends, magazines, or news media. The selection of the best method for a particular couple will entail evaluation of the knowledge, attitudes, and practices of the patient. Although the patient's cooperation is essential, the final judgment can be best made by the well-informed physician who ascertains the patient's anatomic and physiologic status and her motivation.

Surgical methods causing permanent sterility are being used more commonly since family size is more limited. Interruption of the tubal continuity or operation on the vas deferens of the husband should be decided upon only after thorough consideration of the state and function of the uterus. A consideration of menstrual cycles without oral contraceptives is necessary when deciding whether hysterectomy should possibly be the sterilizing operation. If functional bleeding has been a problem and if cervicitis has been bothersome, hysterectomy may be the preferred operation.

Methods used without the aid of a physician or trained assistants are (1) withdrawal before ejaculation (coitus interruptus); (2) condom; (3) douche; and (4) vaginal spermicides in jellies, creams, aerosol foams, or suppositories. Abstinence during the expected time of ovulation (rhythm) may be practiced with or without basal temperature records to indicate that the postovulatory temperature rise caused by progestogens has occurred. If the rhythm method is to be used, instruction supplemented with written instructions will increase the likelihood of effectiveness. The more variation in the length of the cycle, the more essential is temperature recording. It should be emphasized that the day of ovulation cannot be determined prospectively but can be reliably estimated retrospectively; i.e., when a temperature rise of 0.6° F has been noted for 3 days, it can be assumed that ovulation has occurred. It is necessary that this elevation be observed for at least 3 days to avoid the confusion that may result in temperature elevations brought on by other causes.

Observation of the increased watery mucus that occurs just before ovulation is used by some patients in avoiding the fertile time. When there are prolonged proliferative phases and cycles without ovulation this method does not assist the patient.

The effectiveness of the methods already mentioned varies greatly with individual couples but is less than the methods requiring physician's services. The most effective methods are the use of (1) a vaginal diaphragm with a contraceptive cream or jelly, (2) oral medication to inhibit ovulation, and (3) intrauterine devices.

DIAPHRAGMS

In using a diaphragm it is essential that it remain in the proper position, covering the cervix posteriorly and placed behind the symphysis pubis anteriorly. The diaphragm prevents the deposition of the ejaculate into the cervical canal, so that mixing with the spermacide will occur. If the patient has a sizable cystocele—or more particularly a cystourethrocele—and/or the outlet support is inadequate, the diaphragm will not remain in the proper protecting position and should not be used. There are special diaphragms with unusual shapes that can sometimes be fitted successfully in patients with moderate degrees of vaginal relaxation.

To determine the correct diaphragm size, fitting rings (the rubber-covered spring forming the rim) are placed in the vagina, and the size that fits snugly, but not tightly, behind the symphysis pubis and in the posterior vaginal fornix is selected. The technique of placement is demonstrated with or without an introducer to hold the diaphragm. The need to apply the spermicidal jelly or cream on the device is emphasized. The patient should remove and replace the diaphragm so that the instructor can determine that she has learned the method. She must be taught to feel the cervix to ensure that it is properly covered.

The time of placement of the diaphragm can be immediately before coitus or several hours before. It has been advocated that the woman place the diaphragm daily, but more commonly it is placed only when coitus is anticipated. The psychologic aftermath of unrewarded preparation may be distressing. Similarly a cold diaphragm and a cold jelly temporarily, at least, reduce vaginal response to sexual excitation. The annoyance of the exuding jelly or cream during or after coitus can be noted by both the woman and her partner. These annoyances of diaphragm usage, along with the failure to insert the gadget once excitation has started, are probably the most common reasons for failure of this method. Occasionally patients attempt to use the diaphragm without the needed spermicide, and on rare occasions there may be a sensitivity reaction to ricinoleic acid, phenylmercuric acetate, or other spermicides. Among the fringe benefits from the use of this method is the fact that an additional lubricant is needed by some patients, and others find that vaginitis and cystitis are less common using the contraceptive creams and jellies.

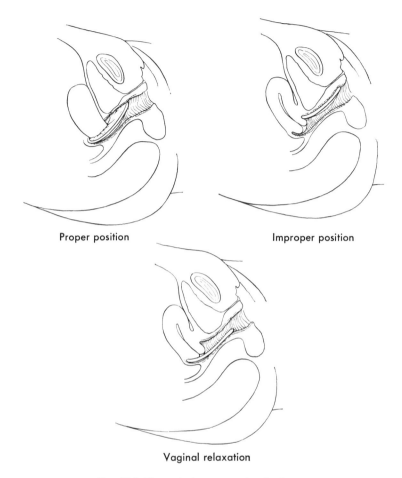

Proper position   Improper position

Vaginal relaxation

Fig. 16-1. The vaginal contraceptive diaphragm.

The pregnancy rate for this method is about 6 to 12 per 100 woman years in family planning clinics. Highly motivated women after proper instruction may attain rates of 1 per 100 woman years.

ORAL CONTRACEPTION

The availability of low-cost oral progestogens to be taken with estrogens has allowed the cyclic employment of these substances in combination to inhibit ovulation. Progestogens render the cervical mucus unfavorable to spermatozoa, and when progestogens are employed with the estrogens early in the menstrual cycle, the endometrium that develops is poorly prepared for implantation. Commonly, to inhibit ovulation the steroids are started on the fifth day of the menstrual cycle and continued through the twenty-fourth or twenty-fifth day. Usually on the third day after the last tablet is taken withdrawal bleeding occurs. When the progestogen and estrogen are combined in the same tablet for the 20 or 21 days of administration, the method is termed combined oral contraception. When the estrogen is given for the first 15 days and combined with progestogen for the last 5 or 6 days, the method is called sequential oral contraception.

The response of the endometrium is quite different in these two methods, and similarly the response in secretion of cervical mucus is different. From the patient's viewpoint the most marked change with the combined method is apt to be diminution in the amount of bleeding at the time of menstruation and in the number of days during which bleeding occurs. The endometrium does not develop to the usual degree of thickness and is less vascular when the progestogen is employed early and throughout the 20 days. When the endometrium is studied histologically, there is a minimal proliferation during the first week of combined therapy; by day 10 there is some subnuclear secretion and slight gland tortuosity; by day 14 of the cycle regressive changes are occurring, resulting in narrowed glands and flat epithelium; and by day 21 some stromal predecidual changes are taking place. Within a day or two after the combined tablet is started the amount of cervical mucus is usually decreased and the viscosity and cloudiness of the mucus become more marked. Sperm motility within the mucus is similarly reduced, and when the mucus is examined for ferning none is noted. Of course, if the patient were to take her basal temperature, the elevation associated with progestogens would be noted with the combined therapy. Withdrawal bleeding usually begins the third day after the last tablet is taken, and this interval tends to vary little in an individual patient. About 2% of patients who continue a combined method over 1 year or more may, at times, notice no withdrawal bleeding when the medication is stopped. Occasionally this occurs in the first or second cycle of administration. If it does occur, the patient is instructed to begin tablets again in 7 days, expecting that at the next time they are stopped withdrawal bleeding will occur. When combined therapy is used the appearance of the cervix is very much like that of early pregnancy, and increased growth of *Candida* in the vagina with the associated pruritus occurs at times in patients.

When the sequential method of administration is employed, the endometrium behaves somewhat like that during a normal cycle in which ovulation occurs. However, since only estrogen is administered through day 20 of the cycle, proliferation continues over this period. On days 23 to 28 of the cycle, pronounced subnuclear secretion occurs with tortuosity of glands caused by the added progestogen. The amount of bleeding is likely to be about what the patient has been previously experiencing. The thickness and vascularity of the endometrium are approximately the same as with an ovulatory menstrual cycle.

When the sequential method is used, the amount of cervical mucus is rather markedly increased 2 days after the estrogen is started, and this continues until the estrogen is opposed in its action by the progestogen. If the patient has an eversion of the cervix and produces excessive mucus, the amount of the thin, watery mucus that is produced with stimulation by the estrogen is apt to be quite annoying to her and, at times, will go through her clothing. This mucus is of low viscosity, is clear, and presents a marked ferning reaction. When the progestogen has been administered for 48 hours, the viscosity is increased and cloudiness and lack of ferning appear. The gross appearance of the cervix with sequential therapy is somewhat like that of pregnancy. If there has been an eversion, the protrusion of the endocervix may be more marked. Without the effect of progestogen over a longer period of time, as occurs with the combined method, *Candida* does not grow as rapidly and there is less likelihood of pruritus that is caused by this organism. In 1976, sequential oral contraceptives were withdrawn from the market because of a reported increased incidence of endometrial carcinoma and breast cancer as determined by retrospective studies.

To inhibit ovulation by influencing the hypothalamus and pituitary so that there is a decrease in FSH and LH secretion, 50 μg of ethinyl estradiol or 80 μg of mestranol is required when given alone to be 98% effective. When progestogens in the following amounts are added, almost 100% inhibition of ovulation occurs: norethindrone, 1 mg; norethindrone acetate, 1 mg; norethynodrel, 2.5 mg; norgestrel, 0.5 mg; or ethynodiol diacetate, 1 mg. When the estrogen is reduced to ethinyl estradiol 30 combined with 0.075 mg norgestrel or to ethinyl estradiol with 0.35 mg norethindrone, ovulation is inhibited in a high percentage of patients. Various dosages in various combinations are available.

Progestogens administered alone in continuous small doses (0.35 mg norethindrone or 0.075 mg norgestrel) inhibit ovulation in about 50% of patients. Although the pregnancy rate is only about 3%, irregular bleeding is common and the "minipills" are not favored. The lower dose estrogen-progestogen combinations cause pregnancy rates to be about 0.2% per year and better regulate the bleeding; however, breakthrough bleeding is common enough to require higher doses in many women.

The progestogens have different progestogenic, estrogenic, and androgenic effects that must be considered in selecting the proper oral contraceptive for each patient.

Oral contraceptives may cause minor disturbances that will concern patients. Nausea with or without vomiting may occur in a minority of women. Some patients will experience nausea to such a degree that the medications must be abandoned. Mild nausea frequently does not require any antiemetic medication and will subside with continued usage. There is frequently sufficient breast stimulation to cause mild breast tenderness. With continued usage of the medication, mastalgia subsides somewhat as it does during pregnancy.

Breakthrough bleeding may occur at times. It is often associated with failure to take medication over a 1- or 2-day period. For some patients it is an indication that the strength of the estrogen and progestogen must be increased. At times when the combined-type tablets are used there is no withdrawal bleeding when the medication is discontinued. This failure is particularly apt to occur after the preparation has been used over many months. Pregnancy does not occur under these circumstances, and the patient should be instructed to resume the tablets on the regular schedule after not taking them for 7 days. As previously mentioned, the amount of bleeding at the time of withdrawal is apt to be less than previously noted when the combined pill is taken. This decrease will concern some patients if it is unanticipated.

A few patients note a tendency toward fluid retention when these steroids are employed. There are some women who apparently have a weight gain related to use of these agents. Estrogens are anabolic, and progestogens are catabolic. Some patients tend to retain more nitrogen when using oral contraceptives. Frequently weight can be lost while taking oral contraceptives and usually weight gain is not a major problem. Patients complain of increased fluid retention, which is associated with administration of estrogens; however, if the dose of estrogen is sufficiently low, fluid retention is not likely to occur or can be compensated for by decreased oral intake of sodium compounds.

For some patients estrogens with progestogens tend to increase deposition of pigment in the skin. Particularly patients who have noted chloasma during pregnancy are apt to have increased pigmentation while taking oral contraceptives. For cosmetic reasons they may desire to discontinue the agents. After discontinuance the pigment is apt to remain. Not infrequently psychoneurotic manifestations are noted after the administration of oral contraceptives and are particularly apt to occur in patients who have had recurrent anxiety for other reasons. The mystery of the pill, along with startling reports by news media, no doubt adds to this problem.

Whereas the disturbances mentioned previously are not of a serious nature, other changes in patients receiving oral contraceptives are of more importance. Infrequently hypertension makes its appearance after the administration of these agents. Study indicates that in some patients angiotensinogen and plasma renin are increased. Perhaps these factors play a part in the hypertension that some patients experience and that subsides after discontinuing oral contraceptives. Rarely patients receiving estrogens and progestogens develop jaundice. In patients with genetic or acquired defects of liver excretion, illness is apt to occur. Sulfobromophthalein (BSP) retention is noted in some patients. In susceptible individuals there may be an increase in glutamic oxaloacetic transaminase (SGOT). Increases may also be noted in glutamic pyruvic transaminase (SGPT) and in alkaline phosphatase. The patients with compromised liver function should not receive oral contraceptives. Recently cases of nodular hyperplasia, adenoma, hamartoma, carcinoma, and vein thrombosis of the liver have been reported. Some patients with diabetes find that regulation of their carbohydrate metabolism is more difficult when they are taking oral contraceptives, whereas others find that they tolerate oral contraceptives well. Examiners should be mindful of the fact that the changes in glucose tolerance that occur in some patients taking oral contraceptives are similar to those changes that occur during pregnancy. Patients with migraine headaches may notice more frequent headaches while using oral contraceptives. Since there may be a confusion as to the possibility of cerebral thrombosis, when there is doubt oral contraceptives should be discontinued in patients with recurrent severe headaches. Some patients with epilepsy tend to have an increase in convulsions while using oral contraceptives; however, the majority of such patients will tolerate oral contraception. When leiomyomas are present in the uterus, they may more rapidly increase in size under the influence of estrogens; however, in many patients with myomas there is no notable increase. To evaluate thyroid function, one must remember that estrogens increase thyronine-binding protein. Accordingly in the evaluation of thyroid hormone determinations one must take this into consideration, as it is taken into consideration during pregnancy. Similarly, transcortin, the protein to which adrenal corticosteroids are bound, is increased.

The most serious consideration in the employment of oral contraceptives is the possibility of vascular thrombosis and embolism. In retrospective case studies it has been well estimated that about 1 in 2000 patients using oral contraceptives will be hospitalized each year. Associated deaths from vascular complications are estimated to occur in patients under 35 years of age using oral contraceptives at a rate of 1 per 66,000 per year. The death rate for women 35 years and over is 1 in 25,000 per year. The infrequency of these complications in patients using oral contraceptives would indicate that the problems are complex and that the steroids employed are but one of many factors involved. Thrombosis in veins can occur and might be accounted for by the fact that some patients have increase in vein size and distensibility, as well as increase in clotting factors VII, VIII, and X, when these agents are used. For some there is an increase in number of platelets and the tendency of the platelets to clump. Investigation indicates that there tends to be an increase in fibrin and fibrinolysis. Studies in laboratory animals and in humans have shown that endothelial hyperplasia and intimal thickening occur in some arteries. Since the complex nature of clotting and the dissolution of clots are incompletely understood, there is little wonder that there is considerable confusion regarding the importance of oral contraceptives as a cause of thrombosis. For patients who have large veins and reasons for decreased venous circulation these agents should be avoided. Those patients with a history of embolism should not receive oral contraceptives. Recent thrombophlebitis of the lower extremity is a contraindication for usage. Since cerebral thrombosis and pseudotumor cerebri have occurred in patients utilizing oral contraceptives, these agents should not be used when there are indications that these disorders may occur.

Growth of neoplasms of the breast, benign and malignant, may be stimulated by estrogens. Benign tumors of the breast should be removed before patients are given oral contraceptives, and patients with breast malignancies should not be given estrogens as a means of preventing pregnancy. When there is any doubt as to the presence of endometrial cancer, these agents should be avoided. From information presently available it is suggested that estrogens and progestogens have no influence on cancer of the cervix.

For the mother who desires to breast-feed her child these agents should be avoided as they tend to decrease lactation.

After discontinuing oral contraceptives a prolonged period of amenorrhea ensues for some patients. This is particularly likely to occur when there have been periods of amenorrhea previous to use of oral contraceptives. When failure of ovulation occurs clomiphene may be given to bring about ovulation. Since this agent is usually effective, postpartum amenorrhea does not cause as much concern as it did formerly; however, the rare possibilities of pituitary or adrenal tumors coincidentally developing deserve consideration.

There are many benefits for the patient receiving estrogens and progestogens for oral contraception. Dysmenorrhea is usually relieved with suppression of ovulation. Frequently premenstrual tension is diminished or abolished. In a patient with irregular cycles of menstruation the regularity associated with withdrawal bleeding of oral contraception affords considerable relief and convenience. When the combined method of oral contraception is used, hypermenorrhea is usually relieved. Acne is usually markedly diminished with use of estrogens. Hirsutism is apt to be improved with the use of estrogenic preparations. Along with the prevention of uterine pregnancy with its complications, ectopic gestation is also prevented by this method. Frequently there is improvement in sexual response. Often the pain of endometriosis is relieved, as there is an associated atrophy of the glandular element and a softening of the fibrous tissue reaction of endometriosis. It is apparent that this method offers many fringe benefits, and it is little wonder that it is the first choice of so many women.

When oral contraception has not been used and the patient has had an isolated exposure to conception, as may occur with rape, estrogens may be administered to prevent pregnancy. Estrogens are usually administered in large doses (at least 20 mg of conjugated estrogens) for 5 days or more. When ovulation is not inhibited, the next menstrual flow is expected to occur on schedule.

INTRAUTERINE DEVICES

It has been known for many years that objects placed in the uterus will prevent pregnancy in humans as well as in certain animals. Previously metallic devices were used. Whereas some of the previous devices were designed to avoid or hinder entrance of spermatozoa into the cervix, the currently used devices function because of their position within the endometrial cavity. When plastics, which cause little tissue reaction and are inexpensive, became available, interests were renewed in employing this method of preventing pregnancy. The devices have been of various shapes and sizes to fit the uterine cavity. Formerly many were designed with a portion projecting through and out of the cervix that would allow palpation by the patient so that she could be sure that the device was in place. More recently devices designed without any rigid protruding portion have a monofilament thread protruding so that the position of the device can be ascertained and it can be easily removed when desired.

Studies have revealed that spermatozoa can traverse the cervix and the endometrial cavity with devices in place. The most commonly accepted hypothesis as to the mode of action of the IUD is that a leukocytic mobilization is provoked. The macrophages destroy sperm and probably act on the blastocyst. Studies in animals indicate that there is an increase in tubal and uterine motility when objects are placed in the uterus. Recent studies indicate that when copper is placed on the plastic there is an increase in the leukocytic response and a decrease in frequency of conception. Intrauterine pregnancies have occurred in about 2% of patients with plastic intrauterine devices in place. Tubal gestation has occurred in about 0.1% of women using the device for a year. When intrauterine pregnancy does occur, abortions are anticipated in 35% of patients with the IUD remaining in place. Incidence of abortion is increased when the device is removed or when soundings are performed to determine whether the device is still present. When pregnancy has proceeded to term there has been no increase in deformities of the fetus. Various types of devices are illustrated in Fig. 16-2. Thus far the Lippes loop, the Safe-T-Coil, and the Cu-7 have been the most popular devices. Adding a possible 200 sq mm of copper appears effective in reducing conception rates to the minimum.

A device is now available with progesterone in the large limb of the T, which will allow for the slow release of progesterone over a period of 12 months. The amount of progesterone is sufficient to affect the endometrium and improve the contaceptive effect of the device. It also appears to decrease the amount of bleeding from the endometrium and diminish the likelihood of dysmenorrhea.

Insertion of an intrauterine device is usually accomplished without anesthesia. In patients who have had a pregnancy it can usually be placed without difficulty at the time of menstruation, when there is less cervical resistance. For the nulligravid individual considerable pain is encountered because of the narrowness of the cer-

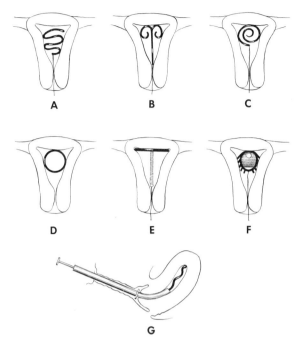

Fig. 16-2. Intrauterine contraceptive devices. **A,** Lippes loop. **B,** Safe-T-Coil. **C,** Margulies coil. **D,** Ring. **E,** Tatum T. **F,** Dalkon shield. **G,** Insertion of Lippes loop.

vix, and this means of contraception is often avoided. There is a danger of uterine perforation at the time of insertion. When performed by properly trained physicians perforation should occur in less than 1 in 1000 insertions. When the device does perforate through the uterus into the peritoneal cavity, it should be removed. The possibility of peritonitis must be considered, and, if a closed ring device has been used, intestinal obstruction may occur. Copper causes a marked peritoneal reaction. Infection at the time of insertion may occur because the endocervix commonly harbors pathogenic bacteria. Such infections have been reported immediately after insertion in approximately 1.3% of patients. If there is any question as to the presence of active cervical infection or pelvic inflammatory disease, insertions should not be performed.

Studies of large numbers of patients have revealed that there is an increased incidence of salpingitis, both gonorrheal and caused by other organisms, with IUDs in place. The severity of infection appears to be increased. A peculiar syndrome of unilateral salpingitis has been found. When early pregnancy and threatening abortion occurs the probability of infection is markedly increased if an IUD is in position. Because of the likelihood of such infection, it is advised that all IUDs be removed when pregnancy is diagnosed and the string is still available.

After the device is inserted there is some trauma to the endometrium that will result in bleeding for several days. Frequently there is some light bleeding in between menstrual periods. The menstrual flow may be increased. Approximately 10% of IUDs are removed because of the amount or duration of bleeding.

Although the devices are designed so that expulsion should not occur, expulsion is apt to occur particularly during the first month. This may be brought about because the device is not placed entirely within the uterine cavity but is allowed to partially remain in the cervix. Expulsions have been reported in 8% or more of inserted Lippes D loops and for 2.3% of inserted shields. Usually the patient will observe the device when it comes from the vagina. On occasion the tie that is left protruding from the cervix will be displaced within the cervical canal or within the uterus. When this occurs the observer may question whether the device still remains in the uterine cavity. Passage of a sound may allow one to "feel" the device with the end of the sound. Ultrasound visualization may allow determination of the position of the device. X-ray examination with another device or opaque object placed in the uterine cavity will allow proper determination. When the tie has retracted, removal of the device can be accomplished with the proper instruments.

As already detailed, IUDs do not entirely prevent pregnancy, and infection or bleeding may occur after their insertion. Before deciding on the advisability of insertion of an IUD the physician must consider the possibility of complication or confusion. If the patient has irregular or excessive uterine bleeding, she should not have a device inserted. If dysmenorrhea or pelvic pain is a problem, the patient should not have a device inserted. If a patient is particularly susceptible to bacterial endocarditis because of congenital heart disease or damage secondary to rheumatic fever, the device should not be used. Patients with blood dyscrasia resulting in defects in coagulation should not use IUDs. When there is deformity of the cavity because of anomalies of development or because of uterine myomas, the devices are best avoided. When bleeding does occur in patients with IUDs, confusion as to the diagnosis of cancer or complications of pregnancy are apt to occur. From the preceding information it is evident that IUDs should be used only for patients who are found to be normal on examination and who have normal menstrual cycles.

SELECTION OF METHOD

For the physician to properly advise a patient on the best method of contraception for her, he must ascertain (1) any disorder requiring treatment that would be benefited by oral contraceptives, (2) technical feasibility of using a diaphragm or device, and (3) any contraindications to use of a method. The attitudes and opinions of the patient as to moral interpretation, degree of effectiveness desired, motivation to employ method, cooperation, and fears of complications must be determined.

When medical reasons do not indicate selection of one method, the patient should be informed about each method and allowed to choose the one she finds most acceptable. At times methods should be changed to better suit a particular patient.

Routine follow-up examinations should be done to determine any difficulties the patient may have in employing the method and any complications of the method. Such routine examinations also provide opportunity for surveys to find evidence of diseases in an effort to better assist women in maintaining good health.

SELECTED REFERENCES

AMA drug evaluation, ed. 2, Chicago, 1971, American Medical Association.

Andrews, W.C.: Oral contraception, Obstet. Gynecol. Surv. **26:**477, 1971.

Cohen, B.J.B., and Gibor, Y.: Anemia and menstrual blood loss, Obstet. Gynecol. Surv. **35:**597, 1980.

Edelman, D.A., Berger, G.S., and Keith, L.: Intrauterine devices and their complications, Boston, 1979, G.K. Hall.

Gall, S.A., Bourgeois, C.H., and Maguire, R.: The morphologic effects of oral contraceptive agents on the cervix, J.A.M.A. **207:**2243, 1969.

Hall, H.H., and Stone, M.L.: Observations on the use of the intrauterine pessary, with special reference to the Gräfenberg ring, Am. J. Obstet. Gynecol. **83:**683, 1962.

Hartman, C.G.: Science and the safe period, Baltimore, 1962, The Williams & Wilkins Co.

Israel, R., and Davis, H.J.: Effect of intrauterine contraceptive devices on the endometrium, J.A.M.A. **195:**764, 1966.

Kahn, H.S., and Tyler, C.E.: I.U.D. related hospitalizations, United States and Puerto Rico 1973, J.A.M.A. **234:**53, 1975.

Lief, Harold K.: The physician and family planning, J.A.M.A. **197:**646, 1966.

Lippes, J.: A study of intra-uterine contraception: development of a plastic loop, Excerpta Medica International Congress Series No. 54, 1962, pp. 69-75.

Mastroianni, L., and Rosseau, C.H.: Influence of the intrauterine coil on ovum transport and sperm distribution in the monkey, Am. J. Obstet. Gynecol. **93:**416, 1965.

Morgulies, L.C.: Permanent reversible contraception with an intrauterine plastic spiral (permaspiral), Excerpta Medica International Congress Series No. 54, 1962, pp. 61-68.

Nissin, E.D., Kent, D.R., Nissen, S.E., and McRae, D.M.: Association of liver tumors with oral contraceptives, Obstet. Gynecol. **48:**49, 1976.

Peel, J., and Potts, M.: Textbook of contraceptive practice, Cambridge, 1970, Cambridge University Press.

Penfield, A.J.: Female sterilization by minilaparotomy or open laparoscopy, Baltimore, 1980, Urban & Schwarzenberg.

Pincus, Gregory: The control of fertility, New York, 1965, Academic Press, Inc.

Oppenheimer, W.: Prevention of pregnancy by the Gräfenberg ring method: an evaluation after 28 years' experience, Am. J. Obstet. Gynecol. **78:**446, 1959.

Sagiruglu, N., and Sagiruglu, E.: Biologic mode of action of Lippe's loop in intrauterine contraception, Am. J. Obstet. Gynecol. **106:**506, 1970.

Segal, S.J., Southam, A.L., and Shafer, K.D., editors: Intra-uterine contraceptive devices, Proceedings of the Conference, New York, April 30 to May 1, 1962, Excerpta International Congress Series No. 86.

Tietze, C.: Contraception with intrauterine devices, Am. J. Obstet. Gynecol. **96:**1043, 1966.

Tietze, C., and Lewit, S., editors: Intra-uterine contraceptive devices, Proceedings of the Conference, New York, April 30 to May 1, 1962, Excerpta Medica International Congress Series No. 54.

Willson, J.R., Bollinger, C.C., and Ledger, W.J.: The effect of an intrauterine contraceptive device on the bacterial flora of the endometrial cavity, Am. J. Obstet. Gynecol. **90:**726, 1964.

Zipper, J.A., Tatum, H.J., Medel, M., Pastene, L., and Rivera, M.: Contraception through the use of intrauterine metals. I. Copper as an adjunct to the "T," Am. J. Obstet. Gynecol. **109:**771, 1971.

Chapter 17

MISCELLANEOUS DISTURBANCES

CLIMACTERIC

The climacteric is a period during which there is a gradual decline in ovarian function. Its onset is before the menopause (cessation of menstruation) and its end is months or years later. It is evidenced by a decrease in ovarian size and by the changes of diminished estrogen stimulation. After the menopause, atrophy of the genitals and breasts is manifested by gross and microscopic changes. In the spontaneous climacteric, menstruation usually becomes less frequent and tends to decrease in amount before cessation takes place.

Causes. Cessation of menstruation may occur in many ways.

Spontaneous. The ovary fails to respond to gonadotropic stimulation. FSH increases in amount after the menopause because there is not sufficient estrogen inhibition.

Hysterectomy. Although endometrial shedding is absent, the ovary will continue to function after hysterectomy. The evidences of lack of estrogen will not be noted until the patient attains her usual age of spontaneous menopause.

Bilateral oophorectomy. When the principal sources of estrogens and progestogens are removed, endometrial bleeding will not occur. Cytologic and histologic changes occur that are demonstrable in the vagina, although in young women estrogens and progestogens are produced in small quantities by the adrenal cortex and nonglandular conversion of estrogen precursors occurs.

Ovarian radiation. External radiation therapy applied to the ovary or application of radium in the vagina and the uterus, of sufficient amount, will cause ovarian atrophy to take place.

Symptoms. The majority of women have some symptoms that are associated with the climacteric. Therapy is required in about 15% of women because of the disturbances that occur.

Hot flushes are sudden waves of warmth that the patient feels passing over her body, particularly in the upper thoracic and facial regions. A redness of the skin may be noted and sweating may follow. These changes are vasomotor in origin and are the most typical symptoms of the climacteric. Hot flushes occur with excess catecholamine release (as with pheochromocytoma) and have been recently found to be immediately preceded by a surge of LH. They may occur in men and in women with regular menstruation. Estrogen deprivation is the common, but not the only, cause. Flushes that awaken the patient at night and are followed by sweats are more apt to be relieved by estrogens. Psychic disturbances can cause flushes and must be duly considered in the evaluation of the climacteric woman. They serve as the most reliable guide to the severity of the climacteric disturbance.

Nervousness and *anxiety* are common complaints. Fatigue, headache, insomnia, dizziness, palpitation, and frigidity are likewise common. It is readily recognized that these symptoms are usually of psychosomatic origin. In evaluating the psycho-dynamics of women during this period one must be aware of numerous factors that often are significant: (1) pregnancy is no longer likely or desirable, (2) physical stamina is decreasing, and (3) the problem of waning physical attractiveness may be coupled with problems caused by (a) children growing up and leaving home, (b) old and perhaps disabled relatives requiring care, and (c) a husband with lost youth becoming unfaithful.

Menstrual irregularities run the gamut from amenorrhea to hypermenorrhea. Short periods of amenorrhea may cause the patient concern as to whether pregnancy has occurred. Although a decreasing amount of menstrual discharge is usual, some patients experience excessive flow. There may be intermittent spotting to cause the patient further concern by activating fear of cancer.

Management. The subjective nature of the complaints of the menopause should not be used as the total means of diagnosis. Physical examination should demonstrate some evidence of decreased estrogen stimulation of the breast, vulva, vaginal mucosa, and uterus. The lack of cornified cells in the vagina with an increase of leukocytes and red blood cells is a typical picture of hypoestrogenism. In examination one not only should search for evidences of decreased estrogen stimulation but also one should completely interrogate and examine the patient lest a more serious disorder be overlooked. When there is hypermenorrhea or intermenstrual bleeding in women of this age a thorough search for cancer is imperative. Routine cytologic studies are in order; frequent endometrial biopsy and diagnostic curettage, when deemed necessary, are the principal methods of investigation. Should no evidence of neoplasia be found, thee management of dysfunctional bleeding is as has been presented in Chapter 14.

Hot flushes, when severe enough to cause annoyance, can usually be abolished with small doses of estrogens such as Premarin administered in a dosage of 1.25 mg daily. Medroxyprogesterone acetate can be given to patients who do not tolerate estrogens and may relieve hot flushes. (Obviously when the uterus is absent this type of administration is not necessary.) Ethinyl estradiol, 0.01 mg daily, may be used. Oral administration is in order. Rarely is a parenteral method justified. Cyclic administration with omission for 5 to 7 days each month is advisable to decrease incidence of endometrial bleeding. Recent reports indicate endometrial hyperplasia or adenocarcinoma is prevented by combining 10 mg of medroxyprogesterone acetate or 5 mg of norethindrone acetate daily with the last 10 estrogen tablets to cause cyclic withdrawal bleeding.

To control the variety of symptoms that are basically psychic in origin it is essential to have an adequate understanding of the patient. Psychotherapy includes "airing" problems, education, reassurance, and guidance in channeling interest into rewarding enterprises such as care of grandchildren, civic organizations, religious work, gainful regular employment, and hobbies. Small doses of tranquilizers or of phenobarbital may do much to relieve the patient's anxiety and to improve her ability to sleep.

In women of this age reactive depressions are likely to occur. When the depressions are of severe degree, proper psychiatric care is in order. Estrogen administration has proved to be of limited value in the management of these patients.

Osteoporosis may occur after the menopause. The administration of estrogens and androgens affords some relief, although the radiologic changes are usually not reversed. To be effective, estrogens must be of sufficient dosage to cause endometrial bleeding; consequently estrogen and progestogen given sequentially to allow monthly control of bleeding are preferred. Pains about the joints have been attributed to the decrease in estrogens; however, one should be careful in administering estrogens solely for this indication.

Cornification may be used as a guide to the need of estrogens; however, symptomatic relief may not occur though vaginal response is excellent. In senile vaginitis the relief of symptoms is correlated with the cytologic changes in the vagina.

Long-term use of estrogens must take into consideration the increased risk of endometrial cancer. Most cancers related to extrinsic estrogens have been Stage IA. To find endometrial, precancerous, atypical, adenomatous hyperplasia or early stage cancer any abnormal uterine bleeding must be investigated by adequate biopsy. There is some conflicting evidence that long-term use of estrogens may increase the incidence of breast cancer. Most studies show no such association. There is no good information to suggest that cardiovascular diseases, including thromboembolic events, are related to estrogen administration in postmenopausal patients.

The decrease or absence of libido is related to so many factors throughout the entire life of an individual that it is difficult to evaluate the influence of the climacteric on this physiologic function. Women may gain in libido postmenopausally. Estrogens seldom prove effective in increasing sexual desire.

Hypothyroidism may occur postmenopausally and respond to small doses of thyroid extract given orally; however, this is seldom a solution to the problem of fatty tissues accumulating in undesired areas. Management is better accomplished by proper diet and exercise.

THE BREAST IN RELATION TO GYNECOLOGY

Examination of the breasts should be done routinely not only to evaluate the endocrine status but also to discover neoplasia of the breast as early as possible.

Anomalies

Rudimentary nipples and small amounts of breast tissue may develop below the normal breast, on the abdomen, and, at times, on the vulva. A portion of the breast may exist in the axilla and not necessarily be contiguous with the other breast tissue. These abnormal locations of breast tissue seldom require excision.

Rarely there is unilateral absence of breast or hypoplasia. After the other breast is fully developed augmentation mammoplasty can be done. Slight asymmetry of the breast is common, and usually no therapy is required. If the asymmetry is marked then augmentation can be performed.

Virginal breast hypertrophy may occur in teenagers. Endocrine studies are usually within normal limits. Reduction mammoplasty may be done.

Mastalgia

Mastalgia is a common complaint of women consulting a gynecologist. Premenstrual breast tenderness of mild degree is considered normal because of the frequency of its occurrence. Persistent tenderness of the breast after menstruation should attract attention to the likelihood of other disturbances. Fibrocystic disease of the breast is common. It increases the nodularity of the breast to give a "shotty" feel. This condition has been shown to be associated with a slightly higher incidence of carcinoma, and one should be mindful of the fact that a cancer may begin in a breast with fibrocystic disease and be ignored because of the diagnosis that has previously been given to the patient.

Minimal breast tenderness is often properly managed by reassuring the patient that no organic breast lesion is present. Adequate support of the breast day and night may afford more relief. Rarely is the administration of estrogens or androgens justified in the management of breast pain. Analgesics and vitamin B complex may be used if a "neuritis" is suspected.

Cysts

Cysts of the breast may be suspected when found within weeks after delivery or when the mass is round and freely movable. Fluctuation may be elicited. Such lesions can be diagnosed by aspiration under local anesthesia. For many patients this constitutes adequate therapy. Residual masses or recurrence requires excision. Cystic areas infrequently occur in association with breast cancer. The probability of cancer should be suspected when the fluid is bloody. Cytologic studies of bloody fluid are more apt to be indicative of malignant cells.

Inflammation

The typical abscess of the breast encountered in the lactating patient is easily diagnosed. However, the differentiation of edema of the skin associated with inflammatory carcinoma of the breast and the edema associated with infection in older women may be more difficult. The redness, tenderness, and skin edema of inflammatory cancer are more likely to be away from the areola and do not respond to therapy for bacterial invasion. When infection occurs localized pain is usually the chief complaint, and when the redness, tenderness, and induration are under or near the areola, one often finds periductal mastitis that will respond to antibacterial therapy.

Fat necrosis

When trauma may have occurred one would clinically suspect fat necrosis; however, since the induration of the breast cannot be differentiated from a neoplasm on many occasions, it is necessary that a biopsy be performed.

Sclerosing adenosis

Sclerosing adenosis, an uncommon lesion, is occasionally seen in postmenopausal women and necessitates biopsy for accurate differentiation.

Paget's disease

In Paget's disease the lesion can be confused with eczema; however, it is usually unilateral and involves the nipple and areola. Malignant cells from the nipple invade the epidermis. The underlying carcinoma of the duct is not usually palpable as a mass. Biopsy and radical excision are in order.

Fibroadenoma

Fibroadenomas, benign encapsulated tumors, are found commonly in teenagers and young adults. Local excision is curative.

Cystosarcoma phylloides

In cystosarcoma phylloides the relatively uncommon localized growth in the breast is usually benign and is considered a counterpart of fibroadenomas; however, it can be malignant. Often total removal of the breast is justified.

Solid masses

Solid masses that persist demand excision lest breast carcinoma not be diagnosed at the earliest possible stage. Adequate excision practically always requires general anesthesia. In some patients with breast carcinoma, particularly those with metastasis, oophorectomy or sufficient radiation to destroy ovarian function may add to the patients' comfort and prolong their lives. Determination of the estrogen and progesterone receptors in the excised tumors can be used to better predict the benefits of oophorectomy. The increased estrogen stimulation of pregnancy or administration of extrinsic estrogens should be avoided. Tamoxifen after ovarian atrophy or removal when the tumor has been recognized as estrogen-receptor–positive will benefit patients with metastases.

Bloody discharge

A bloody discharge from the nipple indicates the necessity for cytologic study and for exploration of the breast to search for intraductal papillomas or cancer.

• • •

Mammography

Mammography using a soft tissue x-ray technique has recently become popular as a means of diagnosis of breast cancer. There has been 85% accuracy. Minute areas of calcification are commonly seen in cancers, and the areas of increased density have an irregular outline with tails or strands. Confusion with benign lesions can occur. When a mass can be palpated and found to be noncystic by attempted aspiration, biopsy must be done in spite of a negative mammogram.

Indications for mammography are the following:

1. Carcinoma of the other breast
2. Indefinite mass in fibrocystic or lumpy breasts
3. Recent nipple retraction without a palpable mass
4. Bloody nipple discharge or Paget's disease
5. Palpable axillary nodes or distant metastatic lesions with an unknown primary site
6. Large breasts difficult to palpate
7. Mass known to be present for many months that appears benign
8. Cancerophobia

BACKACHE

Pain in the lumbar, sacral, or sacroiliac region is a common complaint of women coming for gynecologic investigation. Most of these women do not have any evidence of pelvic disease. The pathogenesis of lumbar and particularly sacral backache in gynecologic disorders has been indicated in discussion of those respective topics. Premenstrual and other types of backache have been thought to be caused by changes in circulation in the pelvis. Vascular congestion, perhaps with edema, may be the primary mechanism. The fact that fatigue and psychic disturbances can be related must be entertained. In considering the possiblities as to the cause of backache in women, one must be ever mindful of osteoarthritis; myositis; increased mobility of the sacroiliac joints; ruptured intervertebral disk with protrusion; poor posture while sitting, standing, and lying; spondylolisthesis; and the shortening of one lower extremity, resulting in scoliosis.

SELECTED REFERENCES

Albright, F., Smith, P.H., and Richardson, A.M.: Postmenopausal osteoporosis, J.A.M.A. 116:2465, 1941.

Haagensen, C.D.: Diseases of the breasts, Philadelphia, 1956, W.B. Saunders Co.

Hulka, B.S.: Effect of exogenous estrogen on postmenopausal women: the epidemiologic evidence, Obstet. Gynecol. Surv. 35:389, 1980

Jimerson, G.K.: Breast. In Romney, S.L., et al., editors: Gynecology and obstetrics, the health care of women, New York City, 1981, McGraw-Hill Book Co.

Montgomery, T.L., Bowers, P.A., and Taylor, H.W.: Breast lesions, Obstet. Gynecol. 1:394, 1953.

Morrison, J.C., Martin, D.C., Blair, R.A., et al.: The use of medroxyprogesterone acetate for the relief of climacteric symptoms, Am. J. Obstet. Gynecol. 138:99, 1980.

Novak, E.: The menopause and its management, J.A.M.A. 110:619, 1938.

Overstreet, E.W.: Endocrine management of the geriatric woman, Am. J. Obstet. Gynecol. 95:354, 1966.

Randall, C.L., Birtch, P.K., and Harkins, J.L.: Ovarian function after the menopause, Am. J. Obstet. Gynecol. 74:719, 1957.

Schniff, I., and Ryan, K.J.: Benefits of estrogen replacement, Obstet. Gynecol. Surv. 35:400, 1980.

Worley, R.J.: The menopause, Clin. Obstet. Gynecol. 24:163, 1981.

Chapter 18

MEDICOLEGAL ASPECTS OF GYNECOLOGY

Although the physician may commit a criminal act for which a government prosecutor moves to imprison or otherwise punish him for causing harm to society as a whole, this chapter concerns the civil wrongs (torts) for which the physician may be sued by individuals. The most common accusations are that the physician has rendered treatment not authorized or that he has caused harm to his patient by failing to provide treatment that meets professional standards. These two torts are known as battery and negligence. He may be sued because of the acts of partner physicians or persons who work under or for him.

Authorization is legally valid if the patient or the parent or guardian of minors or mentally incompetents gives informed consent. This consent is best when written but may be expressed orally or by action. Consent is also implied in an emergency when immediate treatment is needed but the patient is physically and mentally unable to give consent. To give informed consent, the patient should understand the following elements: the nature of his condition, the nature of the proposed treatment, alternative treatment that is possible in his case, risk or consequences of the treatment, and chances of failure of the treatment.

It is sometimes medically wise for the physician to exercise discretion as to what he discloses to his patient. The law recognizes the validity of discreet disclosure if it is consistent with accepted medical practices in the physicians' locality. At times disclosure of diagnostic or prognostic data may be given to the husband or responsible relatives when such information would unduly harm the patient.

The duty of the physician to keep patients' secrets is essential for good medical practice, but such a duty is not absolute. To avoid legal complications that may arise, the physician should never disclose any information about a patient that has been learned in the physician-patient relationship unless the patient has given prior consent; disclosure is expressly required by statute or by a court order; the other person needs the information for the benefit of the health and welfare of the patient; or the information is essential for the protection of society in general.

For negligence (malpractice) to be constituted, four elements in a given set of circumstances must be established: (1) acceptance of a person as a patient, (2) breach of the physician's duty of skill or care, (3) causal connection between the breach by the physician and the damage to the patient, and (4) damage of a foreseeable nature (i.e., injury, pain, loss of earnings, etc. that could reasonably have been foreseen to result).

The most important question of a negligence case involves standards of care. In the trial of malpractice cases another physician ("expert witness") must give testimony as to what treatment meets proper standards. In general the expert witness should be from the same locality or from a community of similar size or have similar training as the defendant. However, since communications and travel are becoming more rapid, standards of care are becoming more similar and these general rules no longer apply.

The very occurrence of an injury may be considered to be evidence of the physician's negligence under the doctrine *"res ipsa loquitur"* (the thing speaks for itself). For this doctrine to be applied the following requirements must normally be met:

1. The injury or damage must be something that does not ordinarily happen unless the physician has failed to exercise due skill and care.
2. The action or conduct that caused the damage must have been that of the defendant physician or under sole control of the physician.
3. The patient must not himself or herself have contributed to the injury.

When the plaintiff's attorney invokes this doctrine, the judge must decide whether it applies and so instruct the jury.

From the previous discussion it is evident that physicians must take care as to which patients they accept for treatment; they must have authorization from the responsible person, who is usually the patient; and they must exercise management that meets the standards of adequate professional care. When the honest, capable, conscientious physician accomplishes these necessities, he usually has the confidence of his patients necessary for the proper physician-patient relationship. As long as this confidence is maintained it is unlikely that the patient will institute a suit.

In recent years in the United States there has been a marked increase in the number of suits filed against physicians. Many of these are nuisance suits; however, they are expensive, time-consuming, harassing, and unpleasant to the physician. The following is a list of rules to avoid the common causes of malpractice suits.

1. Do not criticize another practitioner unless you have all of the facts and even then it would be better to say nothing to the patient.
2. Do not leave a patient unattended during labor.

3. Exhaust all necessary means to establish a correst diagnosis whether it be for cancer, pregnancy, or another condition.
4. Do not promise a cure.
5. Select assistants with great care and supervise carefully the duties delegated to them.
6. In operative cases obtain written consent of the husband and wife in the presence of two witnesses. This should include all work found necessary and advisable at the time of the operation.
7. Be sure to assume personal responsibility for the post-operative care when you have performed the operation.
8. Do not promise a patient that she will be sterile as a result of a sterilization operation.
9. Do not sterilize anyone for other than medical reasons without considering the legal status of such an act in the community and state in which you practice.
10. Do not assume that you are free from liability because the sponge count has been made and reported correct.
11. An attendant should always be physically present or within easy hearing when you are examining a patient.

This list gives some of the essential points but, of course, is far from complete. For further information the reader is referred to the *Handbook of Legal Medicine* by Hirsch, Morris, and Moritz included in the references.

Another category of medicolegal problems deals with the physician as a witness. There are various conditions connected with the genital organs concerning which the physician may be called to testify in court or to give a written opinion. Such testimony ordinarily is simply the recitation of facts in anatomy, physiology, pathology, symptomatology, diagnosis, treatment, and prognosis, with which the physician is necessarily more or less familiar because of his daily work. There are, however, certain things, of little or no value in the ordinary diagnosis and treatment of diseases, that assume much importance when the case comes into court. Therefore, when one is called to attend a case in which there is any probability of court proceedings, the facts that are of medicolegal importance should be given considerable attention.

Medical evidence is ordinarily required to confirm or disprove the allegation of rape. The number of rape cases has increased in recent years; 51,000 rape cases were reported in 1975. Criminologists estimate that up to 10 times more rapes occur than are reported. Few trials end in conviction of the assailant. Some of these cases of false accusation are founded on a mistake, as many happen with infants, children, and persons who are mentally defective. In other cases the accusations are made willfully and are either designed for the purpose of extortion or revenge or come from other ulterior motives. The question for the physician to decide as far as possible from his examination is whether or not sexual intercourse took place or was attempted at approximately the time indicated. Also, evidence of communicated disease is to be noted, and evidence of strong resistance may aid in the decision of the important legal question of consent.

A person trained in the identification of sperm and seminal fluid should make the proper examinations of properly identified specimens in order that he can later testify in court if needed. After proper consent of the patient has been obtained, the history concerning the details of attack should be recorded in the patient's words. Physical examination of the body and the clothes should be made for evidence of injury. Laboratory studies should be made of blood or seminal stains, foreign hairs, or foreign substances. Vaginal material should be examined by wet smears, stained smears, and acid phosphatase determination. Spermatozoa remain in the vagina for varying period of time unless removed by douching.

Follow-up examinations for venereal disease, pregnancy, and psychologic disturbances should be made. At the time of initial examination it may be proper to prescribe estrogens in an effort to prevent pregnancy.

The character of a disease, if present—particularly gonorrhea, syphilis, or chancroid—and the source from which it could have come and whether or not the disease is still transmissible are all questions that may assume medicolegal importance under various circumstances, for example, in suits for divorce, suits for possession of children, suits for alimony, or suits for damages against individuals or corporations.

In coroners' cases and much more so in malpractice suits (before or after death) the following questions may be asked concerning almost any gynecologic disease: What disease is present? What are the principal points upon which your diagnosis is based? In your opinion did the attending physician use reasonable care and skill in the diagnosis? What is the established treatment for the disease? In your opinion did the attending physician use reasonable care and skill in the treatment? One should be acquainted with *one's state* laws concerning which cases are coroners' cases.

The importance of the subject of foreign bodies left in the abdomen is often not appreciated by the physician until he is involved in a lawsuit concerning it. Certainty that no sponge or other foreign body was left in the peritoneal cavity during an operation may be a difficult problem. This important subject in its various aspects is considered in detail by Crossen and Crossen in a monograph, *Foreign Bodies Left in the Abdomen.*

Subjects related to obstetrics are not discussed here. For a complete discussion of medicolegal problems and the reader is referred to Morris and Moritz's book, *Doctor and Patient and the Law.*

Many physicians purchase professional liability insurance to avoid the possibility of financial loss. The policy purchased is a contract in which the insurance company agrees to pay the sums legally obligated for the insured physicians and for the insurance company. In the contract it is stated that the physician must cooperate with the insurer. He should report as soon as practical to the representatives of the insurance company the likelihood of claims being made or of claims presented to him. He should not obligate the insurer by making any settlement or compromise without the insurer's consent. The physician should attend meetings and court sessions in defense of suits instituted. The attorney is chosen and paid by the insurer. If the physician desires to choose an attorney, he should accept the obligation to pay the attorney of his choice.

In the contract the insurer must defend any suit in the name of the insured physician, and usually insurance companies have the right to investigate and settle claims; however, a settlement or compromise of a claim cannot be made by the insurer without the written consent of the insured. It should be noted that in the contract the insurer is not obligated to protect the reputation of the physician and is concerned primarily with the financial responsibility of the insurance company. Most commonly in the United States lawyers representing the insurer and the patient discuss the financial and legal matters without the patient or physician being present. It is important that the physician be informed at all times of any negotiation and discussion that are taking place. The physician has the right and duty to discuss with the patient the claims being made. He can enter such discussions that he deems advisable but cannot legally obligate the insurer to pay any stated amount.

The rates for professional liability insurance vary greatly in the different states of the United States. The variations of rates are related to the difference in the functions of lawyers in various states, the state statutes, the experience of courts as to size of judgments rendered, and the attitudes of patients and the public in regard to professional liability. It is evident that some patients and their legal counselors have little mercy for insurance companies and hospitals, which they consider capable of paying large sums for pain and suffering and disability and financial loss, actual and predicted, even though they admit that the error they allege occurred was in no way intentional on the part of the physician or other medical personnel.

It is likely that patients would have more mercy for individual physicians or hospital personnel. Perhaps when the public is made more aware of the consequences of the large claims that are being made and paid and the increasing cost of liability insurance, with its effects on the cost of medical care and its influences on delivery of care, they will influence change in the state statutes and in the legal procedures used in settling disability claims.

Since 1977 some state statutes have provided for physician panels to review claims before instition of court suits. Failure of reasonably prompt action by physicians and attorneys involved has caused the enabling statutes to be ruled unconstitutional in several states. Several physician-controlled insurance companies have been functioning with elimination of some high-risk providers and educational efforts to decrease risk exposure.

SELECTED REFERENCES

ACOG technical bulletin: suspected rape, Chicago, 1970, The American College of Obstetricians and Gynecologists.

Crossen, H.S., and Crossen, D.F.: Foreign bodies left in the abdomen, St. Louis, 1940, The C.V. Mosby Co.

Hassard, H.: Your malpractice insurance contract, J.A.M.A. **168**:2117, 1958.

Hirsch, C.H., Morris, R.C., and Moritz, A.R.: Handbook of legal medicine, ed. 5, St. Louis, 1979, The C.V. Mosby Co.

Morris, R.C.: Is there a doctor in the court room? GP **19**:190, 1959.

Morris, R.C., and Moritz, A.R.: Doctor and patient and the law, ed. 5, St. Louis, 1971, The C.V. Mosby Co.

Sadusk, J.F., Jr.: Expert witness and advisory panels, J.A.M.A. **168**:2121, 1958.

INDEX

A

Abdomen
  examination, 52-57
    inspection, 52
    palpation, 52-55
    percussion, 55-57
  right lower quadrant tenderness, 107-108
Abdominal pregnancy, 261-262
Abortion, 247-254
  anatomic causes, 252
  bleeding with, 249
  chromosome abnormality and, 252
  definitions, 247
  diagnosis, 250
  etiology, 247-249
  habitual, 252
  hypofibrinogenemia and, 251
  incomplete, 251
  induced, 249, 251-252, 253-254
  induction methods, 253-254
  inevitable, 251
  infection and, 165-168, 249, 251-252
  legal, 253
  management, 250-253
  missed, 247, 249, 250-251
  mortality, 253
  oxytocin stimulation for, 251, 253
  pathology, 249-250
  prevention, 250, 252-253
  prostaglandin stimulation for, 251, 253
  Rh sensitization and, 249-250, 251, 254
  spontaneous, 247-249, 250
  tests for, 85
  threatened, 250
  ultrasonography in, 251
Acetylcholine, 30
Actinomyces, 173

Actinomycosis, 170
Addison's disease, 90, 91
  amenorrhea and, 270
Adenocarcinoma; *see also* specific sites
  clear cell, 120
Adenomyoma, 187, 222, 224
Adenomyosis, 222, 223, 224
Adolescence, 16, 17, 30
  examination methodology for, 101-102
Adrenal function
  amenorrhea and, 269-270
  tests, 90-92
Adrenal hyperplasia, congenital, 118
Adrenocortical hormones, 38-39
Adrenocorticotropic hormone assay, 86-87
Ahumada-del Castillo syndrome, 269
Amenorrhea, 268-272
  adrenal function and, 269-270
  anorexia nervosa and, 268
  chemotherapy and, 272
  congenital abnormality and, 268
  hypothalamic abnormality and, 268-269
  oral contraception and, 303
  ovarian function and, 270-272
  physiologic causes, 272
  pituitary abnormality and, 268-269
  polycystic ovary syndrome and, 270-271
  prolactin and, 269
  radiation therapy and, 272
  spontaneous premature ovarian failure and, 272
  therapeutic causes, 272
  thyroid dysfunction and, 269
Aminoglycosides, 180-181
  adverse reactions, 180-181
Amoxicillin, 174
Ampicillin, 174
Anatomy, 1-46